AF564408

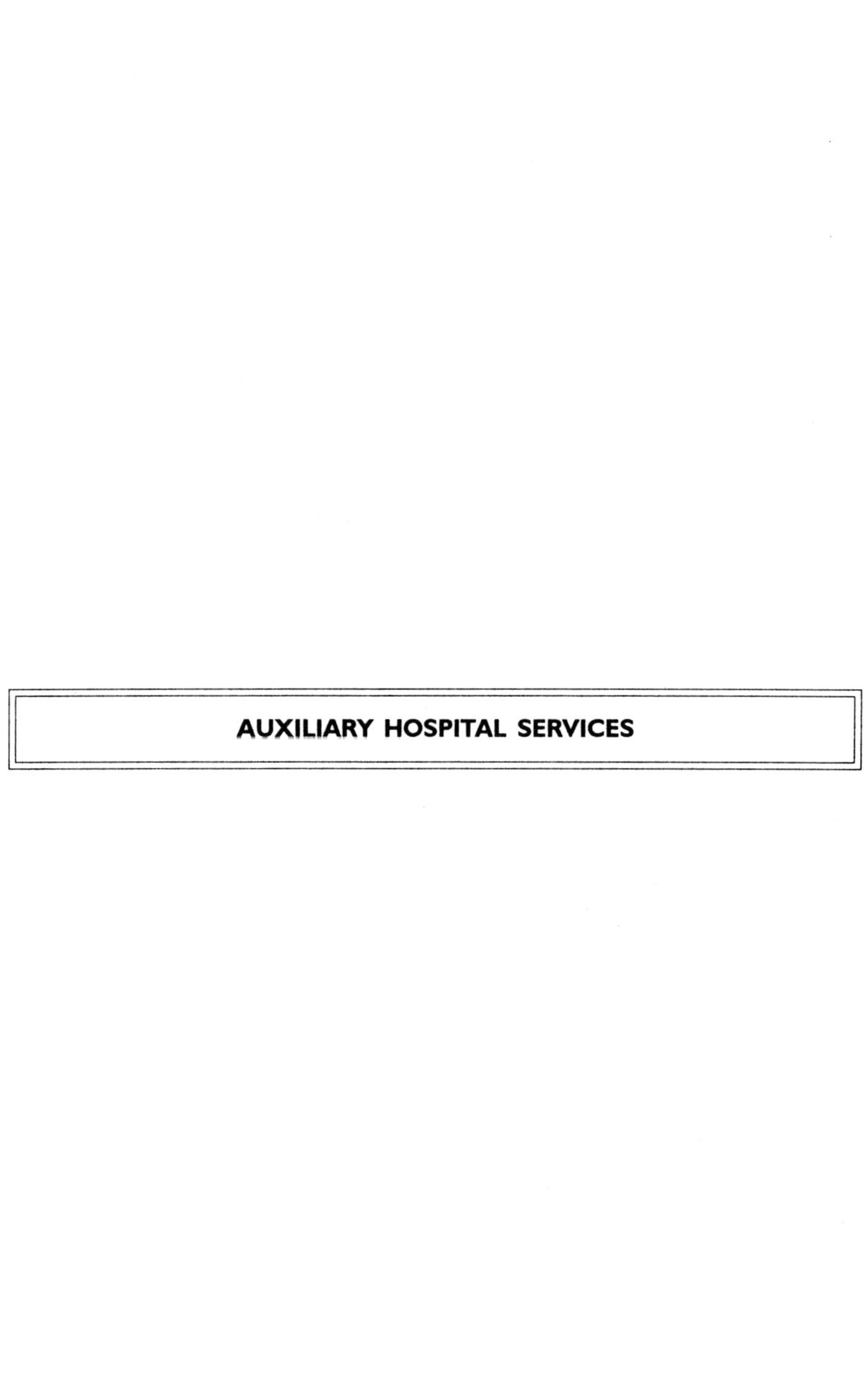

AUXILIARY HOSPITAL SERVICES

AUXILIARY HOSPITAL SERVICES

(Encyclopaedia of Hospital Management—4)

DR. S.L. GOEL

Professor of Public Administration (Retd.),
Panjab University, Chandigarh
Editor, Indian Journal of Public Administration, IIPA, New Delhi
Former Member, UGC, Former Member Distance Education Council
Former Member All India Board of Management, AICTE
Member, Executive Council, IIPA, New Delhi.
Former Vice-President, IIPA, New Delhi.
Emeritus Fellow, University Grants Commission
Former Director, State Bank of India (Local Board) Chandigarh
Former Director, National Horticulture Board, Ministry of Agriculture,
Government of India, New Delhi.

and

DR. R. KUMAR

MBBS, MS, Ex. PGI
President, Chandigarh Ophthalmological Society, 2000-01,
Columnist on Health Education and Management,
Advisor on Health Care and Medical Tourism,
Member Tourism Advisory Forum,
Chandigarh Administration, Chandigarh

DEEP & DEEP PUBLICATIONS PVT. LTD.

F-159, Rajouri Garden, New Delhi-110027

AUXILIARY HOSPITAL SERVICES
(Encyclopaedia of Hospital Management—4)

ISBN 978-81-8450-219-0

Typeset by S.S. COMPOSERS
3190, Mohindra Park, Shakur Basti, Delhi-110034.

Printed in India at MAYUR ENTERPRISES
WZ Plot No. 3, Gujjar Market, Tihar Village, New Delhi-110018.

Published by DEEP & DEEP PUBLICATIONS PVT. LTD.
F-159, Rajouri Garden, New Delhi-110027.
Phones: 25435369, 25440916
E-mail: ddpbooks@yahoo.co.in • ddpubs@gmail.com
Showroom:
2/13, Ansari Road, Daryaganj, New Delhi-110002 • Telefax: 23245122

Contents

Preface

A medical institution is a large and complex organization. Though many of the principles of administration are equally applicable to in its management, some require greater emphasis and some others require modification. There is a perpetual urgency in keeping the supply lines to keep the system working. The maintenance work for essential services must be always actively functional, otherwise an urgent service may have a breakdown. Greater attention is also required in development of skills of manpower and keeping abreast with available technology as otherwise, the institution can no longer be counted amongst the best and above all the institution must have a clear and transparent administration to be able to generate an attitude of fairplay and justice to the highly skilled staff, otherwise their exodus is liable to leave the institution bereft of its skills and thereby, its leadership. In this volume "Auxiliary Hospital Services" we deal with institutional service.

"A patient coming to the hospital gives us an opportunity to serve, by treating a patient we are not doing a favour to him, the patient is doing a favour to us by giving us an opportunity to serve the humanity." The aim of hospital management is to strengthen the preventive, promative, curative and rehabilitation aspects of health care to reach the population in the remotest area of the country, state, district and villages and development of health care manpower resources by proving good quality of medical education.

The Director General of WHO, Gro Harlem Brundland rightly observes that the way hospital systems are designed, managed and financed affects people's lives and livelihoods. The difference between a well performing health system and one that is failing can be measured in death, disability, impoverishment, humiliation and despair.

If policy-makers are to act on measures of performance, they need a clear understanding of the key functions that health systems have to undertake. The report defines four key functions providing services, generating the human and physical resources that makes service delivery possible; raising and pooling the resources used to pay for health care, and, most critically, the function of stewardship-setting and enforcing the rules of the game and providing strategic direction for all the different actors involved.

Science and Technology advancements have provided many opportunities for diagnosis and treatment but the escalating cost of medical services is a cause of concern. Besides, there has been deterioration of quality in all the areas. Prolongation of life has put great pressure on hospital resources and many new lifestyle diseases like heart, diabetes caused by sedative life, alcoholism, accidents, etc. Besides AIDS, HIV, Cancer are also cause of concern.

Auxiliary services reflect the functioning of hospitals. It has been generally observed that hospital authorities do not attend to auxiliary services causing problems to patients and their relatives.

Auxiliary agencies also helps the line agency in the performance of its duties. These are institutionalised services to the line agency. Besides, the auxiliary agency provides expert services in its area of operations economically. Some of the experts make no distinction between staff and auxiliary agency. Others make the following distinctions: (i) Auxiliary agencies are operating services while staff agencies are engaged in thinking, planning, research, etc. (ii) Auxiliary agencies are not directly involved with the major policies of the organisation while the staff is engaged in policy formulation and other advice regarding functioning of the organisation. Such services make the cost of the product cheaper because of large scale operation and expertise developed.

The hospital authorities do not attend to auxiliary services thinking that these are not important. However, take like parking, registration, hospital security, etc. are important and the image of the hospital depends upon their excellent performance. For example, security instead of guiding and serving the patients generally misbehave causing tensions in hospitals. Therefore, hospital authorities must be planned and maintain auxiliary services in a decent way.

There is a need to maintain auxiliary services efficiently so that patients are not harassed and approach the hospital with confidence.

The hospital's admission procedure should be such that the patient is made to feel welcome and secure. Every employee who comes in contact with the patient should make him feel that each one is genuinely interested in his welfare. This experience is the patient's first introduction to the hospital and should be a pleasant one.

Hospitals are not immune from the threat of society's criminal element. Thus, establishment of hospital security force is essential to ensure the safety of patients and the staff. In a teaching-*cum*-research hospital and other large hospitals, the appointment of the security staff has become a matter of great importance. The security officer must be appointed on the basis of his experience either in defence services or police services. Under him, there can be other staff depending upon the size of the hospital. Hospital security department must have active liaison with the local police in the area so that they can supplement each other's effort.

Poor Management of Dietary Services

The dietary unit stands as the second major department of a hospital from the point of view of expenditure. It needs careful analysis and control. Most of the patients always complain of poor and costly diets served in the hospitals. There is a problem of excess diets issued as compared to the number of patients resulting in huge expenditure. Besides, many of the patients do not consume all that is served to them. Patients generally prefer food from their houses as they do not like hospital food. The Public Accounts Committee (1977-78) has mentioned in this connection:

> "The Committee is constrained to note that whereas economy on expenditure on diet is being thought of by reducing quantum of diet, other measures to effect economy without diminishing the quality and quantity of diet such as plugging leakages of diet, have not been given the attention they deserve. In the opinion of the committee, the leakage of diets may be possibly one of the reasons for issue of excess diets over the census figure. Therefore, it is necessary that institutional arrangements are made to watch that leakages of diet and dietary materials do not take place."

Benjamin and Kemppainen have rightly observed that there is a general consensus by trained hospital observers that most physicians do not have sufficient background in dietary sciences to fully serve the best interests of their patients. This statement is not meant as a depreciation of the medical profession, but merely a recognition of the specialised nature of dietary planning . . . Nutrition, particularly as it applies to the healing sciences, is an exacting realm. Most medical schools do not provide extensive training as dietary sciences because it is assumed that a dietician will be available to handle the food selection and planning process. This, unfortunately, is not always the order of the day.

It is suggested that the efficient management of dietary services may be done to achieve economy and quality. The hospital authorities must compare the cost of dietary services with other hospitals' dietary services and thus try to locate the defects and remedy them.

The contents reflect the coverage in this book, "Auxiliary Hospital Services." It is hoped that this book on "Auxiliary Hospital Services" would make a modest contribution to the knowledge and existing literature in this expanding field. Besides, this would help the academicians, national health officials, public health administrators, medical research workers and the policy-makers and planners in the proper understanding of health care delivery system. We will consider our labour well rewarded if the findings of the study are translated to provide decent health care to the millions of people living in rural areas, urban slums and tribal areas. Comments and suggestions from the readers would always be welcome.

Chandigarh

S.L. GOEL
R. KUMAR

1

Registration Process and Patient Access Services

Registration of the patient is the foremost activity in the overall Hospital Information System. Every patient who approaches a hospital has to get registered prior to getting any consultation, treatment, and investigations done from the hospital. Registration of patients involves accepting certain general and demographic information about the patient. The patient is given a unique central registration number (CR. No.). The Patient is also given a patient identification card, known as Registration Card. The authors have been studying the registration processes at the three tertiary care public hospitals at Chandigarh for the last several years. Despite the advent of computers and new technologies, there has not been any tangible improvement in the plight of the patients or their attendants in getting OPD card made after getting the details registered at the central registration counter. However, the process is less arduous at the registration of a corporate hospital situated nearby. There are long and *serpentine queues to get OPD cards made that are never ending. The patients are pushed around like cattle with no respect for their convenience or dignity, let alone their precious time? In fact this part of the hospital services has been found to be the toughest and scaring as and when the need to access hospital services arises. Now another bitter problem has been preceding the foregoing and that is parking a vehicle in the hospital or for that matter transporting the patient to and fro the hospitals. Simple question arises, can we abolish registration altogether and switch on to Pre-registration through the internet? Different categories of Registrations are:

- Normal
- Staff
- Emergency
- VIP/Senior Citizen

Normal registrations are done in the routine OPD timings. Emergency Registration is done round the clock for the patients who require immediate medical attention. The patients getting registered under this category are basically:

- Out-patients whose unit is not working on that day
- Medico-Legal Cases
- Patients requiring immediate medical attention

Patients coming after the OPD hours also are registered as Emergency Patients. Staff Registration takes care of the registrations related to all the staff members of the hospital.

Input/Screen Interfaces

- *Capturing Demographic Details*: The Registration module captures the demographic details of the patient. A patient is assigned a unique 12 digit Central Identification Number.
- *Visit Creation for the Old Patients*: Every time a patient visits the hospital after registering, the visit gets stamped.
- *Change of Department*: This facility is provided to record the change of the department, in which the patient is registered.
- *Duplicate Card Printing*: Since the OPD card tends to get filled there is a facility to reprint this card.
- *Modification Request*: There is a provision to handle subsequent modification requests in registration data.

Reports/Graphical Output

- Printing of Normal OPD registration card.
- Printing of OPD register department-wise.
- Printing a report on number of registrations department-wise.
- Printing a report on number of total emergency registrations.
- Printing a report on number of registrations User-wise.
- Cash collection department-wise on a daily-basis.

Efficiency, productivity and cost effectiveness

The improvements in outpatient registration can lead to improved customer satisfaction, enhanced hospital-physician relationships, and increased revenue from outpatient services. It can also achieve the goal of increasing efficiency, productivity, and cost effectiveness. Each time customers come into contact with a hospital, they develop an impression of its quality. Whether that impression is favorable or not depends on how committed the hospital is to providing quality service to its customers—both its internal customers (physicians and staff) and its external customers (patients, their families, and vendors).

Until recently, quality improvement efforts centered on a hospital's clinical services only. Today, however, the quality initiative is gathering momentum in non-clinical areas as well. By adopting total quality management (TQM) techniques in outpatient registration, hospitals can achieve improved performance and service. These improvements can translate into increased customer satisfaction, enhanced hospital-physician relationships, and higher outpatient revenues.

The team approach

TQM is not a "top-down" management technique. Rather, its foundation is teamwork, with cross-functional employee teams accepting responsibility for improving operations and services. A quality improvement team charged with improving outpatient registration typically would include staff from all areas that are affected by outpatient registration or that interact with the registration process. Physicians and staff from the pre-admission testing area, the laboratory and radiology departments, the ambulatory surgery department, and the information systems department would be on the team. Other points of view that might be represented on the team could include those of staff from the patient accounting, admitting, and marketing departments.

This multidisciplinary team approach offers a broader perspective than can be gained from a team representing only the registration department or finance staff. And, as an added benefit, when changes are necessary to achieve improvement, a broad base of support is already in place. The multidisciplinary approach also recognizes that the registration process has multiple "owners," each of whom has contributed key elements to the registration process. For example, staff in the patient accounting department may have designed the insurance screens, and laboratory staff may have created the test scheduling procedure. But to be successful, all owners of the process need to be identified and included on the quality improvement team. Then, and only then, can effective solutions to registration problems be developed—solutions that will satisfy all key players. But while teamwork and shared ownership can push the quality initiative a great distance, they cannot do it alone. Without executive sponsorship, even the most ardent TQM team can falter. The support of a hospital leader is vital to creating a positive climate for the solutions the team proposes and a belief that change can occur. If the team does not believe that its recommendations are considered important, or if it is not empowered to effect changes within the institution, its efforts may be unsuccessful.

Understanding the process

To improve quality in outpatient registration, the team must first scrutinize the current registration process. To clarify the existing process, questions should be asked. What activities occur daily in the total outpatient registration experience? What roles do physicians, nurses, administrators, and ancillary support staff play? Failure to consider the different functions of those involved can result in incomplete identification of problems. An incomplete understanding of the process may lead to inappropriate or ineffective solutions that will only frustrate other departments and undermine the quality effort. For example, the quality improvement team at one large hospital looked at how patients were referred to the facility. They found that outpatient registration began much further away from the waiting room than they originally thought. Patients could phone the outpatient registration department for an appointment, or they could call an ancil lary department directly. Patients often arrived unscheduled with a note from their physician. Finally, some appointments were made for patients by the physician's office staff. Having a thorough understanding of the many ways patients can enter the outpatient registration system motivated the quality improvement team to improve and formalize its referral methods. The team recommended:

- A new test-ordering form that standardized physician orders for preadmission and improved accuracy;
- A computer link between physicians' offices and the outpatient registration area for physician order entry; and
- An improved phone system to facilitate the handling of incoming calls from patients and physicians.

Brainstorming

Brainstorming is a dynamic process used to identify problems as well as to uncover existing attitudes and perceptions. This process is most effective when a team's facilitator creates a climate of openness. Brainstorming is not always easy; the expression of diverse ideas and opinions—often negative ones—can be very threatening to some team members, particularly if their function or department is being scrutinized. But when brainstorming rules are laid out in advance and executed equitably, the most insightful and creative ideas are sometimes born of the conflict and tension created by the process. Later, in-depth studies of perceived problem areas may prove some early perceptions to be incorrect or invalid, but initially it is important to listen to everyone and to hear all ideas if team members are to be motivated to participate. When brainstorming is used to identify problems, all issues and comments can be laid on the table and considered. For example, brainstorming helped one multidisciplinary group verbalize its perceptions about the outpatient registration process. It uncovered the following problems:

- Difficulty in getting through to register by telephone,
- Long waiting periods,
- Lack of courtesy from registration staff,
- Inadequate hours of operation,
- Poor collection of insurance information,

- Lack of active and functional internet services, and
- Data collection and analysis

Brainstorming gets the teams' perceptions out on the table, but data collection and analysis are needed to validate or discredit those perceptions and, in the process, uncover new issues. Members of the TQM team need to agree on how they will study a specific process, by day of the week, by time elapsed, or by shift, for example. Then, for each perception and opinion to be validated, a data collection tool must be designed. In designing data collection tools, staff members should:

- Ask the right questions during the designing stage,
- Create tools that are easy to use, and
- Develop instructions that are clean and unambiguous.

The team, for example, may have identified waiting times as a crucial measurement of quality. To study waiting times, the team should design a data collection sheet on which to record observations. It is wise to first test the data collection sheet by conducting a small pilot study to determine if those responsible for collecting the data understand how to use the form. The pilot study also will reveal how much time will be required to collect the data in real patient contact situations and what any adjustments to the form are necessary.

At one hospital, the quality improvement team's study of waiting times included measuring how long patients waited before seeing a registration clerk, as well as the total waiting time they spent in the central registration area. Analysis of the data, using histograms, showed that waiting time averages markedly increased during break and lunch hours, when registration staff was reduced. The quality improvement team recommended adjusting staff coverage during these periods to reduce the waiting time experienced by patients. Interestingly, the registration department had been certain that no patient waited longer than 10 to 15 minutes for a registrar, until the study clearly showed that during break and lunch time patients actually waited 30 minutes. In Chandigarh hospitals the authors observed that patients waited for 1-3 hours to get the OPD card made, can it be justified? Other beneficial data collection techniques for studying outpatient registration are interviews with patients, staff, and physicians to collect data on issues of concern and telephone surveys of patients to determine satisfaction levels.

Interviews with physicians can often identify practice patterns that may have a negative impact on a hospital's outpatient revenue. If physicians are dissatisfied with outpatient services, they frequently develop their own office programs for outpatient testing thereby reducing the number of referrals to the hospital. Again, by asking the right questions, the team may identify factors that have resulted in physician dissatisfaction (e.g., the laboratory's failure to send test results to both the surgeon and the referring physician, causing last-minute postponements of ambulatory surgery). This can stimulate suggestions for improving service and ultimately bring dissatisfied physicians "back" to the hospital.

Storyboarding

The ultimate goals of the quality improvement team are to design an improved process and to deliver improved outcomes. To visualize a new process and how it will improve operations and/or services, the team may use storyboards. Storyboards are pictures, charts, or sketches that organize complex ideas and enable team members to develop a common understanding of the process. In one hospital, storyboarding allowed a team to display a redesigned physical layout of the outpatient registration area and to visualize how patients would proceed through the new area. The redesigned registration area introduced the concept of "one-stop shopping" to outpatient testing, where patients could have basic laboratory tests and X-ray studies performed in the central registration area. This concept addressed a major complaint of patients and physicians: ancillary testing was spread out across the entire hospital campus, creating a tiring and confusing experience for many elderly and disabled patients.

Measuring progress

Measuring the improvements gained through TQM is a critical component of any successful outpatient registration project. The quality improvement team needs to agree on measurable goals and determine the methodology for tracking progress. But the monitoring progress should be kept simple. If it takes too much effort, then it probably will not be done.

Benchmarking is an integral component of TQM, and enables an organization to improve by studying how its processes compare with those of other organizations. Benchmarking also can be used internally. To measure quality improvement, outpatient registration can use quantifiable benchmarks that are already available on the hospital's information systems, such as:

- Outpatient revenue,
- Number of outpatient visits per day or week,
- Outpatient days in accounts receivable,
- Average waiting time in registration,
- Number of patient complaints, and
- Number of rejected outpatient bills due to registration errors.

In case of indoor patients, you are expected to receive notification prior to admission, as to what time you should arrive at the facility, where you should register and what items you should have with you. To assist us in keeping our surgeries on schedule, and to allow time for you to get comfortable, please give yourself enough time when coming to register. When there is a patient requiring immediate admission to the hospital due to critical situation, bedside registration needs to be offered. This allows the staff to take care of patient first and, when ready, gather the necessary information needed for proper registration.

In our hospitals, despite giving an appointment no proper arrangements are made to receive the patients or to make arrangements for their being seated or to take care of the minimum basic facilities like water or clean toilets.

Arriving for Appointments in a clinic in USA

If you are an established patient, please arrive 15 minutes before your appointment unless you have been asked to arrive earlier. By keeping the schedule, the hospital and staff can work together to avoid unnecessary delays. When you arrive for your appointment, you will be informed if your physician has been delayed or called away for an emergency. If you have more than a 20-minute wait before being called for your appointment, please check with the receptionist.

New Patients

To help make your visit to the hospital easier, we've outlined some steps. First, if you have never been a patient at the hospital, please check in at the registration desk in the lobby 30 minutes before your scheduled appointment to pre-register. You may be contacted by registration staff prior to your appointment to be pre-registered by telephone. If you have pre-registered by phone, you need to arrive 15 minutes before your scheduled appointment time unless otherwise directed. At the time of registration, they need your medical insurance or billing card and the following information for your file:

- legal name
- current address
- birth date
- social security number
- name and address of person responsible for billing
- name and address for any special billing
- name, address and phone number of the person you want contacted in the event of an emergency
- You will also be asked to pay your co-pay if applicable for your health plan/visit.

Scheduling an appointment

Please schedule routine appointments in advance. Some physicians schedule routine exams months in advance for your convenience. Problems and emergencies will be handled promptly. When you call concerning an emergency, be sure to inform the scheduler of the emergency. Same-day appointments may be worked into the schedule. Please be aware, however, that scheduled appointments do have priority, unless it is an emergency.

When you speak to the scheduler, they will ask you to describe your problem to ensure reserving an adequate amount of time for the appointment, and confirm that you are seeing the appropriate physician for your problem. Anything you tell them is confidential.

Canceling an appointment

If you need to cancel an appointment, please cancel as far in advance as possible.

Innovation

An additional handset and splitter were added to existing phones at each desk in the registration areas so that an over-the-phone interpreter could be readily accessible during the registration process. Families who cannot speak vernacular/English can benefit from the immediate availability of the over-the-phone interpreter, while on-site interpreters are able to focus on other encounters that are lengthy or complex. Increasing Customer Satisfaction through simplification of Registration process, a study of Good shepherd hospital (GSH). It is common practice throughout the health care industry to blame technology or Computer systems when days in accounts receivable and/or patient complaints increase (Kathy Berger). It is not a common practice for a Chief Information Officer (CIO) of an eight-hospital system, recognizing that information systems are not the root cause of the issues, to spearhead an initiative to redesign work processes of the departments utilizing these systems. The GSH project began with a kick-off meeting with selected department heads. This eventually became the project steering committee. Karen Lambert, Vice-President for GSH, presented a crisis situation in the central scheduling department that was created in large part by employee turnover and leaves of absence.

Patient calls were not being answered, physicians were instructing their patients to arrive at the hospital without appointments because they couldn't get through on the phones, and, of course, patient and physician complaints were increasing exponentially. Entering the hospital the very next day, illustrated the crisis situation Karen painted. The main lobby was full with patients waiting to be registered that potentially could have been pre-registered. Central scheduling (or what was left of it) had only 2 staff on the phones with no relief between calls. An outside agency eventually had to be retained to take calls and leave messages for the existing scheduling personnel. Existing personnel, no longer receiving incoming calls, would return the messages and schedule patients in this manner. It was easily recognizable that the assessment had to begin in central scheduling. The pre-registration of accounts, also performed by the scheduling staff, was no longer being done. This contributed to the increased volumes of patients waiting to be registered in the main outpatient registration center and increasing the registration wait times. The first step in the assessment process was to collect the statistics: wait times in outpatient registration, percent of pre-registered patients to scheduled patients, scheduling phone calls answered, the number of abandoned incoming calls, abandoned calls as a percent of the total, etc. These benchmarks statistics established a snapshot of where they were so the affect of change could be measured moving forward. A by-product of the first steering committee meeting was the development of several sub-committees. One of these was the pre-registration committee, whose charge was to enable the hospital to reach a goal of 100% pre-registration of centrally scheduled patients and, eventually, 100% of all scheduled patients, including those not scheduled in the scheduling system. Other committees formed concerned communications and future technology.

The goal of the pre-registration committee was to resolve the crisis situation and design a process that worked for Good Shepherd. This was done through a number or work sessions with key managers and staff. The communication committee was charged with designing vehicles of communication to physicians, patients and staff regarding the progress of improvements. The future technology committee looked at the effectiveness of the scheduling system. In addition, the CEO was holding meetings twice a week to address progress in getting central scheduling staffed again. A perception existed that Central Scheduling was a difficult area to move existing staff into and train from other hospital departments because the scheduling system was too difficult to teach to just anyone, and that the learning curve for new staff was incredibly difficult. After asking probing questions, it was determined that the scheduling system had not been maintained over the past several years because of turnover. Staff was checking as many as 12 detailed sheets of exceptions to consider before scheduling a particular test in the system. The scheduling criteria, such as staff and physician availability, room availability, and equipment needs had to be built into the system to transform the system from a glorified calendar to a true scheduling system. An employee with previous in-depth system knowledge was immediately dedicated to rebuilding the system. Departments were required to document the criteria needed to schedule a test so staff could immediately 'see' when the next available test could be scheduled. Another sub-committee was formed to develop procedures for ongoing maintenance and support for the scheduling system as well.

Over the next several weeks, Central Scheduling was again fully staffed, training was completed, and the system was well on its way to serving as the tool it was intended to be. Central Scheduling personnel were handling all the calls themselves, the services of the outside agency was discontinued, and the percentage of incoming calls that patients abandoned (hung up) before a scheduler could answer dropped from 46% to 22% within six (6) weeks. Establishing a pre-registration area, while scheduling was being 'fixed' was an equally important priority because patients were waiting 13 minutes on average to be registered in the Outpatient Center, which created a lot of congestion in the main waiting area. Good Shepherd Hospital committed to hiring 3 staff to perform this function. The paper flow between Central Scheduling, pre-registration and the front desk was designed, and staff was trained. Removing the pre-registration function from the scheduling staff, allowed both areas to become more proficient in their respective jobs. Registration errors decreased from 35% to 26% and the percent of pre-registrations to scheduled patients increased from 54% to over 80% in two (2) months. Having resolved this crisis, the management at Good Shepherd Hospital began to look at the entire front-end process for each classification of outpatients entering the hospital.

Through flowcharting, it was discovered the registration process had become very fragmented. Different mechanisms were in place for scheduling and registering patients based on the services they received. Many ancillary areas did their own registrations because they did their own scheduling. Some patients went directly to the servicing area, and some went through the Outpatient Center where they waited for a registrar even if they were pre-registered. This fragmentation caused a lot of patient confusion and frustration. Hospital personnel had difficulty-directing patients to their first point of entry. The inpatient admitting process had also become very fragmented, resulting in the Emergency Department or the Admitting office being the place an urgent admission was directed to. If the Admitting Department was not staffed, then the ER was the back up. The entire front-end process has been completely redesigned with centralization of registration as the primary focus. All patients are currently directed to the central registration area. If they are pre-registered, Guest Services personnel obtain signatures and a copy of the insurance card at the front desk, and patients are directed to their servicing area. If the patient is not scheduled, and therefore not pre-registered, the registration process is completed in the central registration or Patient Intake area. Pre-registration and registration are a combined function of all the staff in the central registration area as well as the Emergency Department and report to the same supervisor.

This central reporting structure allows for flexibility in moving staff or reallocating staff to an area that needs assistance during peak times. Implementation is scheduled for late November, and many processes have already been established. Reporting structure changes will be the last step of the re-design process. Good Shepherd Hospital will serve as an example of improvements that can be made to help increase patient and physician satisfaction for all of Advocate Health Care. Through work sessions, processes were redesigned to accommodate the patients and staff was allocated to the areas in support of their patients rather than patients being directed to the different areas in support of the staff. Paper flows were streamlined and redundancy eliminated. Benchmarking statistics are serving, as the report card to measure what is working and identify what isn't. Utilization of an outside perspective (TTG) provided an objective viewpoint and assisted the hospital staff and management in looking at the whole picture and also provided the opportunity to see that picture through the eyes of their patients. The hospital will continue to monitor the success of the redesign through the benchmarking, making adjustments to the processes as needed. This experience will also provide Good Shepherd Hospital with the tools to enhance this process when their new outpatient facility opens next summer. This experience also illustrated that any information system is only as good as the work processes that support it. (Kathy Berger is the Director of Hospital Consulting for The Tintari Group, in Des Plaines Illinois).

A case study of The K.L.E.S 1200 bedded hospital

The patient care services will be executed through the diagnostic and therapeutic services spread over various technical functional areas of the hospital, i.e. OPD, Accident and Emergency department. In-patient Wards, diagnostic services like Hospital lab and Medical Imaging, specialized care areas like Operation 'theatre', Trauma Care Unit and I.C.U, etc. While these are the 'CURE' aspect of the theme of our hospital. The 'CARE' of the patients will be served adequate nursing services, hospital dietary services, and other supportive services like laundry, CSSD and building; maintenance cell. Let us have a look at the OPD and registration processes and policies.

Outpatient Department

OPD will provide health promotion diagnostic and therapeutic services to patients who need hospital services without; the need to be admitted would include references made from outside doctors, patients coming on their own, references from private clinics investigations recommendations and civil hospital references, etc. The outpatient department services will also attempt to reach the door step of it's beneficiaries through peripheral health centres in the hospital's catchments areas, Outpatients services in the hospital premises will be conducted through various specialized clinics in addition to one general clinic (filter clinic). The OPD consists of 18 specific discipline clinics which would be supplemented by further specialized clinics. Such special clinics run by specific disciplines would be on pre-determined, staggered days and timings using the infrastructural facilities as provided for the parent discipline clinic. The peripheral health centres would be in the form of augmenting the three PHCs adopted by J.N.M.C as well establishing dispensaries and medical staffed centres in selected catchment area towns. The OPD will have a medical officer in charge for day to day administration of the department and co-ordination of the department and co-ordination among various clinics and administrative echelon of the hospital. Authority granted to officer in charge of OPD will be given in different section of the document.

Grouping of OPD Clinics

Policy 1: OPD will be classified into six categories:

(1) General OPD (filter clinic)

(2) Specialty clinics
(3) Higher specialty clinics
(4) Special clinics
(5) Pay clinics
(6) Peripheral Health centres

Policy 2: The basic disciplines would run on daily basis, super or higher specialties would also be attempted to be run on daily basis but depending on the availability of 'faculty', hospital authorities may have to run it on fixed periods on pre-decided days and time. Some other special clinics would be conducted once or twice a week depending upon the availability of faculty and flow of patients.

Central Registration

Policy 3: Initially every patient would enter at the central registration counters of the OPD in the main entrance lobby for his/her registration as a new case with central registration number. After registration the patients would be guided/sent to the particular clinic depending upon the nature of ailment judged by the patient or advised at the enquiry counter. The patient will get the clinical case No. at respective clinics. On the subsequent visits patients shall directly report to their respective clinics for follow-up management as advised by the concerned consultant/authorized doctor of the clinic.

Policy 4: The Entrance lobby will have a general enquiry/guidance counter. This counter will assist patient in all respect for their registration and other needs in addition to general enquiry and assistance.

Policy 5: Registration of the new/patients will be done in three categories.

(1) General OPD, maternity and Paediatrics.
(2) Specialty clinics for conventional and broad specialties
(3) Higher specialty clinics.

Policy 6: These categories of registration will have specific counters in the main lobby. Attempt will be made to segregate male and female patients oil each category of the counter. The central registration for special clinics and pay clinics will also be done from same counters and under the parent discipline classification.

Policy 7: The registration fee for these categories of clinics, will be different. The General, maternity and Paediatric clinic registration fee will be the lowest, specialty clinic will be in the middle order and higher specialty and special clinics will be the highest. The purpose of this three-tier registration has been to encourage general practice, make the OBG, and Paediatric services accessible at the lowest affordable registration fee for the vulnerable group of population and also prevent unnecessary flocking of patient to specialty and higher specialty clinics, thus giving more time to the clinic for each needy and genuine patients.

Policy 8: The pay clinic will be giving the registration card with a number, as an authorized documentary permit to the patient to reach his choice consultant for private consultation. The registration clerk will also collect the consulting fee of the concerned consultant as per the pre-fixed rate. The clerk will account for the collected fee for each consultant at the end of the clinic. Registration staff will handover the collected fee to the consultant alter deducting 25% of the same, which he will deposit to the hospital cashier simultaneously with detail account of collection against each consultant.

Policy 9: Registration at a given time will be for a specific ailment or set of ailments at the time of registration. Any subsequent or different ailment not related with the previous ailment will require a separate registration. However this may be modified for a contractual regular patients with the hospital.

Policy 10: In case of professional cross-references, no fresh card need to be made. Cross referral form will be initiated by the referral clinic.

Policy 11: OPD card once made will be valid for one month, after which repeat visit fee of 50% of original registration fee would be charged lo renew it. In case the patient discontinues his/her visit for consecutive one month the card will stand invalid, unless the long gap in follow-up visit is on the doctors advise in writing on Us card.

Policy 12: The registration fee will be in the form of the cost of the central card printed/stamped on the card itself. The registration staff will make registration by collecting the prescribed registration fee directly while issuing the card to the patient and by entering the detailed bio-data and date in the register.

Policy 13: The registering staff will account for the registration card issued and deposit the collected cash at the cash counter at the expiry of his/her duty and return the unused registration cards to the authorized person.

Special Examinations and Investigations

Policy 14: Patients under examination and treatment in various clinics in the OPD may require special investigations or examination which warrant prescribed special fee to be paid for such examination/ investigation. These can be grouped in different categories:

(1) Specific to and thereby Integral to the medical discipline like KEG, EMG to Neurology.
(2) Investigations which are of general nature like X-ray 'Path Lab', etc.

Policy 15: Provision has been made for investigations/examinations which are specific to particular discipline to be provided in the clinic itself. Whereas the general diagnostic facility like pathology lab, x-ray, gamma camera, etc. provision has been made centrally in the diagnostic block of the hospital. The policy would be that the consultant/clinic will be initiate a request form for such investigations/examinations and the patient or lustier attendant would bring the request form to the diagnostic services counter in the main lobby where he/she will be required to get the investigations/examinations cost estimated and computed, deposit the amount at the cash counter and on the authority of the paid and stamped request form he/she will proceed for the required examination/investigation. This policy has been made with full awareness of possible consequences and occasional avoidable inconvenience caused to the patient. But the same has been adopted to avoid multiple centers of cash handling by the functionaries. However tills policy of functioning will be reviewed after giving a justifiable period of trial.

Policy 16: OPD function and timings

Registration

Regular Clinics (Pre-lunch)	Commence at 8.30 AM and closes at 12.30 PM
(Post-lunch)	Commences at 2.30 PM and closes at 4.00 PM
(Special Clinics)	Commences at 2.30 PM and closes at 4.00 PM
(Pay Clinics)	Commences at 4.45 PM and closes at 8.30 PM

Consultation

Regular Clinics (Pre-lunch)	Commences at 9.00 AM and closes at 1.00 PM
(Post-lunch)	Commences at 3.00 PM and closes at 5.00 PM
Special Clinics	Commences at 3.00 PM and closes at 5.00 PM
Pay Clinics	Commences at 5.00 PM and closes at 9.00 PM
Diagnostic/Special examinations/procedures	From 9.00 AM to 1.00 PM and 3.00 PM to 9.00 PM

A retail pharmacy counter will operate from 8.30 AM to 10.00 PM to cater for dispensing of prescriptions from various clinics of the OPD. Cash will be collected on the pharmacy counter and deposited with the hospital cashier on closing of the counter after verification/tally of cash memo with stock quantity sold for the day and balance left at end of the day.

Policy 18: Command and control of OPD

The over all command and contort of the OPD in all respect of its operations will remain with the Director Hospital Services and through this position with Medical Director and Chief Executive of the hospital at par with any other part of the hospital. However for routine day-to-day administration and logistic support, the officer-in-charge of OPD will be the Chief Coordinator. He will function through designated sectional officers and other medical and non-medical categories of staff.

Policy 19: Division of Specialties and their Staffing

Various clinical and para-clinical disciplines will be framed and named as per accepted nomenclatures approved by MCI or established practices in the medical fraternity. The consultants or other specialist appointments in various disciplines will be filled by specialists possessing MCI approved qualifications for respective disciplines, however exceptions will be made for competent faculty trained and having work experience in U.K, U.S.A, etc. The specialty departments thus formed and established will be under overall charge of the designated HOD of respective disciplines and the main faculty resource will be from specialty qualified specialists. The hospital patients will be directed to respective disciplines based on system or organ mobility status. Encouragement would be made for the clinical specialists to refer patients, to the higher specialty clinics based on the principle of specialization. However, the current practice broad or basic specialty specialists with particular organ/system biased experience undertaking management of such patients under their own care will be respected, subject to periodical patient care evaluation to ensure that by such practice the quality of patient care is not being compromised, nor is the patient being deprived of the expertise and benefits of care under exclusive specialist of the respective discipline. Thus, in spite of higher specialty clinic with all their staff, equipment and infrastructure under overall control of concerned specialty will be also made available to the broad specialty specialists making use of such specialty facilities subject to their being found trained and competent to handle those specialty equipments and this would be under overall co-ordination of parent specialty.

Policy 20: Professional Fees

As stated earlier in section pertaining to terms and conditions of medical staff no professional fee other than the registration fee will be charged to the patients except in the pay clinic as explained in the earlier paragraphs.

Policy 21: Diagnostic/Special Examination/Procedure Fees

Registration fee paid by the patients is limited to their consultation in respective outpatient clinic and does not authorize them for special diagnostic/examination/procedure service. Patients will have lo pay as per the approved rates for such diagnostic/examination/procedure. No sharing of such charges will be done with the faculty members.

Policy 22: Exemption from Diagnostic/Special Examination/Procedure Fees

Any exemption/concession on such fee will be done by the Medical

Director or any other staff authorized by him for this purpose. However, the consultants have the privilege to recommend deserving cases based on economic status/exigency of patient condition/and or interest of clinical teaching/research work. The recommendations will not be mandatory but due weightage will be given for the same. The yardstick and parameter for exemption will be as per given in a separate section of the document and as approved by the governing body.

Policy 23: Admission In-Patients

Patients undergoing consultation/treatment in outpatient clinics and advised admission would be admitted as hospital patient either in the general ward/semi private/private/deluxe ward as per patients choice but under the unit advising admission. The detail of payment has been dealt under another section of this document.

Policy 24: Availability of Medical, Para-Medical and Other Staff

Even at the cost of repetition, if is essential to reiterate a firm policy that a particular specialty and or higher specialty clinic including special clinics as mentioned will be conducted without fail on designated days/ timings, which warrants that the faculty and other staff essential to conduct such clinics will ensure their availability on those days and timings without fail. With full-time and exclusive attachment to K.L.E.S hospital all faculty and other staff are obliged to be in the premises during the scheduled hours, however what has to be ensured is that while scheduling any other work in the hospital or in the medical college, the scheduled clinic timings will take precedence and they will not absent themselves on any pretext, without implicit approval of the Medical Director or management staff deputed by him for such approvals.

Policy 25: The General OPD

The General OPD will be as the name suggests a model of general practice clinic or a primary health centre in Government sector, where patients of all ailments will primarily report. Patients requiring attention of any specialist as per the nature and extent of illness as judged by the attending doctor in general OPD. This OPD will be given the faculty support in the form of basic doctors drawn from hospital pool of general duty medical officers, with supporting staff from the department of medicine and general surgery. This OPD will also have the facility for centralized in junction and dressings for the patients. The charges for the same will be deposited at the Counter. Medical record department consists of working area with huge space for storage of medical records which are to be used for Patient, Medical Professionals, various Health Agencies, Legal, Insurance and other hospital needs. These are being preserved for about ten to fifteen years. Department have two sections namely: 1. Out-patient Department. 2. In-patient Department.

Out-patient Department is De-centralized keeping in view of better and quicker medical services to the patient. Thanks to our Medical Director Dr. Col. A.K. Singh (Rtd.) under whose guidance we have successfully changed the Out-patient system from Centralized to De-centralized way. Under this system patient need not wait for a long time either at the Central Registration Counter or in the department where the patient require services. Even filing and retrieval for follow-up is being done in the respective department. For In-patient there are two admission Counters, one at the ground level and another at the Causality. IPD Registration takes place in these two counters. After admission patients are being treated in the ward and no. of forms are used to document the patient's treatment. After discharge such Medical Documents are processed at MRD like assembling and deficiency check, completion of the case-sheets, discharge analysis, compilation of statistics, coding and indexing of diseases and operations, etc. Completed case-sheets are filed for all future needs of the hospital.

Computerization

At present OPD Central Registration and IPD Registration are Computerized and Inter-linked. Computerization at Out-patient Department level and at MRD are under progress.

Registration Process at Credit Valley Hospital

Approximately 5,400 visitors and patients pass through the Credit Valley Hospital in Mississauga, Ontario each day. Each year approximately 20,000 patients are admitted to hospital, and more than 66,000 patients are seen in the Emergency Department. In addition to a quality physician base, Credit Valley prides itself on a strong and innovative IT department. With a keen focus on ROI, the IT staff applies productivity improvements through technology to reduce clerical errors and deliver higher quality health care to its diverse customer base. This pays high dividends as clinicians can focus on provision of care and spend less time with manual tasks that can be automated.

Ensure High Quality Health Care from the Start

Credit Valley realized it needed more efficient and adaptive patient registration processes with its current HIS from MEDITECH. The hospital was resource constrained, yet without an efficient patient registration process, the hospital risked inaccurate patient information and adverse impacts to revenue. Avril Cardoso, manager, application services at Credit Valley, discovered that by using Boston WorkStation, from Boston Software Systems, her facility could administer business rules through the effective application of technology.

Boston WorkStation (BWS) is workflow automation and integration technology that provides an environment for on-demand process innovation and development. Boston WorkStation allows health care organizations to dynamically respond to changing business requirements by automating common tasks, creating complex processes, automating interaction with websites, or integrating new applications, systems and devices.

Using Boston WorkStation, Credit Valley developed an improved registration workflow which applies business rules as part of the registration process. Patient address validation is also included against a postal database. Boston WorkStation, running in the background, can 'watch' the registration screen and 'see' what a user is keying in. This quickly helps users detect errors, increasing address standardization and improving data quality. Through the inventive marriage of technology and process, Credit Valley was able to automate a standardized registration process across more than 40 points of registration. "Registration is the beginning of the health care process, so it is critical to ensure patient information is correct," said Cardoso. "This provides more reliable patient information which is important in maintaining the continuity of care."

Self Registration

The most exciting application of BWS is Credit Valley's automated patient registration process—possibly the first of its kind in North America —which Credit Valley has been piloting with great success. Patients are able to "self-register" at a kiosk in the patient care area, which helps to expedite the registration process. The hospital will soon open five kiosks in the new regional cancer center. Credit Valley will eventually install them in the outpatient and ambulatory care clinics, where the hospital sees the most volume of patients in a short period of time.

Without a keyboard, a patient can scan his/her health card at a wall-mounted computer (soon to be a kiosk). The hospital system deploys a real-time network-to-network connection with the Ministry of Health and Long-Term Care to ensure the patient's identity and validate the card. If they are in sync, the system automatically signs the patient into the MEDITECH Admissions Module and delivers paperwork to the registration desk. If the card is not valid, the system displays a message instructing the patient to see a registration clerk, who will assist them. The transaction takes 30 seconds. Credit Valley has achieved proof-of-concept on this device through a unanimous affirmation by the key stakeholders.

As a result of using Boston Software Systems' workflow automation and scripting software, The Credit Valley Hospital has greatly improved its registration processes, saving time, increasing accuracy and revenue recovery and ultimately improving patient care.

"The Credit Valley Hospital implemented Boston WorkStation to improve and automate processes," said Cardoso. "The Boston WorkStation suite of software is helping us to automate the application of business rules during the registration workflow. It is also being used as one of the application components, to deliver automated patient registration to streamline this workflow and offer better service. The Credit Valley Hospital will also become one of the first hospitals in Canada to implement address validation and residence postal code cross-reference. We will explore every opportunity to deliver safer and higher quality service to our patients," said Cardoso.

Medical Records

Consequent to sound registration process the hospital has a treasure of medical records that are valuable for patient care, teaching and research besides medico-legal purposes. With the computerization of the records it has become much easier to preserve and access the records. Earlier it used to be arduous job to locate or retrieve the records when required. In our modern hospitals still the old method of searching the files is prevalent, to the discomfiture of the patients and their relatives.

Herbert Hoover has rightly mentioned the advantages of proper records keeping when he says: "A business decision is only as good as the facts on which it is based." Records are the memory of the internal and external transactions of an organization. By external transaction we mean the correspondence between the organization and its clients beneficiaries as well as supporters. By internal transaction is meant the dealings on external transactions by persons in the organizations at all levels. Records contain a written evidence of the activities of an organization in the form of letters, circulars, reports, contracts, invoices, vouchers, minutes of meeting, books of accounts, etc. Thus, the records management is concerned with the retaining, submitting and destroying of records. The proper maintenance of these records in right quantity and quality is the essence of records management. The success of this record keeping would be reflected in the timely availability of all the records. In the context of Medical Records, Dr. McGibony had said, "A chronicle of the pageantry of medical and scientific progress is found in the hospital records. There may be found the running story, disconnected it is true, of the drama, the comedy, the mystery, the miracles of medicines and hospital of the Twentieth Century."

The medical record is a clinical, scientific, administrative and legal document relating to patient care in which is recorded sufficient data, written in sequence of events to justify the diagnosis and warrant the treatment and end results. With the advert of frequent litigations increasing super-specializations, numerous investigations based on technology and patients data swelling by the day, the process of record management is becoming complicated and challenging. A patient history and his data of clinical examination and various tests has to be compiled precisely and stored with care. This has to be available by flick of a finger, within a few hours, to all those who are allowed to access the same. With the advent of RTI, such a data has to be concise, comprehensive and reproducible. For the data to be clinically useful and legally supportive, Management of records assumes a great significance.

ESSENTIALS OF RECORDS MANAGEMENT

1. Comprehensive

The records should be such as can be easily understood when retrieved back for planning, policy-making and decision-making. The language used should be simple and understandable.

2. Properly Planned

The records be screened at regular intervals of time to weed out the information not required for future. In this way, we can reduce the paper work to twenty-five per cent. This would indirectly help us in locating the desired information quickly.

3. Economical

We should manage the records economically so that we may achieve more with minimum efforts.

4. Accurate

The records should be accurate otherwise its utility would be doubtful.

5. Timely

The time taken in reprieving the information should be as short as possible. Reducing retrieval time is essential for effective materials management.

6. Classification

Records must be classified to be of practical use. The classification be done either on the basis of subjects or chronology. According to Dr. K. Pennathur, Records should:

- Serve specific needs.
- Have specific objectives and purposes.
- Be kept to a minimum with respects to number, scope and content.
- Be designed for least expensive handling.
- Be up-to-date.
- Be worth their cost.
- Be related directly to tabulations and reports that will stem from them.
- Be available when needed.
- Be considered valuable by supervisors and lines management.

CONTENTS OF MEDICAL RECORDS

The medical record is a clear, concise and accurate history of the patients' life and illness, written from the health and medical point of view. The story of the patient's illness narrated by the patient, observations made by nurses and the comments and treatment given by the doctors are recorded in the medical record. Thus, the medical record comprises three general sections: (i) a general section covering administrative and personal data. The socio-economic record of the patient includes—The Name of the Patient, Father's or Husband's Name, Age, Sex, Religion, Income, Patient's

Address and the Address of nearest relative. Other administrative information's which are included are—The data of admission, The in-patient number, The name of the nursing unit and bed number. This sheet is prepared in the Central Admitting Office; (ii) a nurses section wherein are noted the observations of the trained nurses and the detail of treatment administered. This part of the medical record consists of graphic charts relating to Temperature, Pulse, Respiration, Blood Pressure and any other observations maintained, intake output chart and medicine administered; (iii) a medical section containing statements on the studies, observations, conclusions and activities of the attending doctors or of the intern or the resident working under him. The medical section of the record consists of the entire medical history of the patient. It contains:

- History sheet
- Physical examination sheet—Provisional diagnosis
- All the investigation reports
- Physicians orders sheet
- Treatment, medical or surgical
- Anaesthesia record
- Operation record
- Obstetric record
- Consultancy report
- Progress report
- Final diagnosis
- Discharge summary
- If death—Cause of death Autopsy report.

CLASSIFICATION

The classification of records would depend upon the nature of organization. However, it would be useful to classify records into the following four-fold classifications: (a) Vital records protected and preserved for a long time. (b) Important records not currently in use but are of high value of retain. (c) Useful records currently used correspondence. (d) Transit record useful for only a short period till the subject is alive or active.

MECHANISM OF RECORDS MANAGEMENT

There are two basic instruments through which we create and maintain records, i.e. form and files. Let us discuss in brief about these two mechanisms.

Filing

Filing is the process of classifying, arranging and storing records systematically so that these can be easily retrieved. Neuner and Haynes defined filling as 'the systematic arrangement for keeping of business correspondence and records so that these may be found and delivered quickly when needed for reference in future.' George R. Terry defines, "Filing is the placing of documents and papers in acceptable containers according to some pre-determined arrangement so that any of these when required, may be located quickly and conveniently."

Filing Arrangements

- Alphabetical order
- Numerical order
- Geographic order
- Chronological order
- Subject-wise

Many variations and innovations in these five general systems of filing have been developed, e.g., the use of colours, sound and special visual devices.

In the offices of the Government of India and State Governments, filing system is based on subject system. This system has many defects—lack of uniformity, lack of clear-cut demarcation and time-consuming tracing process.

The question of filing system was examined by the Administrative Reforms Commission and they recommended the functional filing system. The proposed system can be elaborated as follows: (a) The main subjects under the functions, say establishment, common office services, budget, are first listed under functional group headings which are respectively identified by capital letters, 'A', 'B', etc. (b) Each main subject or main head under each functional group is assigned consecutive Arabic numerals beginning with 'I' which may go upto '99'. (c) Similarly, the sub-subjects or sub-heads under each main head are assigned consecutive, Arabic numerals beginning with 'II' which also could go upto '99'. (d) The identifying subject numerals and sub-subject numerals are separated by '0' the group of numerals to the left of '0' refer the main head while that to the right to its sub-head, topic or aspect. (e) Files opened under the same subject, etc. are given serial numbers 1, 2 and 3 and so on and separated from the groups of numerals by an oblique. (f) The year in which the file is opened is shown separately from the file number by an oblique. (g) At the end of each file code number is to be indicated with the abbreviated form of a section or a unit.

File Indexing

File Indexing is a key to locate the files. Index is a reference list used for locating a particular document in the filing equipment. The following types of indexing may be used for locating:

- Vertical card indexing

- Visible card indexing
- Visible book indexing
- Loose leaf book indexing

Centralized and Decentralized Filing System

Centralized filing system is one, where all the filing equipments and personnel are located in a single area of the office, accessible to all departments by messengers, controlled by a centralized plan or index of the filing. Decentralized filing system also called departmentalised filing system is one, where each organization makes its own arrangement for filing.

Advantages

Advantages of centralized filing are:

1. It ensures uniformity and standardisation of the filing equipment and procedure which can help in easy and quick location of records.

2. It eliminates the need of duplication and distribution to all concerned sections. It encourages completeness of related documents.

3. It enhances economy of time for both file users and file personnel because there is only one place to send material to be filed, and one place to find it.

4. Control is exercised more effectively since one person or group alone is responsible, which minimises oversights and loss of valuable records.

5. It promotes economy of filing equipment and floor space. To be most effective a compromise has to be struck between centralized and decentralized filing systems. Decentralized filing should be kept to a minimum.

ADVANTAGES OF RECORDS KEEPING

The records help the management in the following ways:

1. Help in Sound Decision-making

Effective decision-making depends to a great extent upon the adequate information provided by the records and availability of these records in time.

2. Effective Channel of Internal Control

Records are very important to ensure internal control. Records can help in minimising chance of error and prevent occurrence of fraud and corruption.

3. Facilitate Evaluation of Corporate Performance

The records can help in evaluating the performance of an organization during definite intervals of time and different periods. Besides, records can help in comparing the performance of organization in the same line.

4. Promotes Efficiency of Operations

The effective operations of an organization depend to a great extent upon the speed and accuracy of the records. Records keep the wheels of the organization moving fast.

5. Fulfils Statutory Requirement

Records are also kept in compliance with the provisions of different statutes, e.g., maintenance of statutory books under Indian Companies Act, 1956. Besides, records are needed in the event of litigations, disputes or claims.

6. Futuristic Approach

Analysis of records help in ascertaining future trends which can help in better policy-making and planning. The fundamental reason for promoting maintenance of an adequate medical record is its utility to good patient care, to the doctor, to the hospital and towards medical education and research. Besides, the legal requirements of the hospital, medical records are also to be completed.

USE OF HOSPITAL STATISTICS FOR MANAGEMENT

The Medical Records Department in a hospital is mainly responsible for the collection as well as analysis of the date to ensure utilisation of the hospital for patient care. Such date has immense value for the day-to-day management of the hospitals as well as future planning of the hospital services. Let us some mention of the important information which is used by the hospital management to enhance the hospital functioning.

1. Death Rates

Hospital deaths include deaths of patients admitted to the hospital. Deaths are generally classified into two categories, i.e. the Gross Deaths and the Net Deaths. Gross Deaths include all the deaths of admitted patients while Net Deaths exclude the patients dying within 48 hours of admission. Net Deaths in a hospital is a reflection of the working of the hospital. Net deaths rate is calculated as follows:

$$\frac{\text{Number of total discharges during that period of time}}{\text{Number of net deaths during a period of time}} \times 100$$

In an average net death rates range between 4 to 6 per cent. Any gross variations from the normally expected net death rate indicates an abnormal phenomenon which should be analyzed by the hospital management. Such deviation can either be due to natural causes or due to failure on the part of one of the service areas of the hospital. In the case of later event correctives need be applied and death rate brought back to the normal expected range.

The use of net death rates for enhancing the efficiency of the hospital services is not only limited to the overall net death rate of the hospital but also can be split up into death rates of various departments and units of the hospital. As such, the hospital management can keep a track of the performance of each and every unit/department of the hospital by keeping a track of their net-death rates. This is being practised in most of the teaching hospitals but not in district hospitals.

2. Average Length of Stay

The length of stay of patients is another important hospital indices. For purposes of calculations, the day of admission of the patient is always taken into consideration and the date/day of discharge is always ignored irrespective of the time of admission or the time of discharge. Through the process of discharge analysis, the average length of stay of patients discharged during a particular period of time is worked out not only for the whole hospital but also department-wise/unit-wise. The aim of this information is to locate the unnecessary length of stay and to discourage it. By reducing the unnecessary length of stay more patients can be admitted to the hospital and provided services. This information, therefore, is not only important from the economic point of view but is also important from the community services point of view, average length of stay is calculated as follows:

$$\frac{\text{Total length of stay of discharged patients during a period of time}}{\text{Total discharges during that period of time}} \times 100$$

3. Bed Turnover Rate

Bed Turnover Rate indicates the number of patients who have been given services per bed per year. It is calculated as follows:

$$\frac{\text{Total number of discharges during a year}}{\text{Total number of authorized beds}} \times 100$$

Bed Turnover Rate is determined by the Average Length of Stay as well as the time interval between one discharge and successive admissions. This time interval is known as T-interval. Also, Bed Turnover Rate as well as T-interval are important indicators of the planning utilization of hospital resources.

4. Bed Occupancy Rate

Bed Occupancy Rate gives the relationship between the availability of facilities and their utilization. Optimum bed occupancy is treated to be between 85-90 per cent. An occupancy of over 90 per cent means stress is on one or another area of the hospital. When the bed occupancy rate is 100 or more than 100 per cent, it is a case of dilution of hospital facilities and lowering of efficiency. Bed Occupancy Rate can be worked out for the whole hospital as well as for each discipline/unit of the hospital, as on next page.

$$\frac{\text{Average daily census during a period of time}}{\text{Number of authorized beds}} \times 100 \text{ Bed Occupancy Rate}$$

ISSUES AND PROBLEMS OF RECORDS MANAGEMENT IN HOSPITAL

Based upon observation, discussion and analysis we give here the main problems faced by hospital authorities in Records Management and suggest probable solution:

(a) Use of Out-dated Forms

Need of Constant Revision: At present, forms being used in most of the hospitals are not in tune with the improvements in new technology and scientific developments. Some of the columns in the forms are obsolete while many important columns are not available. It is thus essential that forms must be revised constantly to keep them up-to-date. The ultimate purpose of tabulating the date from forms becomes insignificant as the forms do not convey the desired information. It must be statutory for every organization to get their forms reviewed after every three years either by the internal O & M cells or central O & M organization.

(b) Shortage of Experienced Personnel

Need of Trained Personnel: The hospital authorities do not attach as much weightage to records management as is done to other sources. This gives less emphasis in terms of resources to this activity. There is generally shortage of trained personnel to handle records. It is suggested that adequate experienced personnel may be appointed to take care of records management.

(c) Lack of Planning of Storage of In-active Records

Need of Effective Storage and Control of Inactive Records: Storage should be done at a proper place where proper conditions of temperature, circulation of air and humidity are provided. Mostly, we find dirt and dust in this area. After storing the records, indexing is necessary to locate the record for retrieval.

We can reduce congestion and cost through the control of inactive records. This would indirectly help us in finding the relevant record immediately. The Secretariat Training School in its report on Work Study (III) suggested the following improvements to make effective control of the inactive records:

(a) Keep a table of the important contents of a file on the cover or a slip. This will facilitate location of contents which the title of the file or its number may not help to locate speedily.

(b) Keep documents like records, separately from the files. This will reduce the bulk of the files and assist speedier location and use of documents not related to correspondence and notes.

(c) Papers containing information may be carried in a third folder separately from notes and correspondence.
(d) Persons dealing with 'information' should compile the vital elements of information and keep it at hand in cabinets for ready reference. Simple 'Home made' devices can be invented to carry such information and reduce dependence on records.
(e) Keep a small alphabetical register of important files, cases, reports and other documents in your personal custody for more purposeful follow up, records location and speedier disposal.
(f) Need of Effective Handling and Processing of Records.

Handling and processing of records should be simple and should not consume much time and personnel resources. The expert handling and processing of records would depend upon the design of registry and its place in the office layout, rational and well laid out procedures and the training of the personnel responsible for job.

Evaluation of Records Handling: There is a need to check the records frequently. A random checking can be done with the help of the following two ratios:

1. Accuracy Ratio = $\dfrac{\text{Number of references not found}}{\text{Number of references found}}$

2. Activity Ratio = $\dfrac{\text{Number of references found}}{\text{Number of documents filed}}$

If the accuracy ratio is half or one per cent, it is thought to be excellent. If it is three or more per cent, it is in a poor state.

If the activity ratio is below ten per cent, it exhibits that there is too much inactive material. If it is between ten to twenty per cent, it means that there is a need of improvement while it is more than twenty per cent it shows that the records are in bad shape. Such evaluations can help in improving the records.

(g) Need of Determination of Records Retention Period

There is no hard and fast rule that specific record should be retained for specific period of time. The decision regarding the retention period should be decided by the organization basing on its needs, requirements and objectives. The records which help in tracing the history of the organization and help in policy-making should be kept for long. The unwanted records should be destroyed to save time and resources.

Transfer of Records

Transfer of records entail two stages, i.e. (i) Dating of unimportant records for destruction and ultimate disposal, (ii) moving the records from active to inactive files and from there to storage area. In a complex organization we can make use of micro-films. Micro-films can help in space saving, safe preservation and clean and easy handling. Besides, these reduce the risk of fire hazards and chances of loosing document.

(h) Need of Improving Quality of Medical Records

Quantitatively the system of medical records is fairly satisfactory, but qualitatively the medical records need lot of improvements. It is recommended that more efforts should be made by the hospital management, all clinicians as well as medical records officer towards improving the quality of medical records.

QUESTIONS AND ANSWERS

Why Do I Need to Register?

Registration is an important part of your services at Rush North Shore Medical Center. The information gathered at registration is important in order for hospital departments and your physician to provide you with timely, quality care. Governmental requirements are also part of the registration process. This includes but is not limited to: Complete Physician Order, The Notice of Privacy Practices, Medicare Secondary Payor Questionnaire, and your signature. Information about these requirements is provided below:

- Registration staff will ask for, or verify your personal information such as name, address and telephone number in addition to insurance information, and any other insurance requirements on every visit.
- Since each visit is billed separately, you will have a new hospital account number each time you register, except for Recurring Services. Please review the section. "Registering for Recurring Services."
- The information collected during registration becomes part of your hospital record and is also used for billing your insurance company.
- If you do not have insurance coverage or are concerned about your portion of the hospital bill, Rush North Shore Medical Center offers several payment options. Please review the section: "What if I Do Not Have Insurance or Owe a Balance After Insurance." Registration staff will also be able to provide you with information about our programs.
- Please be prepared to pay your co-payment, if applicable, at time of registration.

When Should I Be Here?

If you are scheduled for a test or procedure, please arrive at Registration at least 20 to 30 minutes prior to your scheduled appointment time unless otherwise instructed.

Where Do I Register?

If you are scheduled for any surgical, endoscopic or cardiac procedure, you will register at the Ambulatory Surgery Department located next to the main lobby of the hospital.

For all other services, you will register at the Central Registration Department in the main lobby of the hospital.

What Should I Bring to Registration?

All Services

- Photo identification (this includes driver's license, state ID, or employer photo identification card);
- Your insurance card(s); and
- Written authorization from your employer for services pertaining to Workers' Compensation, if applicable.

Outpatient Services

- Written order from your doctor; and
- If you have HMO insurance, you must bring your referral form completed by your primary physician for Outpatient Services. Your insurance may not pay unless you present this form at the time you register.

What are the different types of service for Registration?

Your physician determines the type of service you are registering for:

Inpatient:	Overnight stay; normally more than 24 hours.
Observation:	An outpatient service; normally one overnight stay or less than 24 hours. This allows your physician to observe your condition in a hospital room.
Outpatient:	Not an overnight stay; service is performed and you go home on the same day.

Examples of Outpatient Services

- Laboratory test
- X-Ray test
- Outpatient surgery/outpatient procedures
- Recurring services (Physical Therapy, Chemotherapy, etc.)

You must present a written order from your doctor. This order must include:

- Patient name

- The type of test or service
- The reason for the test or service (signs and/or symptoms or existing diagnosis)
- Ordering physician's name
- Ordering physician's signature

What are the Recurring Services for Registering?

A recurring service is a series of treatments that occur over a number of days. Registration occurs only once every 31 days. Examples of recurring services:

- Cardiac Rehabilitation
- Infusion Therapy
- Physical Therapy
- Pulmonary Rehabilitation
- Outpatient Oncology
- Speech Therapy

The first time you register for recurring services, you will follow the same registration process listed above for outpatient services. The most important difference in registration requirements for patients receiving recurring services is that you may be required to re-register every thirty-one days or after any inpatient stay, observation stay, emergency room visit, or outpatient surgery if your recurring service will continue. If you have any questions about your recurring services, ask the staff in the department where you are receiving services.

What Does Medicare Require?

As a provider of Medicare services, Rush North Shore Medical Center is required to follow certain Medicare guidelines. This sometimes includes providing you with certain information and other times require that we ask for information from you. Each time you register, Medicare requires the hospital to:

- Complete a Medicare Secondary Payor Questionnaire (MSPQ). This form tells Medicare and the hospital if there is other insurance that would pay the bill instead of Medicare. This could include, but is not limited to, automobile insurance or insurance through an employer.
- Comply with Medical Necessity Guidelines outlined by Medicare. This means that the test(s) your physician orders must follow certain specific coverage guidelines. If the diagnosis, sign or symptom given for a particular test(s) does not meet Medicare's Medical Necessity Guidelines, Medicare will not pay for the test(s). We will inform you about it on a special form called an Advanced Beneficiary Notice (ABN).

If this happens you may choose to do one of the following:

- Have the test(s) or service(s) performed. You will be asked to sign the ABN. By signing this form, you understand that the hospital has informed you about this coverage issue and you will be responsible for payment of the test(s).
- Postpone the test until you are able to talk with your physician.

What Does the Federal Government Require?

A governmental regulation called the Health Insurance Portability and Accountability Act (HIPAA), went into effect in April, 2003. This Act is meant to protect your private health information and its use. On your first visit to Rush North Shore, you will be given the hospital's "Notice of Privacy Practices" brochure, and will be asked to sign an acknowledgement of receipt form.

What Does an HMO/PPO Require?

HMO plans may require you to bring a completed referral form from your primary physician. Some HMO/POS and PPO plans may require prior authorization for certain services. Since insurance requirements vary by employers, please contact your health plan, or the employee benefit department where you work for additional information.

What Does Rush North Shore Medical Center Require?

We require you to sign an authorization form which allows us to release information to your doctor and insurance company, if requested. Please refer to the "What Should I Bring to Registration" section of the brochure for more specific information.

2

Management of Hospital Parking Problems

With the increasing number of vehicles, the hospitals are getting choked and give the look of an old car bazaar, more than a health care facility. The patients have a tough time in parking a vehicle and an ordeal in taking it out every time they visit a hospital; tertiary, district or institutional. Recently a heated argument over a parking problem ended with a patient being shot dead point blank outside a public hospital. A police spokesman said the incident happened about midnight when a businessman was unable to drive his car out of a parking lot as it was allegedly blocked by this patient. "An argument ensued between them which led to a scuffle. At this juncture and the . . . Better management of parking lot could save the life of the deceased patient, who had come for treatment from a distant town."

The car parks at various hospitals are woefully inadequate for outpatients especially, as well as for visitors to the wards. Outpatients risk fines for overstaying should the medicals overrun their time schedules. Waiting times are well known to drag on, sometimes over an hour. But first find a space—if you can.

MULTI MILLION BUSINESS IN UK

Twelve hospital trusts each raised over £1m in charges, figures obtained under the Freedom of Information Act show. The Department of Health said it was up to NHS trusts to decide what to charge, and said charges deterred non-service users from using the car parks. But Macmillan Cancer Relief said it was "morally wrong" to raise revenue by forcing patients to pay for parking. The hospitals earning the most from car parks tended to be the larger trusts treating more patients. The Department of

Health figures suggest that one trust, University Hospital Birmingham, raised £1.5 million from car parking charges in 2004-5. But the trust says this is the revenue from the car parks from three health trusts on four hospital sites; the two sites of the University Hospital Birmingham, the Birmingham and Solihull Mental Health Hospital and the Women's Hospital. A spokeswoman said: "We actually have one of the lowest charges for car parking in the country, this high revenue figure is due to the fact that a lot of people are using these spaces." The two University Hospital Birmingham sites serve more than 553,000 people a year. Of the £1.5m revenue, £1m was pumped into the costs of running the car parks and a shuttle bus from the local train station, while the rest was invested back into patient care.

Flat rate

The Cambridge University NHS Foundation Trust also raises more than £1m from its car parks. The trust's car parks serve two hospitals, the large 1,100-bed Addenbrooke's and the Rosie Hospital for women and charge a flat rate of £2.50. A spokeswoman said the income paid for improvements such as external lighting, walkways, cycle racks and ways, security and improved car park and travel facilities. A spokeswoman said:

"In direct response to local demand, we have considerably expanded the number of spaces available and also ensured a good standard of lighting, security, etc. . . . investing some £1.2m in car park expansion and improvements in the last six years."

A spokeswoman for the Oxford Radcliffe Hospitals NHS Trust, which raised more than £1.2m from its car parks, pointed out it was one of the largest trusts in the country, with approximately 1,200 patient and visitor parking spaces, split across four separate sites.

"The hospital car parks are not run as a commercial operation and all money raised goes directly back into services for patients and visitors."

"The average cost of a three-hour stay at the John Radcliffe Hospital, the biggest of the four sites, is only £1.50."

'Patient exploitation'

A Department of Health spokeswoman said parking charges helped hospitals because they discouraged people who were not using the hospital from taking up the car park spaces.

She added that most hospitals had exemptions from charges for patients, "and hospital staff are generally well trained in advising patients about these exemptions."

"Ultimately, it is a matter for individual NHS trusts to decide whether or not to charge for car parking, and the level of charges in the light of local circumstances."

Macmillan Cancer Relief has been campaigning to end hospital parking charges, especially for cancer patients who make frequent hospital trips for treatment.

The charity's chief executive Peter Cardy said: "Raising revenue by forcing cancer patients to pay for hospital car parking is morally wrong.

"It is shameful that the sickest and most vulnerable people have to pay the most. Hospital car parking costs are often the final straw in a long line of extra costs faced by cancer patients."

Michael Summers, chairman of the Patients Association, said: "We take the view that this is exploitation of patients who are very vulnerable.

"Some of these patients are visiting hospital several times in a week for treatment and a lot of patients' families are also visiting several times. "Those who are genuinely attending for treatment ought not to be charged."

Patient's stories

A few days ago Baldev's mother became ill and had to be taken to hospital. He decided to bring her in his car and he took his young daughter along for the ride also. On reaching General hospital, he left his car along the driveway up to the main entrance, while he took his mother inside—she had difficulty in walking. He left his daughter in the car for the little while he was inside. After he got his mother settled inside—about five to ten minutes later, he came out to move his car, only to find that he had got a parking ticket from the car park patrol. Annoyed, Baldev went to the hut where the patrol staff are based and explained that he had no other option but to leave his car where he did, as his mother wouldn't be able to walk from the car park. He didn't get any satisfactory reply. His story raises a very pertinent question: "What is a driver supposed to do with his/her car while taking an elderly/disabled person into the hospital." There appears to be no place near the hospital where a car can be legally left when helping an incapacitated person in. The whole parking arrangements at the hospital need to be examined—not necessarily a medical examination! Some comments heard on this behalf were:

"I'm totally opposed to these car parking charges, they're disgraceful. "Why should someone have to pay to park when they are just picking someone up" I want to know why they're doing this and where the money is going.

"I want to know if this is just a means to have their own campaign to stop people driving and get them to be more environmentally aware?"

"I totally oppose any members of the public having to pay to park at the hospital."

"Car park attendants are stopping us from parking in the outpatient's car park and staff parking is clearly signposted, to leave as much space as possible for patients, and now we look forward to the new decked car park to improve things further."

Hospital parking system requires surgery!

Nehru hospital at PGI Chandigarh is a frequented place by the patients of the city and others. At least 2000 vehicles are parked in the campus at any one time; most belonging to staff members. Where should the disabled and serious patients go to park their vehicles? Can shuttle service solve the problem for the staff as well as patients and their attendants? The author has a harrowing tale to tell when he had to go to the hospital with his ailing wife in Ambulance. When an ambulance approaches the giant building of this hospital, it is refused entry to that gate, which may be convenient to the patient. Several cane bearers will shoo it away from one gate to another, even before the patient is unloaded. Parking problem is so acute that even serious patients do not find entry. At PGI parking housing estate is congested for over half a mile. Its residents are very upset and are putting wheelie bins on the roadside to deter motorists. These people have no right to make these obstructions. Providing there are no double lines or drive entrances to block, and enough room allowed for passing traffic, motorists have a fully legal right to park on the road—that is why motorists pay road tax. But come on PGI, the need for more and better parking facilities is absolutely essential as the hospital grows larger and our population increases.

A park and ride scheme has been suggested as a solution to parking problems in a Hospital like at PGI Chandigarh. The scheme is to encourage motorists to park their vehicles at designated car parks away from the hospital premises and use the shuttle service, MRT, LRT or buses to travel to other parts of the city. "There is an urgent need for more parking spaces at the Hospital", said one visitor. The space should be underground so that the hospitals look is clean and serene. In Thailand's Bumrungrad hospital; top in the field of medical tourism, the first 10 stories in the 22 storied building are earmarked for parking of vehicles. Vertical growth of buildings can provide more space for parking and other needs in the scarce land scenario.

The demand for parking space is becoming increasingly high. Blue light emergency ambulance routes within hospital sites are frequently blocked by thoughtlessly parked vehicles and car park management is a difficult challenge facing all sites. Parking problems coupled with the threat of workplace parking charges have meant that hospitals are rapidly latching onto the government's requests to develop Green Travel Plans. The main aim of a Green Travel Plan is to encourage users of a particular site, in this case hospitals, to reduce the number of car trips made and to promote the use of sustainable, alternative transport modes.

Delhi on way to park and ride mode

In a new initiative aimed at discouraging use of private vehicles for long inter-city travel, the Delhi Government is going to launch a "park and ride scheme" at all Delhi Transport Corporation (DTC) bus terminals across the city. In addition, private bus operators would be allowed to park their vehicles during the night at these terminals for a certain parking charge.

The idea behind the exercise is not only to ensure better utilization of the vast land available at the DTC terminals but also to generate extra revenue for the loss-making Corporation. This would also ensure proper utilization of the extra staff that is lying idle with the DTC. A number of other initiatives including opening of Pollution Under Control Certificate Centers on commercial basis at these terminals, opening another fitness centre at the Okhla Depot and starting a driving training school at Nand Nagri Depot. "This is part of the restructuring plan drawn up by the DTC and the Transport Department to generate additional revenue and tone up the functioning of related services," the Transport Minister, Haroon Yusuf, told *The Hindu*.

Under the new park and ride scheme, the owners of private vehicles would be allowed to park their vehicles at the DTC bus terminals and depots and then take the DTC buses and the soon-to-be introduced luxury coaches for their respective destinations. Those terminals that are near the Metro Rail stoppages would act as parking slots allowing the private vehicle owners to park and take a ride either on the bus or Metro Rail. According to the Secretary-*cum*-Commissioner (Transport), Rajeev Talwar, the idea is to encourage the people to undertake major part of their journey on one of the modes of public transport system and keep their vehicles off the road for as long a duration as possible. This would also lead to decongestion on city roads and save on fuel and pollution in the long-run.

In addition, Mr. Talwar said the Chief Minister, Sheila Dikshit, had given directions that the DTC should encourage introduction of luxury and air-conditioned bus coaches on the intra-city routes to encourage private vehicle owners to have a comfortable travel to their work place.

Apart from this, Mr. Talwar said that it had also been decided that the private bus owners would be asked to park their vehicles at the DTC terminals or depots during the night. They would be charged a certain amount for this service. It is important that these vehicles are parked at the DTC terminals as these buses are also expected to start and terminate from these terminals or depots.

In addition, the Government has given the go ahead to open a new fitness centre at Okhla in South Delhi. This would put an end to the monopoly of the Burari fitness centre that has come to be identified with corruption and inefficiency and also provide competition leading to better fitness certification. It has also been decided to open a driver's training institute at the DTC terminal at Nand Nagri in East Delhi. This institute will not only provide training to the DTC personnel but also train drivers of other organizations and private bus operators.

Hyderabad's car lift scheme!

They found the solution to the problem on a trip to Tokyo. That's where we saw a car lift. It is a mechanical system that can accommodate two cars in the space required for one car. A car is elevated and another car is accommodated beneath it." With this in mind Paresh and Vijay decided to build similar car lifts and make them available in the city. Says Paresh, "We are basically mechanical engineers and this helped us in mastering the technology. We set-up a unit in Balanagar this February, and began our work. Today we are fully functional and can build a car tower in just four days." Car lifts are being used in Mumbai but these machines are imported and are expensive. "A 50-car tower that is manufactured in Korea costs around Rs. 1.75 crore. But the car lifts we are making are made totally with Indian machinery. This reduces the price to a great extent. A single car lift that we manufacture costs just Rs. 85,000, and can accommodate two cars," says Paresh. This system of hi-tech parking will definitely help in solving parking problems to a great extent. "Even the Mayor was impressed and his response was very positive when we gave him a demonstration. Car lifts are ideal for hospitals, hotels, shopping complexes and business establishments. People just have to be made aware that such machinery is available in the city."

"We have to reduce free parking permits for staff , because primarily we're here to serve patients and they have to come first", a spokesman told. "Priority will be given to those working unsociable hours, for example, those with care responsibilities for children or elderly relatives—or if staff work across various sites. We don't get many complaints about the charges but anyone who visits the hospital knows the main problem is about being unable to park. Patients have missed clinics and appointments and we've even had emergency services struggling to get people in because of parked cars obstructing pavements. People visiting can have all kinds of problems, including mobility and vision, and there are obvious reasons why routes must be clear."

There is no justification for free parking to staff when patients are being charged. In fact the staff should not be allowed to park their vehicles on the campus; they need to come in public transport.

Southampton General Hospital U.K.: A study

Southampton General Hospital is a large teaching hospital and provides specialist expertise to the South of England region. It houses renowned centers of excellence in the treatment of cancer, heart disease, respiratory illness, neurological disease, gastro-intestinal conditions and illnesses affecting children. The hospital is fortunate to benefit from a high number of specialist consultants working in large multi-disciplinary teams and plays a leading role in the development of new and improved treatments for NHS patients.

In November 2005, Alan Whitehead MP sent a survey addressed to approximately 2,500 households in areas surrounding Southampton General Hospital. This included properties served by the Coxford Area Resident's Parking Scheme and those just which lie just outside the scheme. The survey was in response to number of letters from residents complaining of parking problems in the area. There were 225 replies. The survey hoped to shed light on:

The extent of the parking problems How effectively the parking scheme was working Whether there were suggestions to improve or extend the scheme Whether there were suggestions to improve parking generally

The Coxford Residents' Parking Scheme was introduced in the early 1990s after the Hospital introduced parking charges within their site. The scheme solved many of the parking problems in the immediate area of the General Hospital but did also result in over-spill problems in the surrounding area, so it was expanded to its present size a few years later. With the Hospital's continued expansion, parking is again a problem. Staff, patient and visitor numbers to the hospital is increasing. Higher housing density, Houses in Multiple Occupancy and a general increase in car-ownership all contribute. Within the Residents' Parking Scheme area, most properties have one free parking space, a number of visitor permits and the option of a second car permit at a cost of £50. At present the parking bays operate from 8 a.m. to 6 p.m., Monday to Friday, and visitors may use them for a limited time without a permit. In most cases it is two hours, but it has been reduced to one hour in some roads nearest the Hospital. The Hospital has some staff and public parking but this is very limited and there is a charge to park in most cases.

Question 1: How well do you think the Residents' Parking Scheme currently works?

Very well = 24; Well = 24; Poorly = 35; Very Poorly = 40; No Answer = 29.

There were mixed feelings as to the overall effectiveness of the scheme. Some comments included remarks along the lines of "at present I am happy with the parking situation." One person said, "I am not a car owner but I have noticed less congestion since the scheme has been in operation." No one within the Residents' Parking Zone, however unhappy with the scheme, suggested it should be abandoned.

Question 2: Times—At present the parking bays operate from 8am to 6pm, Monday to Friday, and visitors may use them for a limited time without a permit. In most cases it is two hours, but it has been reduced to one hour in some roads nearest the Hospital. Have you any suggestions to alter the timing of the scheme?

Most people (111) didn't make any suggestions to changing the times of the scheme and 79 said there should be no changes. 8 people said the scheme should be one hour and no return but one person said this is not sufficient time for visitors. Another said the key was having no return to any part of the zone and not just the same street. Staff and visitors were reported to park for two hours come back and move cars to the next street. One resident said, "short stays within the two hour limit by non-residents and their visitors cause most of the problems." 5 people said the scheme should discontinue times and introduce residents only parking with visitor permits. 4 people said the scheme should be two hours everywhere—"parking areas are usually vacant between 8 a.m. and 5 p.m.." One person said two hours should be reintroduced where its now one hour. "One hour is ridiculous for patients with appointments." Another said, "two hours are sufficient to prevent long-term hospital workers from parking." One person said reduce the parking time to half an hour. In terms of extending days of the scheme: 1 person thought extending the time to include Saturday mornings (8 a.m.-12 p.m.). 7 people suggested all of Saturday. 8 others thought the scheme should run all week, particularly in roads close to the hospital. Different general suggestions were made for extending hours which the scheme operates: 9-4 p.m., 7.30 a.m.-7.30 p.m., 8 a.m.-4 p.m. Evenings—8 people thought the scheme should run later with 3 suggesting until 9 p.m. Specific changes suggested 24 hour in Dale Road, end of Dale Valley Road—one hour time limit only. 3 people said Vine Road should be made 60 minutes (with one person saying 60 or 30 minutes). Two people said Laundry Road should be one hour only.

Question 3: Do you think the current area of the Coxford Area Residents' Parking Scheme should be extended to include new roads?

We asked if the parking scheme should be extended to include new roads. 85 people gave no answer and 46 others expressed no opinion. This is explained by the survey going both to residents where there is a scheme (who would be less likely to answer) and those who live just outside it. Aldermoor Road—13 replies said the scheme should be extended to Aldermoor Road, particularly by the shops. "We don't have a parking scheme in Aldermoor Road. We tried but the council didn't want to." "Stop all parking in Coxford Road from Lordshill Way up to Aldermoor Avenue and make Aldermoor Close restricted parking." 9 people said Coxford Road especially by the health centre, needed restrictions. Longleat Gardens—"I would like to see parking restrictions by Longleat Gardens/Aldermoor Road (in the slip road). This is filled by hospital staff parking all day." "The junction with Aldermoor Road and Longleat Gardens is absolutely packed with hospital cars, it's a disgrace." Jex Blake Close—"Jex Blake Close is regarded by many hospital visitors as a convenient location to park as there are no parking restrictions in force. Extend scheme." 4 replies called for this Dunkirk Road—2 people called for restrictions. "Dunkirk Road has problems with Hospital and Sports Centre parking." Seymour Road—5 people called for restrictions. Lyburn Close—"Although the first four houses have residents' parking, the Highways Dept will do nothing for us in the last four houses because they say that this part of the road has not been adopted so we always get Hospital cars." Vinery Road, St James Park Road and Vinery Gardens Approximately 9 people calls to extend the scheme to Vinery Road, St James Park Road and Vinery Gardens and asking it was not included previously. "I hope you will be able to help the residents of Vinery Gardens and Road and St James Road to obtain a parking scheme for our area." One resident of Vinery Gardens did oppose extending the scheme in the area. "In Vinery Gardens, myself and other residents do not feel the need for restrictions in our street and would reject any proposals. Our road is mainly clear of traffic during the day." But another resident sent photographs showing these roads full with parked cars and traffic. Medina Road Preshaw Close—numbers 1-7 don't have residents' parking. Malwood Avenue Shalden Close Olive Road—7 people called for restrictions "Why can't we have a permit parking as you have for the bottom of Olive Road. We were promised this." Palm Road—4 people called for parking restrictions. "Yellow lines in Palm Road as it's such a problem for buses." Warren Avenue and Warren Crescent—three people thought a scheme is needed. 7 people said they didn't want an extension.

Question 4. How well do you think the Resident's Parking Scheme is currently enforced?

Of the replies, 18 people thought the scheme was enforced very well, 74 thought it was well enforced, 56 thought it was poorly enforced and 35 thought it was very poorly enforced. 25 didn't answer. "A little sanity should prevail as my husband had two tickets once the pass ran out." "Give residents right to enforce parking." "The Hospital should take more responsibility."

"Enforced very poorly, residents' tickets given to hospital staff. Number given to the council but no action taken." "I always see traffic wardens checking the cars" "More patrols needed especially in Warren Avenue, Jesamine Road and Laundry Road." Two other replies mentioned that Warren Avenue was not well patrolled.

Question 5: Have you any other suggestions to improve the parking situation in the Coxford area?

The Hospital's existing parking. There were a number of calls for the Hospital to change its policy to charging within the hospital. These included suggestions to reduce charges, end charges at weekends, or altogether. "Since the hospital has been charging for parking, residents get problems with staff parking at weekends. This is most annoying as the staff car park is empty at weekends. Staff should be able to use the car park for free in the evening or at weekends."

Many residents also suggest the Hospital could do more to increase its own parking spaces. There were lots of calls for a multi storey car park to be built and adding on levels to existing car parks. One person suggested a site for a purpose-built car park "on the ground behind the Princess Anne Hospital." One person even suggested limiting visiting times to patients.

Disabled parking More than 30 people raised their concerns over disabled badge holders parking near the Hospital on double yellow lines, particularly in Springford Road, Coxford Road and Tremona Road. Descriptions included an "accident waiting to happen", "more hazardous to other road users" and "very dangerous" with many people blaming the hospital for introducing charges for disabled badge holders. People asked this to be discussed with the General Hospital and suggested solutions included getting the hospital to stop charging for disabled visitors, and putting in double red lines to stop parking altogether in the dangerous areas.

Aldermoor Health Centre/One Stop Another area to suffer from serious congestion and parking problems (including disabled badge holders parking) was the area around Aldermoor Health Centre and the 'One Stop' shop. 15 people complained of parking difficulties here. "Outside Aldermoor health centre, cars block the dropped kerb, making access impossible for prams or wheelchairs. You find the surgery car park full with hospital workers. The local bus has problems with getting through. There seems a need for double yellow lines." A number of other people also called for double-yellow lines or restrictions.

Laundry Road Concerns over Laundry Road (just to the south of the hospital) being a 'rat-run'. Suggestions that it should be one way, have speed restrictions speed humps. Calls for the permitted time to be one hour not two hours, and opposition to newly-built flats having residents' permits.

Dale Valley Road A slightly separate issue raised by a number of people was the problem of speeding on Dale Valley Road.

"A more important issue that needs addressing is the urgent need for traffic calming measures on Dale Valley Road. The recent resurfacing has made the road akin to a racetrack—many drivers do not adhere to the 30 mph limit."

"I believe the council gave notice that they were doing more double yellow lines and two hour parking but we've seen no action yet (Dale Valley Road). With the construction traffic as well as buses, it is hideous here. Reducing those who park all day in the area would really help."

Norham Avenue: "Norham Avenue has become a rat-run esp. HGVs, lorries and cars—freedom from traffic lights. Solutions could be weight restrictions or articulated restrictions."

Drop kerb A number of people suggested that they would like to put in a drop kerb "which would mean less car space" but that it was currently too expensive. Possibility of an incentive to get the resident's car off the road. Suggestions for new car park spaces Some residents suggested possible places for more parking spaces. They included:

"Turn the waste land in Palm Road into a car park for the hospital."

"On Aldermoor Road, cut back into the green to make bays deep enough for cars to park their nose in to leave road clear for moving traffic."

"I know some residents allow their drives to be used by Hospital workers during the day, so maybe this could be looked into with the promise of a reward."

"Possible piece of land at Shalden Close could be made into a car park."

"Site of old Alder's furnishing store should be an overspill car park for the Hospital."

"On Coxford Road, remove the bushes and make more diagonal parking."

"Why don't you just build more parking in waste grounds, e.g. the field in Greywell Avenue."

Birch Close—"there is not enough parking for residents, currently approx 11 spaces for 44 flats." Some residents believe the space surrounding each flat would be best used for parking. Eleven people suggested a park and ride scheme should be introduced.

"The staff shuttle to hospital from Sainsbury's is great—but why not try obtaining land—maybe at Nursling Industrial Estate and provide a shuttle service for visitors?" Suggestions for where a park and ride could be included.

Near the B&Q warehouse—on the site of the boat show car park. Car boot sale area opposite Sainsbury's Lordshill. Develop car parking or extend the scheme in conjunction with Sainsbury's Lordshill. Nursling Industrial Estate. Part of the Ordnance Survey site when it moves. Public transport.

There were a number of calls to improve public transport generally. A couple of suggestions to the bus service included "a circular free route from Hill Lane to Winchester Road" and "a bus lay-by at the hospital entrance in Tremona Road to improve traffic flow."

Cost of additional permits 15 people complained about the charge for a second permit. "The residents' parking scheme seems to work well, although I think most residents are upset about the £50 for additional permits."

Visitor permits

Two replies mentioned the problem of abuse of visitor permits.

Summary and suggested action

(1) The high level of parking around the General Hospital clearly impacts on residents within and outside the Coxford Residents' Parking Scheme. This will continue if left ignored. There is a general view from local residents that the Hospital should be more responsible for parking as it expands.

(2) A number or residents outside the Residents' Parking Scheme have called for the scheme to be extended to their roads because of overspill problems from staff and visitors to the Hospital. Roads currently not covered by the scheme, where we have had calls for its extension, should be further consulted with a view to extending the scheme.

(3) The large number of complaints particularly about parking around Aldermoor Health Centre shows this problem needs addressing as soon as possible.

(4) Similarly, the issue disabled drivers choosing to park outside the Hospital needs urgently resolving. The number of concerns over 'accidents waiting to happen' suggests parking shouldn't be allowed in certain hazardous areas near to the Hospital.

(5) Suggestions for time changes to the Residents' Parking Scheme have been made—both in terms of extending the area of the one hour permitted parking limit and the overall times the scheme—

but there are no obvious conclusions from our survey. In future, the scheme may need to be extended to include weekends and evenings but more research has to be done before any timing changes were made.

(6) A park and ride scheme should be investigated as a longer term answer to reducing parking problems. A number of sites have been suggested by residents and should be investigated by the NHS Trust and Council. Sites for smaller car parks have also been suggested.

(7) The University NHS Trust and Council have taken measures—most obviously the Resident's Parking Scheme—which despite highlighted faults, generally works in protecting residents' ability to park near their homes.

(8) It might be logical for the Hospital and Residents' Parking Scheme to come more into line with each other. For example, residents have reported empty Hospital car parks at weekends with staff choosing instead to park on nearby streets. It might therefore be an idea to change or stop Hospital parking charges at weekends.

(9) There is anecdotal evidence of staff and visitors returning to their cars and moving them to a different street to get round the two hour permitted parking limit. This should be investigated with a view to changing the 'no return' to cover the whole zone rather than just the same street.

ParkMed management services

ParkMed is a parking management service specializing in hospital parking and health care industry traffic control and shuttle services. They provide hospital valet parking, front door services, hospital parking management, hospital greeter and traffic control services as well as hospital shuttle services. The management team at ParkMed has many years of experience in the parking management industry and a commitment to excellence which ensures your patients will have a pleasant experience and a good first impression of your health care facility. Valet parking for hospitals helps control the traffic at your front door, provides shorter walks for those with health problems and provides that all important first impression by which so many people judge a business. Valet parking is a "value added" service which your clients will appreciate. Call ParkMed to discuss adding valet parking to your health care facility today. Along with valet parking, ParkMed also offers traffic control services and will act as parking consultants on your health care project. From parking lot management to front door services, ParkMed can provide the answers you need for your specific situation. Their years of experience in the parking management services industry leave them uniquely poised to help you address any parking issue you have.

Parking shuttle service is another parking management option that

ParkMed can provide for your hospital or health care facility. If valet parking is not a suitable option for your facility you might consider a shuttle service from your parking lot to make access easier and less stressful for the patients.

ParkMed offers hospital valet parking, front door services, hospital parking management, hospital greeter and traffic control services and hospital shuttle service anywhere in the continental United States. Regardless of where you are, ParkMed can help you address your health care facility parking problems. Call 1-877-398-PARK today to discuss how ParkMed can help you with your parking situation.

Propark America

Propark America is an experienced medical center parking provider, specializing in full and limited service parking systems for hospitals, medical centers and physician's buildings. We manage parking for primary care centers, children's hospital, cancer centers and full service medical systems, such as Yale-New Haven Hospital, the primary teaching hospital for Yale University School of Medicine. Propark is the right choice for compassionate care and efficient patient service initiatives.

Yale-New Haven Hospital, the primary teaching hospital for Yale University School of Medicine, is a 944-bed tertiary referral center, which includes the 201-bed Yale-New Haven Children's Hospital and the 76-bed Yale-New Haven Psychiatric Hospital. Yale-New Haven regularly ranks among the best hospitals in the U.S. and was accredited by the Joint Commission on the Accreditation of Health Care Organizations in 1999. Relying on the skills of approximately 2,200 university and community physicians, Yale-New Haven, the Children's Hospital and the Psychiatric Hospital provide services for more than 397,000 outpatient and emergency visits and 39,000 discharges each year.

The Hospital Parking System consists of six parking lots, one multi-use garage and two separate point-of-entry valet zones, equaling more than 1,200 total parking spaces. The hospital also administers monthly parking for over 5,000 Hospital employees in the New Haven Parking Authority's Air Rights Garage. Awarded the hospital parking management contract in 1995, Propark immediately improved service, reduced vehicle retrieval cycle time and increased parking capacity. Propark then streamlined the internal parking billing process. Hospital employees interact exclusively with Propark's office staff and monthly parking payments are deducted directly from their paychecks. Propark instituted an upgraded cash and revenue control software package in the hospital facilities to track relevant parking variables including cash shortage control, daily ticket accounting, valet transactions reconciliation and monthly parking payments. An upgraded reporting package was customized for Hospital auditing purposes. Propark designed and implemented a new valet system at the Hospital. Utilizing a stack parking procedure, Propark relocated valet cars to a satellite lot to increase capacity without impacting vital close-in spaces used by Hospital patients. The design of surrounding one-way streets, created a one-mile valet loop from the stack lot to the main entrance valet zone. Propark implemented, and still utilizes, state-of-the-art communication and retrieval systems to efficiently valet park more than 130,000 cars per year at this location. Collectively, these successful programs have doubled the number of cars parked at the hospital since their inception. For more than eleven years, Yale-New Haven Hospital has relied upon Propark America for full-service parking solutions.

Cure for hospital's parking problems at a Birmingham hospital

PLANS were under way for a £1.1 million revamp to solve parking problems and build a new outpatients' department at a Birmingham hospital. Architects have drawn up designs for the new centre at the Royal Orthopedic Hospital, in Northfield, next to the X-ray department. It means patients from across the city, many of them elderly or with knee and hip injuries, will no longer have to be taken nearly a half a mile from the current outpatients' department for X-rays at the other end of the building. Hospital bosses also intend to change the road layout around the site, creating a new parking area, after years of traffic headaches that have seen patients' and visitors' cars clogging up nearby residential streets. Penny Venables, chief executive of the hospital in Bristol Road South, said: "If all goes to plan, the new centre will be open during the autumn of next year.

"We plan to build the new outpatients centre next to the treatment centre and radiology and X-rays, which will be perfect for patients.

"It was awful for patients having to do the long walk from the current outpatients to those departments on crutches and the Friends of the Hospital helped eased this problem with their buggy service, transporting patients."

"This will be a fantastic improvement though and also gives us a chance to redesign the layout around the hospital with new parking."

A lack of parking spaces at the hospital led to gripes from local residents over hospital visitors parking in front of their homes along with patients over not being able to park closer to the wards.

This situation was eased last year when Birmingham City Council created some extra parking spots outside the hospital in Bristol Road South during the day, but there is still a need for improved parking and spaces at the site.

The Orthopedic Hospital has generated money for the project since becoming an independent Foundation NHS Trust last year, enabling it to manage its own finances and pump any spare cash back into improving the hospital.

Residents' demand action over hospital parking chaos

NEIGHBOURS of the University Hospital of North Staffordshire have spoken out about problems caused by motorists parking in their streets.

Residents in Quarry Avenue and Quarry Road in Hartshill say staff and visitors at the hospital regularly park outside their homes, and more than 250 residents have signed petitions calling on Stoke-on-Trent City Council to tackle the problem. A residents' parking scheme was recently introduced in nearby Yoxall Avenue, but drivers who used to park there have simply moved to the other streets.

Yesterday, members of the Improving Communities overview and scrutiny committee visited the area to see the problem and speak to residents.

Randy Conteh, ward councillor for Hartshill and vice-chairman of the committee, said: "The residents' parking scheme in Yoxall Avenue has been a success, but it has impacted negatively on the rest of the streets.

"The hospital, as well as the city council, has a responsibility to try to assist residents with this issue, as a large number of the people who park in these streets are workers from the hospital and visitors."

Seventy residents in Quarry Avenue signed a petition calling for yellow lines and a residents' parking scheme outside homes without drives.

Terry Arnold, aged 64, of Quarry Road, said: "There are about five vehicles that always park here for most of the working day. It means large vehicles have great difficulty getting up here."

"It can also be impossible for people to get into their drives. I reverse into my drive but sometimes I can't do that without going into someone else's drive first.

"It all started when the hospital started charging for parking, but it has got worse over the years."

Dr. John Bridge, who also lives in Quarry Road, said: "Every morning when I wake up there's a car parked outside my gate, and that car will be there until 5 p.m.

"We want yellow lines restricting parking in the morning down one side, and yellow lines restricting parking in the afternoon down the other. That will mean tradesmen visiting residents will be able to park, and if hospital staff want to park here they will have the inconvenience of having to move their car at lunchtime."

Earlier in the year, 177 residents in Quarry Road signed a petition calling for their road to be made 'access only'.

Quarry Road resident Sadia Donnelly, aged 32, said: "As a mother of two young children, I'm scared for them. Today I've had to park right down the road and I have to carry my kids across the road to make sure they're safe."

The hospital has written to employees asking them to be considerate to residents when parking their cars.

I feel sorry for the people living in these streets but as others have pointed out, the hospital has been there for many years (I lived close by 30 years ago) and there have always been parking problems. It will obviously get worse as there are often at least 2 cars per household now and people have become lazier and won't walk very far. I also had parking problems in my last street which wa a cul-de-sac containing 21 houses and because of thoughtlessness from neighbors we had problems getting on and off our drive. My son pays to park outside his house in Pen hull and the restricted parking area is used a a taxi rank during the day and the council aren't interested when you ring to complain as they use the wardens in the town centers and by the time a complaint has been made and they send someone out (if you are lucky!) the perpetrator has gone. The problem is that you cant stop anyone parking outside your property because you don't own the road. In the end we moved so my advice to you is do the same as the problem wont go away even if there are yellow lines or residential parking.

- Most of this problem has been cause by the rip car parking charges introduced on pretext of security issues at the time and the high charges have now driven people on to the surrounding street.
- If there was better parking at the hospitals, i.e. free and more this would not happen, look no further then hospital management.
- The issue is now affecting other emergency services, ignore the factual inaccuracy of the link (Harris Street is in Pen hull not Newcastle). Until parking restrictions are brought in people can park where they want to. Once the 'super' hospital on the City General site is up and running the issue will move onto that area anyway. Springfield residents are already getting a taste of it.
- Beggars belief really doesn't it, how dare people park their cars on the public road in front of someones house. Audacious doesn't really come in to it really does it . . . complete nerve and cheek . . . NOT.

I can imagine that they are now complaining is that the volume of the vehicles parking on the roadside has increased to more than they would have imagined originally or over a period of time. If someone is blocking someone's driveway I would expect a very loud complaint from the aggrieved party, but when the vehicles are parked quite legally on the roadside with road tax, insurance, mot, etc. then there is no complaint to be made, even if it is directly outside the front of your house on the roadside. traffic is a lot heavier than it used to be so the volume of traffic on the road in question would have increased accordingly, the reason why they are now parking in your street is due entirely to the present charging policy at the hospital as it stands today, then there is obviously the fact that on occasions you cant get a space on the car park for love or money, well not on occasions actually on a very regular basis. The doctor that lives on the street I would imagine is all to well informed about that fact as he works at the hospital itself, and he still has the nerve to moan and groan about the present position of the parking etc? . . . peoples attitudes nowadays in certain circumstances does beggar belief, and this is one of those occasions, what do you want the drivers of the vehicles to do, not visit ill or dying friends or relatives in case it causes them to park near your home?, do they want the health care professionals that have to park there not to attend work and leave sick and dying people unattended at the hospital for the same reason? or would they just prefer it if they parked somewhere else and not in their street? . . . the latter I would imagine, hence make the problem someone else's as opposed to their own. . .pathetic and they have the nerve to actually publicly complain about this matter.

If you don't like it anymore, then pay for the residents permit or whatever other manner the local authorities have in place and available to solve the problem, your nothing special and other people have to go about their normal daily and working lives also . . . so yes indeed as stated . . "GET A LIFE".

- Jo Bauld—you obviously cannot read, your poor thing, I do feel sorry for you. If you read my comment properly you will see that I said I AGREE WITH not parking infront of drive ways. As for me needing a life, I am commenting on a story that does concern me, I work at the Hospital, so tell me now it doesn't concern me!

Some comments on internet

- to "gaz" it has absolutely nothing to do with getting a life!! Would you like your driveway blocked for hours at a time and you can't get your car in and out of your drive that you have paid in the price of your property!! Never mind paying for car tax its down right selfish to block peoples drives. Ambulances binmen and firemen cannot not get up and down the roads because people have double parked . I am sure you would be bothered then if you were in that ambulance!!. As for getting a life I suggest you haven't got much of one having time to comment on a story that doesn't concern you so you get a life!!.
- Good on Gaz, Stoke . . . I to pay my car tax. . .and should be allowed to park where I like.within the law . . . I see the residents in the Avenue use cones so people can't park outside there house. Is that legal." " I had to attend the physio dept.I spent ten minutes in there for advice. That cost me £2.00 to park. I wouldn't do it again and parked in the Avenue . . . It's horrendous trying to park at visiting times. What options do people have . . . To those moaning and using parking cones. . .GET A LIFE.
- It is a pity that the powers that be don't take a leaf out of the way its done at Stafford General Hospital. They have a fantastic system for parking for staff and visitors. I don't believe there are any issues for the surrounding residents in regard to parking.
- Oh please, people pay car tax for a reason, it allows them to park where they like and when they like (within the law of

course)—get a life, you chose to live by a hospital so deal with it. If you don't want people parking outside your house, then fork out the money for permit parking each year—the Hospital workers do a fantastic job and I think that these residents are moaning because they have nothing better to do than wake up at and see what cars are parked outside. I agree with people not parking in front of drive ways, you shouldn't park in front of them or across from them. The staff at the Hospital do not have enough spaces to park their cars, so what do you want them to do, "oh no, I must park in that street, the residents will moan, I pay my car tax each year, but I don't care, I wont park there incase I annoy them!" Get a life and stop moaning over something so petty. People park in front of my house ALL the time and there is nothing I can do. If the car was illegally parked or untaxed, then yes, the car can be moved by the police. But if the car has tax, then it can park WHERE IT LIKES. As for the woman going on about her kids and having to carry them over the road, TOUGH, I go shopping and have loads of bags, and I have to carry them over the road in front of cars—big deal. If you are so concerned about parking right on your doorstep, then pay for permit parking out of your own pocket!

- I have every sympathy with the residents in question—I know I would be most unhappy if I lived in those streets. The issue is not the council's nor is it the fault of the staff. The UHNS trust has consistently failed to provide adequate, appropriate parking for Staff and visitors and continues to allow it's parking sub-contract company to enforce draconian measures (tickets for one wheel on grass verges) during the very intrusive Fit for the Future Project works. The council can and may well impose parking regulations on this street however, the core of the issue is people trying to do jobs of a critical nature with inadequate parking facilities. As for the much vaunted park and ride scheme—I assume that the senior management/trust directorate will be the first to trial it? Come on UHNS get your act together and stop letting residents and the council clear up your mess.
- Even if the residents do get their yellow lines there will be no wardens about to ensure the drivers comply—they don't even bother with the cars that are always parked on the yellow lines down the bank near Woolworths.

Northern General Hospital Traffic and Parking Issues

The NHS is the 3rd largest employer in the world. In Sheffield in April 2001 the central campus hospitals (RHH, etc.) amalgamated with the Northern General Hospital to create the Sheffield Teaching Hospitals Trust (STH). At that time, it was the largest hospital trust in England (now second largest) and the second largest employer in Sheffield, employing

12,000+ employees, managing five hospitals carrying out over a million appointments and operations per year.

Parking Charges

In September 2006 STH created parity in parking charges across all their sites. This meant for the first time staff based at the Northern General Hospital (NGH) were required to pay to park, and at the same time the STH applied stricter criteria to gain a parking permit. This was seen as a step in the right direction in terms of the Trust reducing their travel and transport impact.

Why Charge for Parking?

There are national, regional and local policies—supported by the City Council, to reduce congestion, improve air quality, tackle health problems and reduce carbon footprints. This will only happen if there are attempts by organizations to level the playing field in terms of travel to/from work, as well as mitigating other travel impacts (e.g. visitors, out-patients, supplies etc).

A parking space does not come free. Regardless of construction cost, a space in a surface car park can cost between £400-£800 to maintain per annum. A space in a multi storey can be anything up from £1000 to maintain. Therefore, staff who are allowed to park at zero cost are being rewarded, while staff who use public transport, cycle, or walk receive no reward. Car users are being subsidized. The cost of a parking permit for staff at the NGH are not massive—in the region of £200 per annum or less than £1 a day. Car parking at the NGH is costing the Trust over £1,000,000 a year. They are not fully covering those costs from staff permit charges. This resulted in a significant number of staff parking off site on Herries Road, Norwood Road, Barnsley Road and the Crabtree Estate. This caused serious access issues primarily for buses and refuse vehicles, but also for residents accessing drives, or simply walking along footways/pavements. Buses were diverted away from Norwood Road, so the issue was affecting not only pedestrians in the area and car users, but also residents using the bus and staff and visitors to the hospital.

SCC and NGH Action

The initial issue of restricted access for buses and refuse vehicles along Norwood Road and Herries Road was improved by the implementation of a temporary traffic regulation order along Herries Road, and the west side of Norwood Road (Monday-Friday, 8.30-18.30). This kept one side free for parking and restricted parking through the day on the other. The bus operators are happy with the current situation. At the same time the STH relaxed their parking permit criteria to allow on-site parking for all those who applied for a parking permit, while maintaining the charge. To tackle the issue of resident drives being blocked, white H markings were laid down to reinforce the dropped kerb. This was jointly funded by the City Council and STH.

The Burngreave Area Panel considered this problem at he meeting in October 2006 and asked that it be considered as a priority by the relevant City Council Scrutiny Board. The trust were called in to Culture, Economy and Sustainability Scrutiny Board in November 2006, and agreed to participate in a liaison group co-ordinated by this Area Panel with residents and Sheffield City Council officers. To tackle the issue of pavement parking and obstruction, South Yorkshire Police were invited along to the Liaison group to explain what they could and could not do re: enforcement. Problems still remain today with drives being blocked, cars parking with in private developments and footway parking.

Permit Parking Scheme

Progress is now being made in respect of rolling out permit schemes beyond the city centre peripheral parking zone. There is still a significant amount of work to be carried out. The Hillsborough trials (agreed in November 2006) have not yet taken place and it will be approximately 18 to 24 months before the result will be known. As part of the City Council's programme of developing permit parking schemes it will be some time before a scheme could be formally consulted on in the area around the NGH. However a scheme may be brought forward as part of the management of hospital parking and the development of the Multi Storey Car Park (MSCP).

Multi-storey Car Park proposal

NGH has had plans for a 900 space multi-storey car park for a number of years. A planning application was initially received on 3 March 2006. It has been submitted to cater for current demand from patients and visitors, and also to cope with increased development the hospital is planning. It will also act as a subsidy for the much needed MSCP at Weston Park Hospital—which does have planning approval. The MSCP is being built to accommodate patients and visitors only. There has been ongoing discussion for two years focused around the application and supporting documents. STH travel and transport consultants have been informed of the requirements needed to satisfy the travel plan condition. The planning application remains invalid, as the supporting information remains inadequate; primarily for the purpose of this report the site specific car park management strategy needs to be incorporated into the existing Trust travel plan. It looks hopeful that this will be addressed in the next fortnight.

Travel Plan

STH have produced a trust wide travel and transport strategy. This was received by SCC in the summer of 2006, discussed with the Liaison group in December 2006 and approved by the Trust Board in January 2007. A site-specific plan is being developed to accompany the MSCP planning application. A travel plan coordinator has been appointed and was due to commence employment on 9th June.

The Trust

- Have improved the shuttle bus service between the Royal Hallamshire Hospital and the NGH. It runs on a half hour basis with a one small bus and one medium size bus, and often runs at capacity. Trust staff travel for free, and prices for visitors and the general public are competitive.
- It have developed a private group within the car share database
- It has carried out a staff travel survey the results of which show some promise as the number of vehicles accessing the site has dropped by 9% over a 4 year period. This equates to approximately 500 vehicles. The survey also highlighted that more than 200 staff park off site.

The trust can enhance the travel plan and with the new coordinator employed engage staff more actively, promote the measures they have implemented. It is hoped that the Trust will learn form what others have done; for example Nottingham had similar if not the same issues, poor facilities for those not driving, poor security for those driving, 70 vehicles a month stolen, poor links between sites, lack of patient and visitor priority. All have been addressed over the last few years with commitment and a relatively small budget. Shuttle bus running a 10 minute frequency, buses entering the site, pedestrian priority on site, priority to patient and visitor car parking, improved public transport information, staff pay to park.

They can also look to their central campus neighbours—University of Sheffield—who had significant success with their travel plan reducing car use by 500 vehicles from a much lower number—1900 to 1400. In brief the following needs to be looked into:

1. Issues remain primarily a significant amount of off site parking affecting drives and footways. A suitable parking solution needs to be found, the Trust have plans to manage their car park better, but if staff do not want to pay they will seek free spaces off site.
2. The travel plan will need more investment in terms of time and resources to reduce the number of vehicles accessing the site.
3. Parking problems at Tauranga Hospital will be a thing of a past when the new Clarke St carpark opens towards the middle of the year. Construction of the carpark began in January. It will accommodate around 300 vehicles and will be used by both staff and the public during the refurbishment and construction programme. It will also serve as the hospital's main carpark when the redevelopment programme is completed in 2009.
4. People will make their way to the main hospital campus via a lift, which will provide access between the carpark and the hospital. The site will also house the helicopter hangar and helipad.

5. Project director James Crawford says once construction begins there will be limited public car parking available on the hospital campus. Existing car parks will be closed and then re-opened as construction activities permit. When the project is completed, there will be some public carparking on the main campus. "By building the Clarke St carpark before the main construction programme begins, we are ensuring that staff and the public will have access to a purpose-built car park both during the project and when the new hospital is built," he says.
6. Out-patients visiting Jersey's General Hospital could have more parking spaces reserved for them. Concerns have grown after several out-patients cancelled appointments because they could not find anywhere to park.
7. Car sharing "I think we are going to have to make sure there are dedicated parking spaces for people who have to come into hospital. "There are 59 spaces on the lower ground floor of Patriotic Street car park for out-patients." "The survey will show how many that will be extended by in order to cater for those people." Options being considered include encouraging park and ride schemes, car sharing and cycling.

Simple solution to NHS parking problems

NHS Greater Glasgow and Clyde says NHS workers and hospital visitors are being charged to park on hospital grounds in order to stop fly-parking and to reduce road and traffic congestion in the board area. Two simple questions: who on earth appointed NHS GGC to manage the roads system and why should legitimate car users be punished because of a number of anti-social drivers who abuse the system? The board's arguments for the introduction of these charges are spurious and insulting to hard-working staff and visitors who are often under emotional and financial stress with relatives and friends in hospital.

A simple display permit scheme for workers and visitor passes for medium-to long-term in-patient stays would halt the abuse of hospital parking spaces, and better agreements between SPT and NHS GGC for regular public transport both within and outwith normal working hours would save the planet without the low-paid and those on fixed incomes having to carry the costs. This, however, is a blatant money-making exercise by Greater Glasgow and Clyde which I shall call for to be investigated when the NHS inspection is carried out in October this year. If the car parks are being used by non-hospital users-patients, staff or visitors—then there is a simple and easy way of preventing this. Make the charge £10 per hour unless the user has authorization from the hospital to be there. I had the occasion to use St Luke's hospital in Kansas City in the US. It is not an organization known for its generosity. It had a simple system for dealing with this problem which seemed to work.

On entering the car park, the user obtained a ticket which had a date and time stamp. When leaving the clinic or the ward that had been visited, a member of staff stamped the ticket. When presented at the exit gate, the user went free or a charge was levied. The cost to casual non-hospital parkers was $10 per hour (in 1996). As far as I could see (I was acting as chauffeur to my sister who was having daily chemotherapy) there were few if any non-hospital users in the car park but, then, the car park and the system were for the convenience of patients, visitors and staff and not a revenue-raiser. Greater Glasgow and Clyde and other hospital boards that charge for parking should try a similar scheme.

Hospital parking should be free but controlled. I wish to make the following points which are based on considerable experience as an in- and out-patient. First, entry and exit from NHS car parks should be barrier-controlled. After being given an appointment for treatment at the hospital, the patient should be issued with their appointment card and advice on available parking. This card should have room on it to enter the time and date of a visit by car to the hospital. This data should be examined when the car is leaving the parking area to ensure that no abuse of the facility is being made.

There should be at least three times the amount of disabled parking available and this should be placed close to the entry to the hospital.

Hospital staff should have their own free reserved parking but this does not require to be at the entrance as the staff are usually fit enough to walk to the middle of the parking area. When a patient is admitted to hospital as an in-patient, he or she should be given one free visitor's pass which can be used to monitor the parking of their visitors. This pass should also advise on parking space and visiting times. Remember that one car can hold up to five visitors, so it is up to the card-holder to organize who visits the patient and when. This would avoid the common event of one patient being responsible for two or three cars at a time.

Anyone found to be abusing the parking rules should be charged by the police and, if guilty, made to pay a fine which should cover the cost of the prosecution.

The police should be monitored to see if they are doing their duty in applying the laws of our country. If they are not, they should be fired, or the laws should be changed. Anyone requiring emergency parking should be allowed to park close to the hospital entrance where close surveillance of those parking can be maintained by the attendants. Of course, ambulance set-down and pick-up areas should be close to the hospital entrances.

All areas of NHS care are being affected by these outrageous charges. A member of staff earning just around £30,000 will pay £40 per month for a permit, whereas a consultant who is earning three times that will pay the same. It seems to me that someone somewhere is not very good at maths? Why not charge staffs a nominal £24 per year? At the Royal Alexandra Hospital there are more than 1000 staff—surely enough to recoup some money/losses?

There has been no mention if Tom Divers, Greater Glasgow and

Clyde chief executive, and his managerial team are exempt from charges and/or have reserved parking. If anyone deserves such a perk, it is the lower-paid staff and the doctors to whom the public are most indebted. Charging patients and visitors amounts to a stealth tax on the sick. What next? Charges for a glass of water?

The traffic warden is now probably the most detested public servant on our streets today, as they are literally on the streets patrolling to make sure that no one has parked illegally such as on a double yellow lined street or dangerously such as immediately outside of a school gate. The trouble is that many of us fall victim to a 'meter maid' at some point in our driving lives and feel slighted because they didn't understand that they could not park there. Many motorists feel that some signs and instructions are deliberately confusing and aim to catch them out and earn themselves a ticket and a parking fine. A recent survey of motorists found that 60 percent of them were under informed about where they could and couldn't leave their vehicle. One in ten of those questioned had received a fine for parking at a hospital when visiting a sick friend or relative or when they were in the hospital themselves!

The survey was carried out by a car insurance company who found that with most parking enforcement policies it's now local authorities and councils that handle the policing of the streets instead of the police. Whilst a parking fine isn't likely to affect your car insurance quotes it can certainly add to the cost of motoring and this is something people are being more conscious of with expenses like petrol rising in cost many people are finding that they don't want to be caught a foul of some malicious parking attendant.

Other driving convictions such as running red lights or speeding are likely to affect insurance policies so you still need to be careful when you're driving as you may get a fine or penalty in the short-term but in the long-term you also have high insurance costs to deal with, as well as the prospect of a tougher time finding an insurer who will take a chance on you. If you are looking for car insurance or need to find a better deal then check online with many insurers to find the best car insurance quotes for your particular needs. Check with your motor insurance to see if you can make a saving on your car insurance. Roads near Maidenhead's St Mark's Hospital have become heavily congested, following the Berkshire East Primary Care Trust's (PCT) decision to introduce car parking charges at the hospital. There has been at least one collision in the area since the charges kicked in earlier this month, when a hospital user's car was clipped by a bus, while it was parked on St Mark's Road. Diana Crawcour, who owned the car, said: "There were no parking restrictions on that road. I was attending an antenatal class as I am eight months pregnant and this was going to last for three hours." The resident from Wellington Road added that she had four children, with another on the way, and could not afford to pay the fee for parking in the hospital.

What makes the hospital parking miserable?

Let's get to the real reason these greedy parkers make Carleton Glen residents' lives a misery. There are three adequate car parks all half empty. However, they are all pay and display car parks. So, to the thoughtless, selfish, penny pinchers—stop illegally parking and pay the parking charges then you would make everyone's life easier. MORE than 600 parking notices have been slapped on windscreens of motorist's illegally parked or caught abusing spaces at a busy Swansea hospital car park. The tough line is being taken by trust bosses in an attempt to curb parking problems that they claim have been made worse by students leaving their cars at Singleton Hospital.

Parking on the site was said to be so chaotic at the start of the week that queues of traffic were lining up to get into Singleton Hospital. Many drivers found it impossible to find a parking space, and some even missed their appointments.

Hospital bosses have confirmed they are identifying an average of 10 students a day taking up parking spaces, and are asking them to leave. A token system is coming into force in the next couple of weeks to tackle the problem. The scheme would see patients having to prove they had been to a particular hospital department before being handed a token.

He said: "Parking continues to be a major concern for us, and an unwanted frustration for our patients." "Sick patients are depending on these spaces but are being left to look elsewhere and have even missed appointments." He added: "We will be introducing a barrier and token system in the next couple of weeks."

No doubt a well managed hassle free parking in a hospital is a pleasure for the patient and essential part of hospital management. It entails minimizing of the traffic in the hospital, may be for handicapped or serious cases only. It also entails computerized parking where there is no interaction with any person. The parking is managed, including payments through computer and there is no exposure to a foul mouthed attendant.

3

Hospital Security Management

Hospitals have always been considered sacred, in the past. Earlier it was inconceivable that anyone would violate the sanctity of a hospital and commit a crime. Unfortunately, hospitals are no longer immune from criminal assault. Crime continues to find its way into our hospitals at an alarming rate. Why does this happen? Well, for one thing, hospitals are institutions of tradition, and historically have resisted becoming bastions of security. The emphasis has always been on providing open and friendly access to the public. Part of a hospital's image has been to maintain an open door policy for anyone and everyone that wished to visit a sick family member or love-one.

As crime continues to grow in this country, we find that even hospitals are not safe. All of these places have become targets of criminal assault, and as a result, we have been forced to increase security in every facet of our public and private life to keep crime away. Even today, many hospitals have the same open door policy they have practiced for decades. Most hospitals in USA, now have security personnel on site to handle any problems they may have with disgruntled, emotionally charged or mentally unstable patients or visitors. Some facilities employ security only at night, while others have them on site 24 hours a day. Their job is to monitor the facility and the area around it for any suspicious behavior and respond to requests for security by nurses, doctors and other employees. The pay for security personnel is $7.15 to $15 per hour.

Hospitals are targets because they are open to the public 24 hours a day, seven days a week. These public access facilities have been conditioned over the years to allow scores of people from all walks of life to enter these institutions unchallenged. The definition of "public access" means that all persons that enter a hospital seeking treatment, or to visit a love-one, have the right to come and go as they please...and for many facilities, this is still is the practice. This mind-set does not take into consideration there are people in our society that hold no institution sacred, and their sole reason to enter a hospital is to commit a crime against a person, or the hospital, or both.

Unfortunately, because of the continuing criminal threat against hospitals, it's no longer possible to practice an open door policy. For a hospital to be safe in today's world everyone coming into and going out of the facility has to be identified and their access controlled. This is essential to prevent unauthorized persons from entering a hospital to cause harm. Access control has been extremely difficult in the past because of unrealistic and misinterpreted fire codes. Strict enforcement of fire codes have prevented hospitals from securing fire doors that lead to the outside. An unsecured fire door leading to the outside provides an escape route for anyone that has committed a criminal act against a hospital. After what seems like forever, old fire codes are now being replaced with new codes which will now allow fire exits to be locked and alarmed by a time-delay lock and alarm system. This type of "lockdown" capability can prevent unauthorized persons from entering or leaving the hospital undetected.

Another significant problem with providing security for hospitals is their inherently open design which makes them more difficult to secure. Traditionally hospitals have been designed for patient and family convenience. Security was never taken into consideration during the design and construction phase. Because of this inherent problem, retrofitting security protection in older facilities is a security nightmare, not to mention unbelievably expensive. Now violence, theft and vandalism are putting hospitals and health care facilities at risks, with potential impact on patients, staff, medicines and expensive medical equipment. The hospitals need to set-up various physical and electronic security solutions that can help increase security in hospitals and health care organizations. Protecting the life of medical and para-medical staff against assaults and damage to hospital property is essential in the new scenario.

Hospital Security is a Unique Challenge

Consider the variety of people who make up the typical hospital environment—patients, staff, vendors, physicians, visitors and even their enemies. Consider the place—many different rooms and spaces, high-value equipment, accessibility to drugs, many entrances and ease-of-movement around the building and premises. Consider a typical hospital—an open feeling, many managers, politics, autonomous physicians, and what Norman calls "big desires and limited budgets."

It all adds up to a need for different approaches to security. Hospital managers base their security decisions on law, costs, and fear of litigation, and to protect their facility's reputation. But the critical assets of a hospital—its people, property, information and reputation—must be protected with good security.

Civil Hospital Ahmedabad

The Civil Hospital, the site of the bloodiest of bomb blasts in Ahmedabad was before guarded just by home guards. They are in effect untrained volunteers.

SP Jakhwal, security officer at Civil Hospital, said, "Prior to Saturday's events we were using Home Guards they were ineffective as they did not have the required training so it was decided to outsource security services. The tender was issued and around 15 bids were received. The tender was under some kind of dispute regarding taxation and there was apprehension of some of the bidding parties might go to court, so it was decided to just a few days ago to re-issue the tender." "The procedures for awarding this kind of work is very long. We have awarded the contract for sanitation just a month ago. We had to go to the high court to fight, just to award this tender. The security tender was found to have some defect in it and it was decided to re-issue the tender."

On the existing security at civil hospital Dr. Anchalia said, "We have been caught unawares as this is the first time that a hospital has been targeted, even in wars the red cross is spared. We have 110 cameras which were installed about two years ago. Our security was more oriented towards preventing pilferage of supplies, theft and staff duty enforcement. The blast occurred in a blind spot which is not covered by the cameras. We do not have any camera's covering the gates to the campus." "After the blast we have to rethink our security requirements. Since Saturday the CRPF and police have been deployed. Now I think we will need at least 150 security guards for Civil Hospital alone. Since this is a 110-acre campus the total figure will be much more. We will need to re-issue the security tender with Saturday's events in mind," she added.

Police investigators of the serial blasts are yet to ask for the footage of the trauma centre. The hospital authorities also have little knowledge whether the CCTV at the trauma centre was working. "We have not been able to check if the CCTV of the trauma centre, where the twin blasts took place, was working. We have been busy with attending patients after the incident. Police also have not asked us for the footage or the CCTV cameras as yet," said Civil Hospital authorities.

Recent terror attacks at Mumbai targeted several hospitals, resulting in death and destruction at several places. Could adequate security save the situation?

Infant Protection System

A state-of-the-art infant protection system thwarted an infant abduction from Presbyterian Hospital in Charlotte, N.C. An infant protection system sounded an audible alarm when a baby was snatched from the hospital nursery. The high-tech "Hugs" infant protection system is part of an elaborate security management program designed to protect the hospital's patients, visitors, and staff.

The kidnappers were immediately arrested and identified as the mother and father of the recovered, 4-day-old baby boy. In less than a minute the mother and father were able to snatch their son from a seventh-floor nursery, place him in a duffel bag, and run from the hospital.

A quick response by an alert staff set into motion a well-rehearsed plan that lead to the immediate recovery of the missing baby. Suspecting child abuse, the Department of Social Services had earlier taken the couple's other children into custody. Believing their youngest son would also be taken, the couple made a frantic attempt to steal their baby from the hospital. The community was outraged that someone would enter a hospital nursery with the intent to steal a baby. Decades ago this type of crime would have been unheard of in a hospital setting.

Futuristic Approach

Even though hospitals are faced with enormous downsizing and decreasing revenues as a result of "Managed Care", hospitals do have options. First, they can accept the risk and hope that nothing ever happens. Or they can reduce the risk by developing a plan that incorporates physical security, access control, and staff education into a state-of-the-art security management program. The Joint Commission for the Accreditation of Health Care Organizations requires that organizations develop a written security management plan as well as conduct annual security assessments to identify security vulnerabilities.

Security Assessment

How secure is your hospital? What security measures do you have in place to insure that the security of your patients, staff and visitors meet National norms, JCAHO and CMS Standards? What is your hospital doing to prevent infant abductions and mother/baby mix-ups? How well does your hospital manage and address emergency department, pharmacy, and pediatric security issues? If you find these questions troubling you may need to invest in a security assessment.

The Purpose of the Hospital Security Assessment

The purpose of a hospital security assessment is to assist hospitals in the protection of patients, employees, and visitors by identifying organizational strengths and weaknesses in their physical protection and security practices. The security assessment analyzes existing protocols, policies, and procedures, in addition to evaluating physical security vulnerabilities and threats. Findings are analyzed, evaluated, and written recommendations made to control these threats.

All security management programs should be developed using the security assessment concept. A hospital's program should be designed to teach, implement, monitor, assess, and improve components that are part of the hospital's existing program. Security is a system concept which requires on-going training, corroboration, monitoring, and swift attention to problem identification. The ultimate success of a security program will depend upon a renewed commitment by hospital administration to support this most important process.

The assessment should be designed to identify environmental deficiencies, hazards, and unsafe practices. The professional security assessment can serve as a tool in assisting hospitals in developing their own self-assessment. An annual self assessment is required to meet the new JCAHO Standards, as well as CMS Regulations. New standards require hospital to collect information about security deficiencies and provide corrective action to improve the environment of care.

The initial security assessment of a facility should be conducted by a health care security professional with experience in evaluating hospital security programs. Organizations should use only health care security professionals with industry credentials and professional certifications. In addition, the consultant should have hands-on experience as a manager, director, or security administrator in the health care industry. A qualified consultant can better evaluate your hospital's security management program based on industry norms and the 2005-06 JCAHO Environment of Care Standards, as well as CMS's "Condition of Participation."

The security assessment should evaluate JCAHO standards as well as compliance issues that require:

- Hospitals to collect and analyze information to identify safe patient practices and implement changes to reduce the risk of future sentinel events.
- Changes are made and evaluated to ensure that expected outcomes are successful,
- Programs are monitored for effectiveness.

Security Management Plan

The written Security Management Plan (SMP) is designed to provide a proactive approach in the protection of patients, visitor, staff, and health system assets. This is accomplished by identifying security threats in all areas of the facility which could have an adverse impact on persons and property. This is accomplished through the security assessment which is also designed to reduce the occurrence and severity of security incidents and promote security education and training for hospital employees and staff.

Hospital Security Officers

The Security Officer is under the direct supervision of the Shift Supervisor. A Security Officer serves during one of three (3) eight hour (8 hr.) shifts and may be required to work overtime hours on occasion at the discretion of the Security Services/Account Manager. The Security Officer is directly responsible for the security and safety of all client facilities, property, assets, patients and staff located at the respective post to which they are assigned. Security posts within Children's Hospital and Research

Center may involve interior or exterior building and grounds patrol or some combination of interior and exterior patrol. Security Posts may also involve fixed interior or exterior personnel and/or vehicle access points on owned or leased property under the control of the Security, Parking and Transportation Department. Other Security Posts may involve driving a client patrol vehicle and conducting periodic Security sweeps/visits/inspections by vehicle or on foot after exiting the vehicle, at the Main Hospital Campus and at various off site locations at the direction of the client Security Director and the Security Services/Account Manager. The Security Officer will also be tasked to provide a variety of additional services including but not limited to: personnel escorts, parking enforcement, crowd control, responding to various Hospital Emergencies, interacting with and assisting patients, their family members, hospital staff and the general public while they are on the Hospital Campus; and other duties as assigned.

The duties

(1) Patrol all areas to which assigned utilizing a combination of foot or vehicle patrol as directed.
(2) Provide personal safety escorts proactively or as requested.
(3) Provide vehicle services (i.e., jump-starts, tire re-inflation or calling for off-site tow services) for employees, visitors and patients as requested.
(4) Proactively provide Security Service checks for off site facilities.
(5) Maintain public order through proactive customer service and the enforcement of Hospital rules and protocols.
(6) Respond to all Hospital Emergencies as required.
(7) Observe and report all unusual occurrences on client property. Provide written reports, take photos as necessary and accurately record all instances of crime, threats of crime and public disorder occurring at the Hospital.
(8) Coordinate and cooperate with local law enforcement, fire and other emergency agencies responding to calls for assistance at the Hospital.
(9) Perform additional duties as required.

Threats in a Hospital Environment

Norman lists the main threats in a hospital environment as insider/employee theft, outsider gang members, and visitor thefts, threats against patients or staff, and crimes of opportunity.

To analyze security needs, begin by listing the departments, reviewing the business culture of the hospital, determining the threat levels in each department, interviewing department heads about threats and crime, and planning possible countermeasures for each department. Then develop a master plan and review it against a "reality check" on the basis for the plan and the tools that will be needed. Don't forget, Norman says, that you have options in security—high-tech, low-tech, even no-tech.

Among the no-tech options, he says, policies and procedures can be developed to enhance security. Training and supervision keep those policies and procedures at the forefront. Programs help promote security awareness in the staff. And Norman suggests having an anonymous 800 number for reporting crimes and slips in security.

Low-tech options include locks, barriers, good lighting and landscaping), says Norman. High-tech choices include alarm systems, access control systems, photo identification, CCTV, two-way voice communications and weapons screening systems. But new tools such as patient locators, video pursuit software, delayed egress hardware, active asset control systems, enterprise-wide systems, digital video and pager alarms can enhance security even more.

Norman says professionals should look at the threats likely in specific areas:

- The emergency/trauma department (gang fights, vendettas, domestic conflicts, child custody conflicts, VIP patients);
- Infant care area (infant abduction, need for CCTV and infant security);
- Pharmacy/drug storage area (alarm and access control systems);
- Prisoner care area (receiving, elevator lock-off, surveillance, command center);
- Operating rooms (access control, delayed egress hardware, CCTV),
- Labs (access control, duress alarms, CCTV);
- Nuclear medicine area (access control, CCTV);
- Geriatric care area (patient locators, CCTV);
- Psychiatric care area (lock-down capability, access control, staff duress, solitary room);
- Morgue (decedent services area, access control, alarm system, CCTV); and
- PBX area (late-night security, rest room security, door release, duress alarm).

Don't forget such places as the parking lot (lighting, access control, CCTV in stairwells, duress alarm at fee collection booth), food service area (duress alarm), gift shop (burglar alarm, duress alarm) and shipping/receiving areas (CCTV, patrol). And study the threat potential of biohazard waste storage and disposal (CCTV, access control).

New products such as alarm pagers, infant abduction detection systems, patient wandering systems, CCTV video pursuit systems, people trackers and asset protection systems can each enhance hospital security, Norman suggests.

Indeed hospital security is unique, but with good planning, protection of its assets can be enhanced.

New Ways to Prevent Hospital Security Problems!

Would you agree that every hospital does not need a fully-qualified security management team running its security program on a full-time basis? Would you also agree that every hospital, whether large or small, does need the guidance of a security professional several times in the course of a year?

Why do all Hospitals Need Security Expertise from time to time?

The answers are many. They include reducing the probably of security-driven litigation. There is also the need to optimize the protection of patients, visitors and staff as cost-efficiently as possible. Hospitals also must meet the ever-increasing demands of regulatory bodies such as JCAHO, OSHA and the States. Hospitals are slowly beginning to see the need to stop the out-flow of supplies and equipment as a result of theft and fraud. Hospitals are beginning to have their data bases penetrated and patients' rights to privacy are threatened. Infants and children are being kidnapped while under the care and control of the medical facility. Assaults are occurring in emergency departments and parking facilities; at the same time, staff are either inadequately or improperly trained to cope with these threats. Finally, when there are security problems, hospitals often respond in a knee-jerk fashion. These responses are often inappropriate and costly.

Many hospitals are operating under the false assumption that the way to solve their security problems is to hire an ex-police officer who has little or no expertise in security and loss prevention. Through no fault of their own, former police officers tend to apply police solutions to security problems and do not understand the budgetary constraints of the private sector. These types of security managers often operate on the assumption that all security problems can be solved by hiring more uniformed personnel because they do not understand how to use security hardware and technology. There are huge philosophical and operational differences between policing and security, especially in the health care arena. Most hospitals don't find this out until the security budget is out of control, the security program is ineffectual, and/or the hospital is slapped with a lawsuit. The police are primarily reactive; security professionals are pro-active. In the next few paragraphs we will briefly highlight some examples of the security challenges that are best addressed by a security professional.

Security Litigation

Hospitals are being sued because of parking lot assaults, infant kidnapping, as well as attacks on patients by third parties. They are also being sued for intentional torts such as false arrest, false imprisonment and use of excessive force by security personnel. Litigations are often spawned in the emergency room because staff has been either improperly trained or inadequately trained in dealing with aggressive behavior. In some cases, staff are injuring patients or being injured themselves because they do not know how to control aggressive behavior. Bill Nesbitt understands these problems. He has been retained as a security expert in over 150 lawsuits and has testified as to adequacy of security and use of force.

Regulatory Agencies

In Indian conditions there is no regulatory agency for hospital security personnel. In fact there is no proper security system in various hospitals. The so called security personnel only boss over the relatives of the patients, who are ever eager to mark their presence with the patient, more as a social obligation and less as a welfare attempt. In America JCAHO, OSHA and State regulations are all raising the bar as to what is considered reasonable hospital security. Now HCFA has announced patient protection standards that should have been implemented by August 2. Hospitals have a much higher standard of care than most businesses when it comes to defining adequate security. Hospitals that do not meet and/or exceed these minimal standards are inviting negative press, a loss of confidence by the public it serves, as well as litigation.

Fraud and Theft

Research indicates that hospitals are suffering losses of as much as $3,500 per/bed per/year. It further indicates that 1/3 of all employees will steal or commit acts of deception such as the submission of ghost hours. Criminals can walk into most hospitals and help themselves to computers, linens and medical equipment. Despite these realities, most hospitals have no pro-active asset protection program.

Sensitive Areas

In addition to general security concerns there are the very special security needs in the emergency department, L&D, pediatrics, food service, parking facilities and the business office, to name just a few. Those hospitals that wait for the problems to get out of control before acting may never gain the upper hand.

Security Vendors

Hospitals that decide to combat security threats often turn to an array of security providers whose services may range from good to extremely poor. Some security agencies may actually raise the liability factor for the hospitals they are ostensibly hired to protect. Hospitals that do not have the expertise to deal with security vendors may be buying problems instead of solutions. There are choices to be made between contract guards or proprietary officers. Should the hospital use CCTV? How much and where? Should the hospital go with a conventional lock and key system or use a card access system? Is the lighting up to standard? These are all tough questions and require thoughtful responses. The bottom line is if the hospital does not conduct an annual security audit, the security program will continue to flounder and will lack direction and purpose.

Hospital Security Guard

As one of the largest privately held firms in America, Yale Enforcement Services is dedicated to providing our clients with the leading physical security, life safety and remote video intrusion detection solutions. Our security, technology and managed services capabilities afford immediate solutions for today's fast-paced business environment. Our goal is to provide reliable managed services that propel customer success thus allowing you to do what you do best—concentrate on your primary core business.

Yale Enforcement is looking for unarmed security officers to work at area hospital. Must possess good people skills and be customer service orientated while possessing a strong background in security. Looking for 10 officers and a Site Supervisor. plus incentives and bonuses. Benefits.

Security Officer Basic Qualifications

Hospital experience

- Candidate must be customer service-oriented!
- Must be at least 18 years of age.
- Must be at least 18 years of age or older as required by applicable law or contractual requirements or older as required by applicable law or contractual requirements.
- Must have a high school diploma or GED, or at least 10 years of verifiable employment history.
- At least one verifiable employer.
- No criminal convictions as specified under Yale Enforcement guidelines.
- Ability to communicate effectively both orally and in writing for the purpose of public interaction and report writing.
- Authorized to work in the United States.
- Ability to perform essential functions of the position with or without reasonable accommodation.
- Negative result on pre-employment drug screen.
- Ability to maintain satisfactory attendance and punctuality standard.
- Neat and professional appearance.
- Friendly and professional demeanor.
- Ability to providing quality customer service.
- Ability to handle typical and crisis situations efficiently and effectively at client site.
- A Yale Enforcement Security Officer.
- Valid drivers license and a clean driving record are a must
- Florida D or G License required.
- Comes to work; is on time and completes shift assignments (including overtime, if assigned).

- Has a neat, professional appearance and comes to work in complete and clean assigned uniform.
- Has a friendly and professional demeanor and provides quality customer service.
- Is a good communicator (both verbal and written) and is capable of handling typical and crisis situations both efficiently and effectively.
- Understands and successfully executes his/her post orders including enforcement of client and company policies, rules and regulations.

Benefits

Yale Enforcement Services, Inc. is committed to being the employer of choice in the security industry. We offer a vast array of industry-best benefits so we can attract and retain the finest people. Our benefits include:

- Supplemental Health Insurance
- Supplemental Dental Insurance
- Monthly Bonus Incentives
- Paid Vacations
- Paid Holidays
- Equipment and Uniforms Provided
- Direct Deposit
- Uniform Maintenance Allowance

Service Health Care Jobs

While most individuals think of doctors, nurses and other specialists when they consider careers in the health care field, there are actually many more jobs in health care facilities that individuals must fill in order for the appropriate care to be administered and provided to patients.

Ever wondered where the food, clean bedding and the smell of health care facilities originate from? Usually from an individual who is working in a service job or position in a health care facility. These individuals perform common tasks such as cleaning, cooking and laundry for the entire facility, as opposed to one person like a home health aide does. In addition, they have limited or no contact with patients or individuals seeking care and treatment.

The SMSI Solution?

SMSI has the low cost answer to all these questions and many more. SMSI has a team of health care security professionals. SMSI is able to provide your hospital with the security expertise it needs to develop effective security programs that protect patients, staff, visitors and property. This offering assumes that every hospital needs competent security expertise sometime throughout the year, if not on a full-time basis. Hospitals already know the benefits of outsourcing expertise. Now is the time to apply that experience to security. Where does SMSI fit in? SMSI will provide customized security management support to any hospital in the country for as little as $2,950 per year. The annual charge will be predicated on the number of staffed beds. This one low annual fee, plus expenses, will be based on a three-year contract and will include one two-day visit per year. SMSI will provide additional support by offering their clients unlimited phone and/or e-mail consultation. On the first visit, SMSI will conduct a basic security audit and will review any contracts presently in force with security vendors.

Throughout the course of the contract, SMSI will provide guidelines for RFPs (request for proposals) from security vendors. They will also provide expertise in the vendor selection process. SMSI will also provide expertise to those hospitals facing JCAHO review. For those hospitals implementing a recommended computerized incident program, SMSI will provide semiannual trend analysis reviews, thereby keeping the security program contemporary. These services will ensure that limited security dollars will not be wasted. This program will reduce the probability of security-related lawsuits as well as reduce asset losses.

Any hospital wishing to retain SMSI for a more extensive consultation or other security management services will be provided service at a rate 20% below the standard billing rate. All clients will be provided a complimentary subscription to The Hospital Security Reporter. Clients will also receive an additional insert to this publication, The Hospital Security Tip Sheet. This additional publication will provide innovative, cost-saving solutions to tough problems and will share methods that are working at other hospitals.

If you are interested in this innovative approach to the provision of hospital security, ask for a proposal for your hospital. The cost of this service will easily be returned to your hospital through a reduction in security costs and/or a reduction in losses. You may leave a voice mail message at 800/306-8344 or e-mail at smsiinc@aol.com. An effective security program enhances the image of the hospital to the community it serves. Families want the assurance that the hospital is a safe and secure place. There are also positive benefits to employee morale when the workplace is safe and free of crime. One serious security incident may literally take years to overcome. Breeches in hospital security, such as an infant abduction, often reach the national news media. Adverse publicity can result in thousands of dollars in loss and severely harm the reputation of the hospital for years.

Health Care and Hospital Security Consultant and Expert

How do you balance your need to be an open, accessible, welcoming facility against your duty to properly and reasonably protect your people, assets and reputation?

How do you provide a properly secure Environment of Care in an Open Campus with a patient centered and family friendly culture?

Is your health care security program a strategically planned and synergistic system that cost effectively prevents and mitigates your real threats and risks, or is it a relatively random collection of measures applied over the years as a reaction to particular incidents and concerns?

Hospitals, and other health care facilities such as nursing homes, psychiatric hospitals, clinics, assisted living and retirement communities, medical office buildings, etc., are, by nature, relatively porous. They are also complex operations and their security is typically more involved and challenging than other types of facilities. Developing, implementing and managing a health care security program that provides the needed levels of control and protection while maintaining or improving the desired levels of accessibility, service and patient satisfaction is a challenge.

We have extensive experience providing a wide range of security and workplace violence assessment and planning services for health care facilities throughout the U.S. Our hospital security consulting and expert services are always focused upon your unique culture, values, history, location, composition, risks, vulnerabilities, threats and budgets. We know it is particularly essential to elicit the support for, understanding of, and involvement in security by all departments and staff.

Also please see the attached page of Health Care Security Advisories that discuss recent health care issues.

Critical assets to consider in your health care security planning may include:

- Children and Infants
- Staff, Patients, Visitors and Families
- Elderly Patients and Residents
- Supplies including Linens, Scrubs and Food
- Private Information
- Pharmacies and Pharmaceuticals
- Equipment
- Patient, Visitor and Staff Property
- Tenants and their people and property
- The Buildings and Furnishings (e.g. against vandalism and graffiti)
- Vehicles—Parking Lots and Structures
- Cash
- Reputation
- Chemical Storage
- Nuclear Medicine
- Labs
- Loading Docks
- Gift Shops, etc.

Our support to hospitals, medical centers and other health care facilities, that meets the latest JCAHO Environment of Care. IAHSS

Standards and HIPAA Requirements, includes:

- Health Care Security and/or Workplace Violence Assessments or Surveys (see "Assessments" page). Such Assessments can be hospital-wide and comprehensive, addressing all functions and departments, or can be targeted in which there is a focus on particular departments or functions (e.g. Security Staffing/ Management, Physical or Perimeter Security/Access Control, New Construction, Emergency Planning and Response, Maternity/Pediatrics, etc.).
    - o During the assessments or surveys we will typically interview representatives of Security, Safety, Nursing, Maternity/L&D, Pediatrics, Psychiatric, Emergency, Geriatric Care, Supplies, Food Service, Maintenance, Facilities Management, Pharmacy, Risk Management, Human Resources, Parking, Shipping and Receiving, IT/IS, Home Health Care, etc. on all shifts
    - o We will tour and observe the facility functioning at all hours, including the grounds, parking lots/structures and outlying buildings
    - o We will review relevant materials including policies and procedures, emergency and crisis plans, incident and activity reports, post orders, contracts, past security audits and assessments, staff communications, security plans, etc.
    - o We also consider Crime Prevention through Environmental Design (CPTED) in our reviews and planning
    - o We benchmark the latest best practices against similar facilities
    - o We can optionally distribute a questionnaire or survey to all or selected employees to elicit their concerns, issues and suggestions
- Staff Health Care Security Awareness Training and Penetration Testing.
- Health Care Workplace Violence Prevention and Response Processes and Training to include safely dealing with and de-escalaing confrontational, aggressive, irate and threatening behavior and response to robberies.

Development of Hospital Security or Workplace Violence Policies, Plans and Procedures, including Security Management Plans that meet and exceed Joint Commission (JCAHO) expectations.

- Enhancement or Development of Hospital Security Officer/ Police Programs, whether contract, proprietary, sworn officers or hybrid, including Training Programs; creation of Post Orders; development of RFP's, Contracts, Scopes of Work, Job

Descriptions, or Specs;, etc. Note that security staff is typically the most costly, and sometimes problematic, aspect of the security program. There is much that can be done to better assure a more cost effective and consistently professional and customer service focused security force.

- Reviews, Benchmarking, Development and Enhancement of Hospital Security or Police Departments.
- Incorporating Security and Workplace Violence Response into existing Emergency, Crisis and Disaster Plans and Training.
- Serving as a hospital and health care expert witness in related litigations.
- Development of Self-Assessment and ongoing Hospital Security Audit Methodologies.
- The providing of ongoing security support on a retainer basis (The Virtual Security Manager).

We can optionally provide various CAP Index reports geared to your particular location(s) that could include:

- A database report that provides "Past", "Current" and "Projected" CRIMECAST™ scores relative to the national, state and county average of 100. We provide the CRIMECAST™ scores for the ten (10) different crime categories, and a total of ninety (90) crime risk scores per location. This report identifies not only the types and trends of crimes in the area and the frequency with which they are occurring, but it also represents the areas of crime in a graphical format (spatial and temporal analysis).

Most hospitals and clinics have found that it is worthwhile and cost effective to periodically obtain an objective outside perspective on their security program to confirm that it still properly and effectively addresses the true risks, threats, vulnerabilities and liabilities.

What SAI consultants say!

The security assessment covers all physical security components including: locks and alarms; access control; CCTV/CCDV surveillance; infant security and mother/baby mix-ups; personnel identification and badging; asset tracking; nurse call; parking area security; staff and parental education; security policies, protocols and procedures, emergency preparedness, and drills. IT security audits are conducted at the level required by your hospital's IT department administrators. IT audits can target only HIPAA compliance issues or as comprehensive in scope as necessary to insure that every element of your hospital's IT security infrastructure is secure. Your hospital's Security Management Program should include: appropriate security policies, protocols and procedures, security drills, incident reporting, performance monitoring and improvement, staff and parental education, and annual risk assessments of the seven areas of the Environment of Care©. SAI consultants also provide litigation avoidance and expert witness services.

JCAHO* accreditation requires hospitals to provide a secure and safe environment of care for patients, visitors, staff and employees. Effective management of the EOC includes processes and activities designed to:

- Identify security and safety risks and vulnerabilities;
- Reduce and control environmental hazards and risks;
- Prevent accidents and injuries;
- Maintain secure and safe conditions for patients, visitors, staff and employees;
- Maintain an environment which is sensitive to patient needs for comfort, social interaction, positive distraction, and self-control;
- Maintain an environment which minimizes unnecessary environmental stresses for patients, visitors and staff; and
- SAI is not affiliated with the Joint Commission on Accreditation of Health Care Organizations.

SAI's consultants are qualified to perform a wide range of JCAHO related tasks.

— JCAHO Mock Surveys—Environment of Care © Risk Assessments
— Statement of Conditions Preparation (SOC)—National Patient Safety Goals Education
— SOC Electronic Filings—Annual JCAHO Readiness Updates
— Tracer Reviews Inpatient Care—Terrorism Preparedness
— Emergency Management Plans—Policy, Protocol and Procedure Audits?

"Hospitals must insure that the condition of the physical plant and overall hospital environment is developed and maintained in a manner to insure the safety and well-being of patients." This mandate includes developing and implementing appropriate emergency preparedness plans and capabilities. Additionally, hospitals must identify likely risks to their facility (HVA—Hazard Vulnerability Analysis), and develop a coordinated security preparedness effort in cooperation with Federal, State and local emergency preparedness authorities and planners.

AI's mission to empower hospitals to protect their patients, staff, visitors and property from harm embraces the entire spectrum of the Security Management Program [SMP]. A comprehensive SAI security assessment and vulnerability analysis covers all facets of the hospital's physical security. When included in the Scope-of-Work, IT security audits are conducted at the level required by your hospital's IT department administrators. They can target only HIPAA compliance issues or be as comprehensive in scope as necessary to insure that every element of your hospital's IT security infrastructure is secure.

An exit briefing for senior level administrators is consucted at the conclusion of the on-site portion of the assessment. Preliminary findings are presented and discussed, and a formal written report of Findings with detailed Recommendations is then prepared to assist administrators in meeting needs of their facility for the security and safety of its patients, visitors, staff, and employees.

Level of Physical Security

- Physical design and layout of campus and surrounding property
- Local criminal demographics report [CAP Index Report]
- Facility buildings and infrustructure
- Access Control
- Locks and Alarms
- CCTV/CCDV systems
- Asset tracking and inventory control
- Parking Area Security

Security Management Program

- Quality of the Security Management Program
- Previous security Sentinel Events
- Preparedness for terrorism and mass casualties
- Employee security awareness associated with on-going educational programs
- Administration and management support

Policies, Protocols and Procedures

- Administrative Security Policies
- Security Protocols
- In-place Security Procedures

JCAHO Standards and CMS Requirements

- JCAHO Mock Surveys
- Statement of Conditions Preparation and Electronic Filing
- Tracer Reviews Inpatient Care Areas
- Environment of Care©Risk Assessments—Seven Management Areas
- National Patient Safety Goals Education
- Emergency Management Plans and Terrorism Preparedness

It is important for hospitals to develop a comprehensive Security Management Program (SMP) to effectively support and maintain physical protection for patients, staff and visitors. Central to that development is the completion of a comprehensive threat assessment and an evaluation of the security protocols, policies, and procedures unlerlying the SMP. These vitally important elements of the SMP should be well-defined, unambiguous and reinforced with periodic staff education and training. SAI consultants help facilities identify their organizational strengths and weaknesses in physical protection and security practices. Our expertise and experience in hospital security is applied during a comprehensive audit of your physical security measures. We assist risk managers in analyzing existing protocols, policies, and procedures. Our findings are analyzed and evaluated and we provide specific, realistic recommendations to improve over-all security and achieve a total security solution.

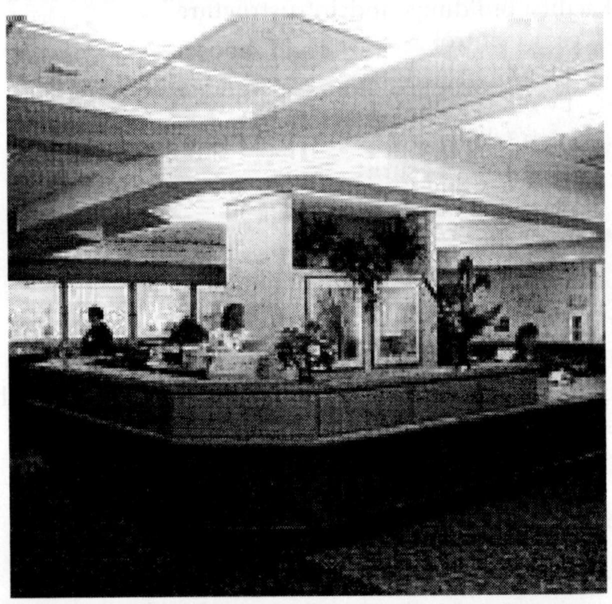

Security Assessments International's consultants can evaluate your existing security and risk management activities and provide recommendations to assist your efforts in providing better protect for patients, staff, visitors and your facility's assets. Consultative assessments are performed within a reasonable time frame at an acceptable cost.

The health care industry's focus on medical privacy and compliance has fostered a lack of awareness around the frequency, cause and seriousness of patient identity theft, according to the 2008 HIMSS Analytics Report: Security of Patient Data commissioned by Kroll Fraud Solutions, a leading provider of data protection and identity theft response services. The report reveals a significant blind spot that hinders hospital efforts to contain the problem and reduce risk.

"Health care facilities are complex environments where information is stored and shared in a number of ways that are critical to patient well-being," said Brian Lapidus, chief operating officer of Kroll Fraud Solutions.

"Until health care organizations expand their data security measures to address the threat of data compromise as well as privacy and compliance, patients will continue to be at risk."

Key report findings include

- Regulatory loopholes in data management standards allow data breaches to go unreported, preventing an accurate measurement of frequency.
  - Only 56 percent of breached organizations surveyed notified the patients involved.
  - On average, respondents ranked their familiarity level with the Health Insurance Portability and Accountability Act of 1996 (HIPAA) at a 6.53 (on a scale of 1-7, with 7 being the highest) and nearly 75 percent claimed a familiarity level of 7.
  - The high level of HIPAA familiarity stems from the commencement of audits and the resulting penalties for non-compliant facilities. The issue: HIPAA compliance is an insufficient proxy for risk mitigation.
- Security policies place a greater emphasis on preventing violation of privacy than preventing fraud and malicious intent.
  - Of those respondents who experienced a fraud-related breach, 62 percent identified the type of the breach as unauthorized use of information, while 32 percent cited wrongful access of paper records.
  - Noticeably absent were breaches attributed to malicious intent (i.e., stolen laptops/computers, deliberate acts by unscrupulous employees, and cyber attacks through the Internet).
- Health care organizations lack appreciation for the costs of a breach + Only 18 percent of breached organizations surveyed believed there was a negative financial impact, even though the average cost of a breach is estimated to be as high as $197 per compromised record and $6.3 million per incident.

"The number one priority of U.S. health care institutions is saving the lives of those in need and rightly so, I might add," said Lisa Gallagher, senior director of privacy and security for the Health Care Information and Management Systems Society (HIMSS). "But patient safety extends beyond clinical care. This data tells us that organizations must also broaden their data security and risk management measures to address the threat of patient data breach." Among the 13 percent of respondents who revealed that their facility had experienced a data breach:

- 48 percent indicated that 'reprimanding the employee' is effective breach response, while 11 percent offer 'education' as a solution.
- 35 percent said that they did not change the organization's security policy after the incident.
- Identity theft is three times as likely to happen at a larger facility (more than 100 beds) than a smaller facility (under 100 beds).

The report also indicates that health care organizations are focusing their security programs on employee education with nearly all respondents reporting that their organizations educate employees about the importance of maintaining patient data security. Almost 50 percent cited reprimanding or terminating the employee as an element of their organizations' breach response plan and 35 percent of breached organizations surveyed did not change their security policies after the incident.

"There's a dangerous assumption in the health care industry that education leads to policy implementation and change." said Mr. Lapidus of Kroll. "Best practices in data security cannot be achieved by employee training alone. Organizations must make data security a part of their DNA, reflected in every aspect of business operations."

Survey Methodology: A total of 263 health care industry professionals participated in this research conducted in January 2008. They included IT professionals (50 percent), Health Information Management (HIM) managers (21 percent) and chief security officers (12 percent), among others working in the area of information management. Most respondents were small to mid-sized health care facilities, i.e. Health Insurance Portability and Accountability Act of 1996 (HIPAA), Sarbanes-Oxley Act of 2002 (SOX) and Payment Card Industry Data Security Standards (PCI)

About Kroll

Kroll, the world's leading risk consulting company, provides a broad range of investigative, intelligence, financial, security and technology services to help clients reduce risks, solve problems and capitalize on opportunities. Kroll Inc. is a wholly-owned subsidiary of Marsh and McLennan Companies, Inc. (NYSE: MMC), the global professional services firm. Kroll began providing identity theft solutions in 1999 and created its Fraud Solutions practice in 2002 in response to increasing requests from clients for counsel and services associated with the loss of sensitive personal information, and related identity protection and restoration issues facing organizations and individuals.

Since then, Kroll's Fraud Solutions clients have included Fortune 500 companies, non-profit organizations, and government entities dealing with health care, financial services, insurance, consumer service, and any activity involving the collection and use of personal information. Kroll's Fraud Solutions team presently serves over 10,000 businesses and millions of individual consumers.

Hospital Security for Patients and Visitors

Are you a Hospital Administrator? Are you in need of trained security personnel? Then you have chosen the right company for your facility. Since your personal safety and security are very important to us, our security officers will patrol your hospital around the clock. Hospital security is a top concern, and Knights Protection is ready to solve the problem.

Consider the variety of people who make up the typical hospital environment—patients, staff, vendors, physicians, visitors and even their enemies. Consider the place—many different rooms and spaces, high-value equipment, accessibility to drugs, many entrances and ease-of-movement around the building and premises. Consider a typical hospital—an open feeling, many managers, politics and autonomous physicians. It all adds up to a need for different approaches to security. The critical assets of a hospital—its people, property, information and reputation—must be protected with good security guards. The main threats in a hospital environment are theft, gang members, threats against patients or staff, and crimes of opportunity.

Knights Protection Security provides hospital security services throughout New York. When it comes to protecting hospitals, Knights Protection security officers are at the top of their class.

Responsible Hospital Security

SECURITY LIABILITY is one of the newest problems and trends facing all safety and security directors, whether employed in the health care field or other industries. The problem is so new to some that it just now is being discussed in professional journals and presented at conferences. It will be a major topic at the Hospital Association of Pennsylvania Fall Conference this October in Hershey, Pennsylvania. I am sure you are familiar with the most common liability issues that face you as professionals who specify, install, key, retrofit and repair hardware. But are you following the most recent security liability trends, as well?

The failure to provide adequate security has caused businesses, including hospitals, to pay some rather large awards over the past several years. Among the list of reasons for these problems are ineffective patrol patterns by security audits or self surveys that identify security hazards, inadequate lighting and perimeter security issues—in many cases these issues were identified but not resolved. Whether an issue involves doors and hardware or anything else on the above list, if it is proven to have been foreseeable, there is usually liability.

When it comes to specifying hardware, there seems to be an extremely difficult balance between code and law compliance issues and security needs. A college I attended erected a large building in the mid-1970s. The hardware consultant on that job specified expensive mortise locks with a classroom function for nearly all doors. He specified levers rather than knobs on the inside of the doors to accommodate handicapped students, and he undercut all doors by approximately one inch for air handling purposes.

The school did not have a safety and security director at the time, and neither the consultant nor the college representative foresaw the impending problems with the specification. Following a long series of unexplained thefts, it was determined that students were using wires to access the inside door handles and steal expensive equipment. This job might meet the criteria of a liability case. The immediate options were to retrofit the hardware to eliminate the problem or saw off the end of each handle. Due to budget constraints, the college maintenance staff was directed to perform surgery, and to this date the brass is visible at the end of the 26D finish of these levers.

To reduce liability, architects, architectural hardware consultants, contractors, locksmiths, hospital maintenance and engineering staffs and security departments must work together. This eliminates problems at the end of the job, and people generally support what they help create. All have some role in specifying the hardware, and frankly, no one, no matter how well-trained or experienced, is capable of foreseeing all potential problems in a health care setting. And, hardware applications vary from hospital to hospital, based upon location, local crime rates, types of services provided, hours of operation, security philosophy and other factors.

In keying conferences, you should speak with individuals from each department of the hospital. It may take 15 minutes with some departments, but questions and concerns over the application of specific hardware functions will be addressed and a consensus can be reached. Also, it gives the hardware specifier a chance to talk the hospital staff out of making or duplicating mistakes from previous projects. Please keep in mind that you are intimately and totally familiar with hardware and, in most cases, know what is best for the application—but will never use the product after it is sold. Hospital staff members, on the other hand, will be the ones who use the product and really know little about it. Share your knowledge before a costly mistake is made.

At the March meeting of the Northeast Chapter of the Hospital Association of Pennsylvania, 17 safety and security directors representing some 175 years of combined health care experience in northeast and north central Pennsylvania discussed hardware, and we agreed on many of the items that follow.

Hardware Selection

Often—with good intentions—styles, finishes, keyways/keying and lock functions are selected by individuals who will never operate the hardware. In many cases, the locks are chosen without consulting those who will use them, maintain them and rekey them (assuming there is an in-house locksmith). Lack of communication on the part of the hospital contributes to the problem, in other words, expectations are not made clear about who will be involved in the hardware selection process. In other cases, hardware specifiers assume they understand the applications and fail to involve all of the required parties. Sometimes, time constraints are factor. Rather than install temporary locks until the desired hardware arrives, some make compromises in quality. These rushed jobs can result in less than sufficient quality or locks not being consistent with the hardware plan.

In some cases, light-duty hardware is used, because it is available or because the supplier wants to purge old or unwanted materials, compromising security and standardization. I am reminded of the adage, "The bitterness of poor quality remains long after the sweetness of low price is forgotten." Just because it is available and cheap does not mean it is the right product to use. Our hardware supplier, White Brothers in Williamsport, Pennsylvania, has recognized our hospital as a customer with special hardware needs and has regularly stocked the products that we most often use. Otherwise, we would be forced either to stock our own spare hardware or compromise quality, because our hardware manufacturer processes orders too slowly to keep pace with our needs.

Setting aside aesthetics, the issues that impact most upon security, as determined by polls, are quality, lock functions, the choice of keyway/ keying and expandability.

We all look for a quality product. If the quality of a keying system we have used for years begins to deteriorate and we have long-range plans to standardize everything, careful consideration must be given to changing hardware vendors. For example, many hospitals and locksmiths have begun to notice that plugs from one vendor have been hand-filed to the point where the smallest master pins actually spin with the plug and get lodged elsewhere in the cylinder. It became such a problem that we had to create our own special masterkey system, avoiding certain keying combinations. To this day, the factory has not acknowledged to us that they are the cause of the problem and has not accepted our offer to provide evidence. Please discuss these quality issues with your customers before you assume that they want to standardize, and if a vendor change is in order, make sure that the decision-maker understands that everyone is not bidding the same quality product. A more expensive system up front sometimes will save the customer money down the road and provide better security.

Expandability must be addressed well in advance of projects in order to consider the condition of the existing keying system and to determine whether it is in the best interests of a facility to expand an existing system or to start over. Frankly, some individuals in charge of key control are misplaced—they fail to understand their responsibility to the integrity of the keying system and do not have the authority to issue keys on a need-only basis. If high level master keys have been issued inappropriately to individuals because of their status, and/or if key control record keeping has not been maintained, it might be tough for you to make a recommendation about expandability.

Key control is a serious problem for some facilities. It complicates planning, because a system not well controlled, if expanded, will continue to provide a minimum of security protection. Newly constructed areas are violated before the building is opened. If a new multiplex masterkey system is sized for a building project with the intention of expanding into existing areas (for the purpose of regaining key control), and then is controlled as poorly as the first system, a new person must be placed in charge of key control or the system will again be compromised. We believe it is the responsibility of the keying planners for the new construction to advise responsible building owners, managers or security directors of these problems and options. In some cases, all of these people fail to understand the responsibility to carefully control an expensive masterkey system.

Keyway and Keying

The issue of keyway and keying always strikes a nerve with knowledgeable security directors. Sure, many of us would prefer our own keyway for which only our facilities are able to obtain blanks. But we know this, for many of us, is practically impossible. It often is difficult to get hardware when requesting standard keyways, and we accept the fact that obtaining hardware with special keyway is unrealistic. However, sectional keying is a form of control and expansion that many of us feel is necessary. And, many directors would like to know all the options before making decisions in a keying conference.

Not all security directors are locksmiths or are fortunate enough to employ locksmiths in house. Many facilities do employ locksmiths in their security or maintenance departments because of the frequency of key duplication and rekeying work and because it saves money. However, training, knowledge, experience and commitment to key control varies from hospital to hospitals, and you should explore the locksmiths' capabilities to determine whether they understand keying options available within any given system. Some of us will surprise you. Some create and maintain our own systems so that keying records are absolutely confidential.

Offer the customer removable core options for high-security areas. For example, in pharmacies, where it is good procedure to rekey more often than other departments, the additional money for removable core cylinders will save rekeying costs over the years, because backup cylinders can be keyed and ready to install at any time. The actual rekeying of doors can take minutes, and then the old cylinders can be rekeyed at your leisure. If the customer cannot afford this type of keying throughout (and most cannot), offer suggestions for other sensitive applications, including research areas, some building entrances and large storage areas.

Most important, the control keys should be kept well secured or the system will be compromised. Sure, you know this, but often the customer either does not know or simply forgets. Remind them: Occasionally send your customers a checklist or ask if they would like a keying audit to determine their vulnerability. Some will say yes and you will gain customer loyalty.

Keyway Lock Function

This must be correctly specified to assure the maximum protection with a minimum of effort required by employees, physicians and others. Specifying lock functions for a project without considering security needs often will result in an inadequate security situation (overprotection, in some cases). Depending upon the location of a facility and the quality of its security program, these types of situations may go unnoticed until a serious or potentially serious incident occurs.

For example, some doors should remain locked at all times. However, hospital employees and physicians are issued keys and are required to turn a key one way to unlock and the other way to relock. Because of different locking functions specified over several years and used throughout a facility, the key is not turned the same way in each lock to gain access and, consequently, some doors that should be locked are presumed to be relocked, because the user repeated the same procedure used on other doors. Sometimes a door remains unlocked, compromising security. This is an ergonomic issue that could easily be designed out of most projects by determining before starting the project the type of hardware and functions that exist and by specifying "like hardware functions."

Many hospital security directors are concerned about the keying of new building projects occurring without their input—without balancing convenience (fewer keys) and security issues—and the master keys being issued by anyone other than the security department or other responsible party. Some directors feel that the hardware specifiers actually should coordinate all of this activity before the materials are ordered.

Electronic Access Systems

These are being specified for more and more hospitals because of the increased security they afford. Once again, however, the hospital users are introduced to the system after it has been ordered or installed. Consequently, valuable input has been forfeited, and the system will probably not meet all security needs. The major problem cited by security directors is that central system is seldom planned or even considered, which usually results in a multitude of electronics from a variety of vendors. Control of these systems becomes extremely difficult. For many of your health care clients, you are considered to be the experts. We look to you for advice not only on the current job, but for the long-range planning necessary to assure continuity in our protection systems. I have presented the above concerns to encourage dialogue with hospital safety and security directors. Some of you will find that this input will make your jobs easier, promote customer satisfaction and reduce the possibility of security liability lawsuits for everyone involved.

J.C. Wolverton, *"Responsible Hospital Security."* Doors and Hardware, FindArticles.com. 03 Dec. 2008.

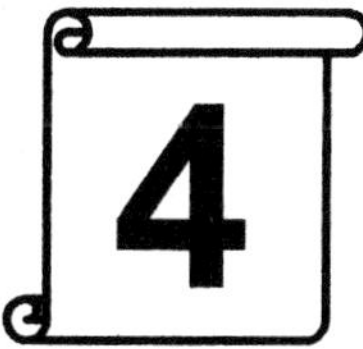

Hospital Ambulance and Transport Services

Ambulance service is the cornerstone in the patient care, so rightly called as the backbone of a Hospital. A prompt and quality ambulance service plays a very important role in management of critical patients. Similarly large hospitals have multifarious needs of the transport services viz. ferrying of staff, guests, visiting professors, examiners, etc. Appropriate management of transport services is essential. Early focus areas are the training of ambulance drivers, development of a transport policy, and implementation of basic transport management tools to record data such as fuel consumption and maintenance costs. The policy covers issues of vehicle security, completion of log-sheets, health and safety, and maintenance. The Hospital ambulance service runs 24 hours a day throughout the year. There should be sufficient number of ambulances to give service to the patients. The access to ambulance should be easy, simple, prompt, and affordable and hassle free. All the ambulances need to be equipped with oxygen cylinders and necessary equipments viz. monitors, ventilator, defibrillator, suction machine, auto loading stretcher, Spinal stretcher and other life saving emergency drugs. Whenever there is call for critical care ambulance a doctor and nurse need to accompany to take appropriate care of the patient during transportation. There is need for networking of ambulance all over the city as well as to various other adjacent areas.

Hospital ambulance should be utilized as efficiently as possible so in turn, it can service the community with optimum effectiveness.

AMBULANCES ARE SCARCELY AVAILABLE AND ILL EQUIPPED

Sanjay Gandhi hospital Delhi, run by city government, is yet to get its act together. The blood bank still remains non-functional after 4 pm and is closed on holidays. Also the ambulances continue to carry patients without the essential life saving equipment. The hospital that started its round-the-clock emergency wing gets about 15-20 accident victims every day from Rohini, Shalimar Bagh, Nangloi, Narela, Mangolpuri and Jehangirpuri areas. Recently, 85-year-old Hari Ram was brought to the hospital by an ambulance. He was grievously injured and after administering an intravenous drip, the doctors decided to movc him to sushruta trauma centre. Being a Sunday, the blood bank was closed. A hospital ambulance without any emergency medicines and equipment arrived and ram was on his way to the trauma centre. But the man died before he could reach there. A doctor at the hospital said: "the man was very seriously injured and some more time was wasted in first bringing him to sanjay gandhi hospital, which already has very little to offer to a patient with multiple injuries." Hospital medical superintendent Dr. Khanna said: "We try to do our best. Ideally every emergency wing should be well-equipped so that there is no need to refer a patient elsewhere and waste precious time." "But we would need more staff and equipment before we can reach this stage," he said. A few days after the times of India published a report on the death of an accident victim, Dilip Arora, who reached the hospital after the blood bank had closed, the hospital bigwigs issued directions that the "key" to the bank should remain accessible even after it closed for the day. The official circular spelt out the working schedule of the blood bank. It said: "blood for donors will be collected during routine duty hours on all working days. Blood will be issued during routine working hours." The circular also said after routine working hours, requisition slips for blood may be sent to the technical staff of the pathological laboratory that would make the required blood units available after carrying out the necessary tests. Though hospital authorities insisted that the blood bank did not become inaccessible at any hour of the day or night, the facts tell a different story. The bank was inaugurated in December, 2001, and since then only about two or three units of blood have been made available in non-working hours. The two ambulances, one of which was used to transport a patient who died on his way to sushruta trauma centre on February 26, are still without the essential equipment. Dr. Khanna said: "our ambulances are not fitted with equipment. But then we have all the required medicines and equipment in the casualty and every time a patient is moved, the equipment usually accompanies." It has now come to light that along with Arora, another girl was transported in the same ambulance to the trauma centre. A source in sanjay Gandhi hospital said: "when arora was being taken, another patient sapna (8) was also put in the same ambulance. This is against all norms and ethics. Quite obviously, the accompanying doctor had to sit next to the driver and had no clue when arora died."

Kailash Hospital, Noida

This hospital offers 24 hours round the clock ambulance services, geared to meet any emergency—surgical or medical. An ambulance that can take care of the patient, right from the site of the accident, or illness, and can make available to him, at his doorstep all the medical expertise and advances inpatient care.

The ambulance, which is a Mobile Critical Care Unit, provides the patient, the same care as would be available in any well-equipped intensive care unit, during his/her transit to the hospital. Designed along the lines of the modern hi-tech ambulances, it has all the fitments for an emergency unit including a two-way communication system.

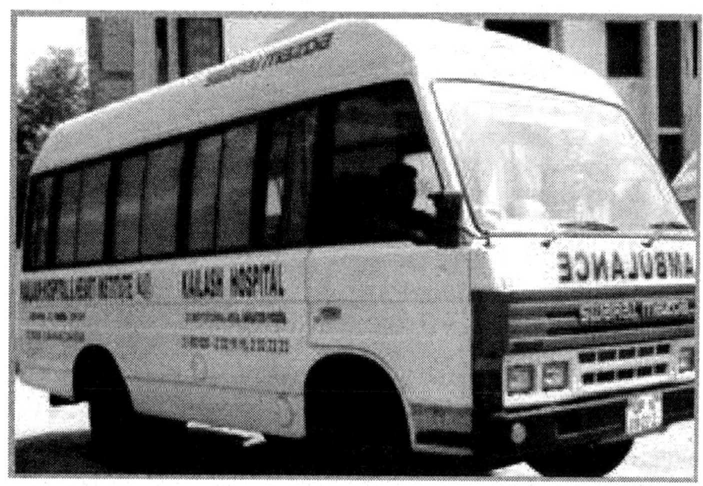

It is manned by a doctor and trained para-medical personnel. A telescopic stretcher, which doubles as a trolley, minimizes the effort for transfer of the patient. Special shock absorbers on the vehicle allow for a smooth journey. Moreover, the unit being air conditioned, it provides maximum comfort to the patient while travelling.

Following are some of the unique facilities available with the Ambulance—

The Mobile Critical Care Team

A doctor, trained in Intensive Care, will always be on board. Tc assist him with the patient, will be a male nurse and a ward-boy, apart from the driver, who would also help in the shifting of the patient.

Ventilator

This is a breathing machine. It supplies oxygen to all patients, whether adults, or children.

Defibrillator

This is used to shock a diseased heart to bring it back to normalcy.

Suction Machine

To take out secretions (sputum) from the lungs.

Emergency Kit

This is a light-weight aluminum suitcase, containing all emergency drug, equipment and infusions (drips). It is carried by the Mobile Critical Care Team to start emergency treatment on the spot.

Two-way Communication System

The unit is equipped with a wireless system, to provide for communication between the hospital and the mobile care unit and *vice versa*.

This is to help provide information regarding the patient to the hospital authorities, so that various specialists could be kept ready for the patient.

Also expert advice could be sought from various specialists, as the patient is being transported to the hospital.

SMS Hospital, Jaipur

SMS Hospital, Jaipur has five ambulances for patients. The ambulance has one driver, one stretcher bearer. The office dealing with the Ambulances is Inquiry office of SMS Hospital.

- The direct telephone number is 102 or 0141-2564222 or 2560291 extension 222,422.
- Ambulance can be provided on telephonic/person request to patients within city of Jaipur limits. A fee of Rs. 40 minimum for a distance of nine kilometers (to and fro) is charged. Beyond nine kilometers, a fee of Rs. 10.50 is charged per kilometer.
- If the ambulance is to be taken outside of Jaipur city, due permission from General Administration Department of the Government of Rajasthan has to be obtained.
- Shortly, three well-equipped critical care ambulances are to be added to the existing fleet of ambulances.
- Medical officer incharge of SMS Hospital ambulances is Dr. Narendra Lodha.
- The Inquiry office dealing with the ambulances has the following team on round the clock duties

Ambulance Services have a Great Role in Saving Disaster Victims

"I saw trauma patients dying in front of my eyes despite the best efforts of doctors. It was an exercise in futility in trying to save lives of these patients brought hours after the 'golden hour'." recalls Dr. Prakash Kasbekar, while sharing his experience as a resident doctor in the casualty ward of Lokmanya Tilak Municipal General hospital Mumbai in 1985. More than fifteen years down the line, ambulance services in the country has not made much progress. Around 30 per cent of the emergency patients die before they are rushed to the hospital and over 80 per cent of the accident victims are denied emergency medical care during the 'golden hour'.

According to World Bank, 30 per cent of the deaths occurring due to accidents could be avoided. if better EMS facilities are provided. Analysts lament that even though technical advancements have made a breakthrough in many disciplines in critical care, emergency medical services (EMS) is the most neglected aspect of health care sector in India. Ironically the basic framework of a successful EMS, i.e. vehicles equipped with life saving equipment, infrastructure required to reach the accident spot, trained paramedics and networking with hospitals has become the greatest hurdle. While the establishment and operational costs of an EMS amounts to at least a couple of crores, the hospitals are currently charging only about Rs. 150-500 per call. With around 100 to 150 calls per year, private hospitals question the viability in investing in EMS. Also, the mundane medico-legal problems associated with accident cases have kept the private hospitals at bay.

Scraped EMS Projects

While EMS started as early as 1966 in the US with the help of both private and government sector, India lags far behind and is only in its nascent stage. Only few cities like Mumbai, Hyderabad, Pune, Bangalore, Delhi and Coimbatore have developed EMS on a small scale. A few of the government run EMS projects are either scraped, lying in the cold storage or functioning without proper infrastructure. Paucity of funds has been the major deterrent in such ventures. For instance, luck has refused to smile at the Rs. 2.5 crore EMS project of the Brihanmumbai Municipal Corporation (BMC) which was conceptualized three years ago. The project had proposed a three tier system of referral, whereby ambulances were placed under the fire brigade. Dr. R.G. Shirahatti, former dean of KEM hospital and head of professional services, P.D. Hinduja hospital, the man who conceptualised this project scoffs, "Why cannot BMC invest Rs. 2.5 crore as the establishment cost and another Rs. 1.8 crore as operational cost annually from its health budget of Rs. 680 crore? It just reflects that they do not understand the importance of EMS."

In 1996 Life Guard Medical Foundation developed a Rs. 40 crore EMS project for Mumbai, incorporating the use of helipad and expensive technology, which was shelved because of unavailability of any sponsers. Rationalizes Dr. Vivek Desai, MD, HOSMAC (Mumbai), the man who planned this project, "Why would anybody invest so much money when EMS is a non-profitable venture? Most of the EMS patients are accident victims of hit and run cases from the lower strata of society who cannot afford to pay."

According to insiders, the Centralized Accident and Trauma Services (CATS) under the Delhi government, with an annual budget of Rs. 3 crore, is faltering in the absence of proper infrastructure and manpower. The dying CATS project was revived recently with the introduction of 35 ambulances each costing Rs. 20 lakh with funds from the Japanese government, says Rakesh Wadhwa, Public Relations Officer, CATS, Delhi. "With around 80 calls a day, we definitely need a better infrastructure." An extended project proposing 400 ambulances and 200 staff member is lost in bureaucratic red tapism. Even the same financial crunch has hampered the EMS project as proposed by American Association of Physicians of Indian origin (AAPI) for the city of Mumbai, Ahmedabad and Pune. Not much progress has occurred in this project, except for Pune. Reveals Dr. S. Balasubraminum, chairman, task force, disaster and trauma management, AAPI. "We need funds for the project."

EMS—A Social Service?

A few private hospitals which have started EMS projects reveal that it is nothing but a social service for them. According to Rajesh Talwar, CEO, Bhakti Vedanta hospital, Mumbai. "EMS is purely social service for us. Charging only Rs. 150 and around 70 calls a year we hardly earn from EMS." Bhakti Vedanta hospital has spent more than Rs. 2 lakh on training its cadre of 70 volunteers, a team of medical and non-medical personnel and printing literature about its EMS facilities for better awareness in the public. The hospital has developed a unique system of having a cadre of volunteers as an integral part of its EMS. Explains Babita Seli, EMS co-ordinator, Bhakti Vedanta hospital. "Merely having ambulatory service is not enough during emergency. Our volunteers, who are local people, reach the place before the ambulance to ensure proper cure."

Viability of Air Ambulance Service

While few hospitals are weighing the pros and cons of developing EMS, what is the viability of having air ambulance facility, which charges anything between Rs. 50,000 to Rs. 1,00,000 per hour? Few experts scoff at this expensive proposition, a concept essentially borrowed from the defense services, whereby helicopters pick up patients from the accident sites. The service providers of air ambulance do not hesitate to admit that their project is viable only because their target audience is the affluent class. For instance Indian Aero-medical Service (IAS) Pvt Limited is already working in this area, catering to Nepal, Bhutan, Malay and a host of other countries. Confesses Dr. Anil Mehra, medical director, IAS. "With the expensive aircraft and the cost of the medical team, air ambulance facility as of now is affordable to the higher strata." He is quick to add, however, it can be made affordable to the middle class with the aid of right policies from the insurance sector.

The upcoming Akshaya Apollo Hospital (Ahmedabad) and Nitu Mandke Heart hospital (Mumbai) have plans to have their own helipads. For Akshaya Apollo Hospital the helipad to be build in the terrace of the hospital was incorporated as an after-thought after the Gujarat earth quake. The hospital plans to hire the services of an agent for the air ambulance, as when the service is required. According to C.D.D. Reddy, managing director, Akshaya Apollo Hospital. "It is not a fancy project. However, we might face difficulties in acquiring land to build helipads in various places."

Networking

Experts say that a stand alone hospital in a city offering EMS is not viable. Instead of one hospital offering its posse of ambulances, hospitals should come together and network so that an emergency patient can be rushed to the nearest hospital. Pune has been a success story of networking of hospitals. The EMS project in Pune was initiated by the formation of Pune Heart Brigade by Sanjeevan Hospital and Rotary Club of Pune South in 1999. Already the EMS facilities is in place with four hospitals and a few more are in the pipeline. According to Dr. Prasad Rajhans, Jt secretary, Society of Emergency Medicine in India (SEMI), and the man behind forming Pune Heart Brigade and chief intensivist at Dinanath Mangeshkar Hospital. "Pune has the best EMS in the country because of good networking between hospitals. We have divided Pune into different zones with each zone being handled by a particular hospital." Pune Heart Brigade is trying to rope in both the private and public sector. "We are having talks with Kamla Nehru Hospital (municipal) and Sasson hospital (government), so that we have an integrated system", says Dr. Rajhans.

However, networking of hospitals for EMS in other cities has met with innumerable obstacles. For instance, Apollo hospitals Group which started four years back its first EMS system in Hyderabad met with lukewarm response from the other hospitals in the city. Recalls Dr. K. Hari Prasad, Vice-president, Apollo Hospitals, Hyderabad and Director, National Network of Emergency Medicine. "We literally begged other hospitals to join us but they were not interested. Hence we went ahead and set-up facilities ourselves across Hyderabad." Based on this successful model of Apollo hospitals Hyderabad, Apollo had spent Rs. 6 crore on various components of EMS including ambulances, communication systems, personnel, emergency rooms, creating awareness, affordability and accident insurance. This has also resulted in the formation of National Network of Emergency Medicine (NNEM), an NGO. NNEM is now functional in Hyderabad, Chennai, Delhi, Madurai and Bilaspur and is supposed to take off in Pune, Karimnagar, Kakinada and Bangalore within a month.

How to make EMS sSlf-sustaining?

It is observed that EMS can made financially viable if hospital concentrates building both its pre-hospitalization and in-house component facilities. If 50 to 60 per cent of the patients availing the pre-hospitalization facility is rushed to the hospital, then the hospital does make profit. "It is only when EMS is split into pre-hospital and in-hospital components, pre-hospital services become capital intensive and non-viable", avers Dr. Prasad. Even NNEM as a policy does not involve any institute which limits itself either to pre-hospital or in-hospital EMS. With corporatisation of health care sector, experts say that the perception of EMS as a social service has to be altered. "EMS must be perceived as any other hospital service." says Dr. Prasad. With the insurance sector paying compensation for accidents, experts say hospitals can make money by taking in accident victims.

Also, a new concept gaining ground is that of a agency who stabilizes the accident patient at the accident site, settles the medico-legal hassles associated with accidents and then switches him to the hospital. A joint venture by Maharashtra State Road Development Corporation (MSRDC) and Sterling hospital is already functioning on this line on the 96 km long Mumbai-Pune Express Highway since the year 2000.

Driver Training

The training covers the following topics:

- Basic Vehicle Handling
- Defensive Driving Techniques
- Advanced Driving Techniques
- Driving at Night or in Poor Conditions
- Attending Road Traffic Crashes
- Completion of Log Sheets and other Administrative Duties
- Daily Vehicle Inspections

The system should allow for the collection and analysis of the following 7 Key Performance Indicators (KPIs):

- Kilometers traveled per vehicle
- Fuel utilization per vehicle
- Running costs per kilometer
- Availability
- Utilization
- Needs satisfaction
- Safety record

Over time, with the appropriate interventions successful use of the system will deliver the following benefits:

- Greater vehicle utilization—less vehicles doing more
- Reduced maintenance costs
- Reduced maintenance time
- Reduced expenditure on fuel
- Faster response to vehicle demand
- Longer vehicle life

The benefits of the training for the drivers will be:

- Reduced Fuel Consumption
- Reduced Maintenance Costs
- Reduced Number of Road Crashes
- Reduced Downtime for Vehicles

Some Studies to Evaluate the Advantages

In a study, St John have discovered that the most common cases of patient transfers using the ambulance are maternity cases which involve transporting pregnant women to hospital. They have also used the vehicle to attend a number of road traffic accidents. St John can now determine the average running cost of the vehicle which enables them to charge the correct fee to users. The data collected has shown that there is a significant amount of unused capacity to help the local community and St John will now focus on increasing utilization of the vehicle. The vehicle has suffered no damage since they began using it and recently underwent its first service. Effective management of the ambulance will serve to enhance and prolong the impact which this vital asset can have upon health service delivery—increasing capacity and giving more people access to health services.[1]

It is clear from several large studies that rapid diagnosis and application of thrombolysis reduces morbidity and mortality rates. Strategies that improve time to treatment in the pre-hospital setting are therefore of fundamental importance in the management of this fatal disease. The advantage of 12 lead electrocardiography use by paramedics to diagnose AMI and reduce time to treatment is discussed. Moreover, paramedic application of thrombolysis in the pre-hospital environment is examined. Several studies conducted worldwide support the notion that ambulance services can play a role in minimizing time to treatment for patients with AMI. The contribution of early intervention by paramedics trained in critical care is potentially considerable, particularly in the important chain of survival that is often initiated by pre-hospital intervention.

Emergency Pre-hospital Management of Acute Asthma Patients

Little is known about the management of acute asthma prior to hospital admission. Pre-hospital treatment of patients referred to hospital with acute asthma was therefore studied in 150 patients (by A.J. Simpson *et al.*) divided into three groups: those in the Edinburgh Emergency Asthma Admission Service (EEAAS) who can contact an ambulance and present directly to respiratory services when symptoms arise (n = 38), those under continuing supervision at a hospital respiratory outpatient clinic (n = 54), and those managed solely in primary care (n = 58).

In each group airflow obstruction had improved upon arrival at hospital, the effect being most marked inpatients transported by ambulance ($p<0.001$) and in those receiving nebulised â2 agonists prior to admission ($p<0.005$). However, 25% of patients arrived without having nebulised â2 agonists and 37% without having glucocorticoids. EEAAS patients were least likely to receive nebulised â2 agonists before arrival at hospital ($p<0.05$). This observation was attributable to a tendency for these patients to travel to hospital by car rather than by ambulance.

Ambulances equipped with nebulised bronchodilators provide the optimal mode of transport to hospital for patients with acute asthma. In Edinburgh ambulances are not being used by a significant proportion of the population with asthma, possibly because of the mistaken belief that personal transport arrangements reduce journey time to hospital.

The service has acted as a model for similar services elsewhere and has been shown to be both efficient and effective.[2] However, relatively little is known about patients' contact with medical services and implementation of treatment for severe acute asthma prior to admission to hospital. The present study compared pre-hospital management in three distinct groups of patients admitted to hospital with acute asthma—those registered with the EEAAS, those under continued supervision at a hospital respiratory medicine outpatient department but not registered with the EEAAS, and those managed solely in the community.[3]

MODE OF REFERRAL AND TRANSPORT TO HOSPITAL

The median duration of symptoms prior to admission was 14 hours for EEAAS patients, 12 hours for clinic patients, and 10 hours for primary care patients (no significant difference, $p = 0.67$). Of the EEAAS patients, nine (24%) requested a visit from their general practitioner which potentially delayed admission to hospital while the remaining 29 (76%) presented as self-referrals. Self-referral was used by six primary care patients (10%) and five clinic patients (9%).

Twenty five EEAAS patients (68%) used transport to hospital with no access to emergency treatment and approximately one third of primary care patients and a quarter of clinic patients traveled to hospital by car.

Discussion

In a small proportion of patients with asthma life threatening airways obstruction develops unpredictably and precipitously. For these patients delayed specialist treatment is associated with increased morbidity and mortality.

The early administration of oral glucocorticoids and bronchodilators is considered to be necessary in acute asthma, and the benefits of nebulised bronchodilators given in ambulances are now well described. In view of this, EEAAS patients are encouraged to self-administer oral glucocorticoids and to contact the Respiratory Medicine Unit early in the course of an attack. The fast track system encourages the use of ambulance transportation to hospital, and all attending ambulances are equipped with nebulisers and oxygen to allow â2 agonists to be given. Potentially, the system offers optimal speed of access to hospital as well as effective first choice treatment for severe asthma prior to arrival, and has provided a widely accepted model for admission of patients with severe asthma.

As such, patients not traveling by ambulance are denied nebulised bronchodilators and supplemental oxygen. In this study ambulance transport and use of nebulised â2 agonists were both associated with highly significant improvements in airflow obstruction upon arrival in hospital.

District-based Transport Management

Transport is not only an expensive resource, but is also critical to effective health care delivery. A lack of transport and the poor use of existing vehicles can lead to problems such as poor supplies of drugs to clinics, inadequate supervision of clinic staff, difficulties in referring patients between facilities, infrequent visits to schools by the school health team, and a lack of community outreach health services or mobile clinic services.

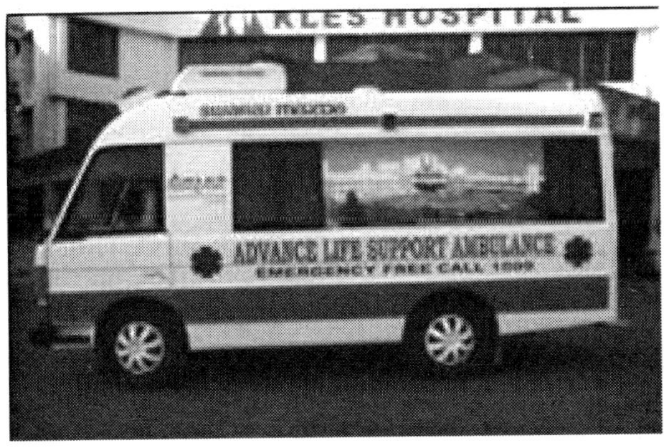

It is imperative for district health services to focus on developing good management for transport. It is one of the most important functions of a district health management team (DHMT), and adequate time must be spent improving performance and educating users. One advantage of the district health system is that it helps to bring together all the available resources within a well-defined geographical area, so that they can be used in a way that will make the biggest impact on health care. One of the first tasks for any newly established health district should therefore be to develop a system for coordinated planning, use and maintenance of all the available vehicles in the district.

In some health districts all vehicles may be under the single authority of the provincial Department of Health, which makes things much easier. In some districts, vehicle management and control will be fragmented—for example, some vehicles may be controlled by the district office, some by local authorities, some by hospitals and some by an independent ambulance service. However, it will always be possible to develop a coordinated district transport management system that will pool all the vehicles within a district, so that there can be co-ordinated planning and more efficient use of vehicles by sharing tasks and trips.

An important requirement for developing a district transport management system is therefore the establishment of a DHMT, an interim DHMT or (in districts where health services are still fragmented), a district-based co-ordinating team where the different authorities within a district can come together to discuss collaboration and joint planning.

Poor Transport Management, Poor Health Care Delivery

The transport problems of a health district may be the result of poor coordination of transport—different facilities and authorities within a district having control of their own vehicles, resulting in inefficient planning; lack of vehicles—especially in rural areas where health services are under-resourced, the roads are bad and the population is widely dispersed; theft, indiscipline, drunk driving and the abuse of government vehicles; and the poor maintenance and repair of vehicles.

Step 1: Conduct a rapid situation analysis of transport in the district

The first step in resolving any problem is to describe and analyse the current situation. This means finding out about the existing transport resources, identifying un-met transport needs, and pinpointing other transport problems in the district. Find out how health workers make transport requests, and how vehicles are allocated. Describe how vehicles are controlled: is there a person in charge of regulating the use of vehicles, and is this person able to prevent the abuse of vehicles?

Conduct an inventory of all vehicles in the district, and document what these vehicles are used for, their mileage and whether they are in a good state of repair. Describe and assess the procedure for the maintenance and repair of vehicles.

Step 2: Develop a district "transport task team"

The situation analysis should be conducted by a 'team' of senior district personnel representing the various authorities and institutions that control vehicles, the users of transport and the drivers. The team should include senior personnel because they will continue to work together to develop the district's transport policy and management system.

Step 3: Identify a district transport officer

One of the first tasks of the task team is to identify a person within the district to be responsible for overall co-ordination and day-to-day management of vehicles.

The Transport Officer may be a senior person who is part of the DHMT, but should be someone who is able to devote at least half his or her time to running transport. Ideally, the Transport Officer will have some previous transport experience, but must be able to undertake administrative and analytical tasks, be able to manage drivers fairly and firmly, be senior enough not to be intimidated by the transport users, and have some background knowledge of the delivery of health services. Depending on how the district is composed and structured, there may need to be assistant transport officers based at each institution at which vehicles are kept. For example, in the Mount Frere health district of the Eastern Cape, vehicles are divided up and spread between the two hospitals. In the Tsepho district of the Free State, vehicles are spread between the Department of Health and seven different local authorities.

Step 4: Establish the concept and idea of a district-based vehicle pool

It is critical that from the very beginning, all the stakeholders and authorities within the district understand the purpose and need for the co-ordinated planning and management of vehicles. The idea of the exercise is so that vehicles based in the district are not allocated to specific authorities or institutions, but belong to the district as a whole. Although vehicles that are normally used by specific institutions or authorities can continue to be based at those locations, the vehicles should be used in a way that serves the needs of the district as a whole.

Step 5: Develop transport policies for the district

Appropriate local transport policy is one of the keys to successful transport management. As the transport task team conducts its situation analysis and begins to co-ordinate vehicle transport planning and management, it should develop the rules and guidelines for transport control and use. These should be based on provincial transport policy, but there will have to be detailed operational policies and guidelines which are based on the local situation and specifics of each individual district. Policy areas should include:

1. determining who in the district is allowed to request the use of vehicles, and who is responsible for signing trip authorities;
2. clarifying the roles, responsibilites and lines of accountability of all those involved in transport management and use; and
3. the mechanism and procedure for the issuing of vehicles; and what should happen to drivers and transport users who continually return vehicles late, or who persistently fail to keep to their schedules.

Step 6: Develop an appropriate information system for transport management

Good quality information is the key to effective transport management. The transport management system is based on regularly filling out a number of forms for collecting this information. These forms include:

1. the vehicle log-sheet or logbook (which should be completed by the driver for each trip taken); and

2. vehicle issue and return forms which are completed when vehicles are issued out by and returned to the transport officer (recording the condition of the vehicle, quantity of fuel in the tank, log book and petrol card numbers); and monthly vehicle report forms which summarizes the use and performance of each vehicle for the preceding month, including information related to accidents and maintenance, service or repairs. In addition, a file should be opened for each vehicle. The file should contain the vehicle registration document, the completed monthly report forms, completed vehicle log sheets, and any other correspondence relating to that vehicle.

Step 7: Identify priority services that rely on regular transport

The DHMT should identify the basic priority health activities and services that should be regularly and routinely allocated a vehicle. This should include the regular allocation of a vehicle for:

1. the supply of drugs, equipment and sundries to clinics (for example, at least once a week there will be a vehicle routinely visiting each clinic in the district);
2. the support and supervision of clinics; and
3. mobile clinic services.

Step 8: Develop a system for making a monthly transport schedule

Before the beginning of each month, a monthly transport schedule should be drawn up by the district transport officer. This will show the allocation of vehicles to those activities and services mentioned in Step 7, as well as the allocation of vehicles to other activities. Therefore, by the 25th of each month, all requests for planned trips in the following month should be submitted to the transport officer. These requests should include the number of people and places to be visited, and whether the dates are fixed or flexible. It is important that dates are kept as flexible as possible so that different trips can be combined, but without making wide detours.

As there are no individually-allocated vehicles, no one can assume that there will always be a vehicle available. All potential transport users will quickly learn the importance of planning their transport needs ahead of time and preparing a travel itinerary. Once the monthly transport schedule has been completed, a copy should be issued to the district manager, and displayed in the transport office and other major institutions of the district.

Step 9: Develop a system for handling unplanned transport requests

Not all trips can be planned a month before. Other transport requests should therefore be made through a transport request form as soon as the need for a vehicle becomes known. Therefore, on each Thursday, the transport officer should prepare a more detailed weekly plan for vehicles for the week ahead. This will be based on the monthly schedule but will be updated daily to include any new requests for transport or any changes. It should be possible to determine the location of all vehicles at any time by looking at this form. If there are insufficient vehicles to meet the planned programmes, or an emergency should arise, then the district manager or designated person should assign priorities. Vehicle allocation should be determined according to the health care priorities of the district, and should not to be issued according to seniority or rank.

Step 10: Develop a system for monitoring performance

At the end of each month, the transport officer should review the allocation of vehicles in the past month and note any failures and problem areas. He or she should keep records on the number of transport requests that were made, and how many of them were satisfied. Major problems should be brought to the attention of the DHMT. Various transport efficiency indicators can be calculated from the data collected from the vehicle log sheets to help assess performance and efficiency. These include: kilometres travelled per litre of fuel (fuelutilization), maintenance costs per vehicle per year, running cost per kilometre (fuel plus maintenance). The calculation of these factors will aid the preparation of budgets for future years and the identification of uneconomic vehicles.

Ambulance Diversion

The practice of telling EMS services "don't bring patients to our ED by ambulance right now, we are too busy/full to care for them adequately."

Condition Yellow: "The Emergency Department is busy but not overwhelmed. Patients presenting to the Emergency Department via EMS may experience significant delays in treatment due to the current volume and/or acuity of patients already in the Emergency Department. EMS personnel should inform the patient of this situation and consider transporting the patient to another facility if the patient consents.

Condition Red: "All of the usually available resources in the Emergency Department are overwhelmed such that receipt of additional patients will result in the inability to care for them safely. Patients may not be brought to the Emergency Department unless EMS personnel perceive the patient to be suffering from an immediately life-threatening illness or injury."

It is critical that hospital personnel and administration be guided by a formal hospital policy on ambulance diversion. Having such a policy will:

1. Minimize uncertainty, anxiety and staff conflict when having to decide 'on divert' status.
2. Provide decision-makers with criteria to ensure they are making an appropriate and defensible decision.
3. Provide hospitals with a guide to appropriate actions to take when 'on divert'.

4. Allow hospital administrators to demonstrate their planning to accrediting organizations, to local, regional and state Emergency Medical Services councils, and to county and State health departments.
5. In Pennsylvania, since February 2002, by order of the state health department, every hospital is required to have such a policy.

Criteria for "divert" status has, in different places and times, been based on different criteria:

(a) the number of beds available (e.g., one area in Florida reportedly requires 110% occupancy prior to diversion),
(b) the number of beds of a particular type available (e.g., ICU beds),
(c) the number of beds that can be adequately staffed by nurses, or
(d) the status of the Emergency Department.

Stabilization and Transfer; Specialized Beds

1. Once a patient Comes to The Hospital, and has a Medical Screening Exam, the patient can be transferred, based on insurance or other payment issues, or based on the patient's special needs, once the patient has completed his or her Medical Screening Exam and once his or her Emergency Medical Condition has had Commencement of Stabilizing Treatment, sometimes called Initiation of Stabilizing Care. The hospital must also ensure that the patient is Stable for Transfer.
2. The patient can be transferred, even before the Medical Screening Exam is completed, and even before the hospital has initiated stabilizing care for the Emergency Medical Condition—but only if the hospital doesn't have the capacity to care for the patient. Examples include an unstable trauma patient at a non-Trauma Center, or a patient who needs an ICU bed at a hospital whose ICU beds are all full.
3. Therefore, for purposes of inter-hospital transfer of stabilized patients, information on availability of specialized beds can be useful. However, based on a clear reading of Federal EMTALA law, this information cannot be used to refuse ambulance patients ('emergency patients') from the field. When an ambulance is en route to an Emergency Department with the capacity to accept additional patients in the ED, it is not lawful for the hospital to refuse a patient because initial assessment suggests the patient may need specialized inpatient care. The current interpretation of EMTALA also requires hospital-owned ambulances to transport patients to their 'home' hospital. The only exceptions are when ambulance redirection is in accordance with Regional EMS Protocols as described below.

Content and Format of Hospital Ambulance-Diversion Policies

A. A Hospital Ambulance-Diversion Policy must answer the following specific questions:
   - Who makes the decisions?
   - How are these decisions made? Are there objective criteria for making these decisions?
   - How are these decisions recorded?
   - Once these decisions are made, what actions are taken? Who is responsible for implementing these measures?

B. The Hospital Ambulance-Diversion Policy should be part of the hospital's Disaster Plan. In particular, if an ED is crowded enough that patients must be placed in the hallways, in excess of the ED's licensed capacity, then Pennsylvania state law requires the hospital activate its disaster or emergency plan. When the Emergency Department is overwhelmed with patients, it doesn't matter whether the overload is from a multi-casualty incident, a major disaster, an influenza epidemic, the closing or "Condition Red" of a nearby Emergency Department, a blue moon, or no discernible cause. The hospital's response should focus on the emergency department patient overload situation, regardless of cause."

   "Condition Yellow" should be integrated in the Disaster Plan as a low-level disaster plan activation. This means that the hospital should institute aggressive actions to improve the situation, and to avoid a "Condition Red" situation. This should be the same as the measures the hospital takes to deal with a multi-casualty incident that expected to briefly overwhelm the Emergency Department's capacity.

   "Condition Red" should be integrated in the Disaster Plan as moderate-level disaster plan activation. This means the hospital should institute immediate aggressive actions to alleviate the situation. This should be the same as the measures that the hospital takes to deal with a large multi-casualty incident that is expected to overwhelm the Emergency Department's capacity for an extended period.

Standard measures for multi-casualty incidents generally include some or all of the following:

(a) Calling in additional housekeeping staff,
(b) Calling in additional nursing staff,
(c) Calling in a backup emergency physician,
(d) Opening closed units, and
(e) Canceling all elective admissions and elective surgery.

Canceling elective admissions and surgery is an administrator's tool, and should be listed as an option in the hospital's diversion plans. Usually, such cancellations will not improve short-term ED congestion, and this drastic option will seldom be needed. Yet, a hospital's plan should provide thoughtful and graded provisions for dealing with "Condition Yellow" and "Condition Red" disasters. The decision for diversion should be made by the emergency physician in the emergency department in coordination with nursing and/or administrative staff.

Condition Yellow Actions

There are many recommendations for dealing with hospital and ED overcrowding and the nursing shortage. Many of these recommendations focus on long-term "fixes" for making EDs more efficient, for recruiting or retaining staff, or for fixing the health care system as a whole. The literature shows that "ED overcrowding" is actually a problem that has its roots outside the ED, and reflects hospital crowding and systemic health care system problems. The literature also shows that patients boarded in the Emergency Department have a longer length of stay than those admitted directly to the floor, and that inpatient care provided in the ED is understandably inferior to that provided on an inpatient floor, which has recently been a powerful stimulus to decrease ED "boarding." Others focus on persuading the hospital administration that they should be proactive in dealing with the Emergency Department in general.

Notes and References

1. EMTALA
   - 1.1. A detailed tutorial on EMTALA is available at http://www.pitt.edu/kconover/ftp/emtala-draft.pdf
   - 1.2. The official Interpretive Guidelines put out by HCFA in 1998 are available online at http://www.hcfa.gov/pubforms/07%5Fsom/somap_v_001_to_012.htm and an excerpt is provided as an appendix below.
   - 1.3. Published EMTALA materials, especially the November 9, 1999 document put out by HCFA, are available on the websites.
   - 1.4. On May 9, 2002, CMS published proposed modifications to EMTALA policies in the Federal Register (67(90): 31470 et seq, available at http://www.access.gpo.gov/su_docs/aces/aces140.html). Even though they are "proposed" they offer insight into official CMS thinking, which may be of use now.
   - 1.5. The EMTALA forum at www.medlaw.com contains wide-ranging discussions of EMTALA issues.
   - 1.6. Frew's book on EMTALA containing past forum discussions is available at the above website.
   - 1.7. Dr. Dan Sullivan's EMTALA website at www.thesullivangroup.com contains a variety of cases and other references about EMTALA.
   - 1.8. The book "Providing Emergency Care Under Federal Law: EMTALA" (Robert A. Bitterman, M.D., J.D., FACEP) is available through the American College of Emergency Physicians (www.acep.org).
2. Pennsylvania's Emergency Health Services Council (north-central PA EMS region)

has a diversion plan available online at: http://hospitals.ehsf.org/hospitalstatusprogram.pdf

3. Hospital and ED Overcrowding
   3.1. Responding To Emergency Department Crowding: A Guidebook for Chapters. A Report of the Crowding Resources Task Force, American College of Emergency Physicians (American College of Emergency Physicians, August 2002) is available online at http://www.acep.org/download.cfm? resource=681. EMTALA Interpretive Guidelines. The Emergency Medical Treatment and Active Labor Act specifies that hospitals can refuse an ambulance only when hospital facilities are overwhelmed. The Office of Inspector General Interpretive Guidelines state: INTERPRETIVE GUIDELINES—RESPONSIBILITIES OF MEDICARE PARTICIPATING HOSPITALS IN EMERGENCY CASES, Tag 406, Rev 2., 05-98, p V-18 and Tag 411, Rev. 25-98, p V-34 100 Simpson, Matusiewicz, Brown, *et al.*

References

Asplin BR, Magid DJ, Rhodes KV, Solberg LI, Lurie N, Camargo CA, Jr. A conceptual model of emergency department crowding. *Ann Emerg Med* 2003;42(2):173-80.

Bazarian JJ, Schneider SM, Newman VJ, Chodosh J. Do admitted patients held in the emergency department impact the throughput of treat-and-release patients? *Acad Emerg Med* 1996;3(12):1113-8.

British Thoracic Society, National Asthma Campaign, Royal College of Physicians of London, *et al.* The British guidelines on asthma managment: 1995 review and position statement. *Thorax* 1997;52 (Suppl 1):S1–21.

Campbell IA, Colman SB, Mao JH, *et al.* An open, prospective comparison of â2 agonists given by nebuliser, Nebuhaler, or pressurised inhaler by ambulance crew as emergency treatment. *Thorax* 1995;50:79–80.

Clark K, Normile LB. Delays in implementing admission orders for critical care patients associated with length of stay in emergency departments in six mid-Atlantic states. *J Emerg Nurs* 2002;28(6):489-95.

Corbridge TC, Hall JB. The assessment and management of adults with status asthmaticus. *Am J Respir Crit Care Med* 1995;151:1296–316.

Crompton GK, Grant IW, Chapman BJ, *et al.* Edinburgh Emergency Asthma Admission Service: report on 15 years' experience. *Eur J Respir Dis* 1987;70:266–71.

Crompton GK, Grant IWB. Edinburgh Emergency Asthma Admission Service. *BMJ* 1975;4:680–2.

Fergusson RJ, Stewart CM,Wathen CG, *et al.* Effectiveness of nebulised salbutamol administered in ambulances to patients with severe acute asthma. *Thorax* 1995;50:81–2.

Fields WW. Calculus, chaos, and other models of emergency department crowding. *Ann Emerg Med* 2003;42(2):181-4.

General Accounting Office. Hospital emergency departments: Crowded conditions vary among hospitals and communities. Washington, DC: General Accounting Office; 2003. Report No.: GAO-03-460.

Graham VAL, Milton AF, Knowles GK, *et al.* Routine antibiotics in hospital management of acute asthma. *Lancet* 1982;i:418–20.

Harrison BDW. Acute severe asthma. In: Brewis RAL, Gibson GJ, Geddes DM, eds. Respiratory medicine, 1st ed. London: Baillière Tindall, 1990: 674–90.

Kolbe J, Vamos M, Fergusson W, *et al.* Differential influences on asthma self-management knowledge and self-management behavior in acute severe asthma. *Chest* 1996;110:1463–8.

Lipworth BJ. Pharmacokinetics of inhaled drugs. *Br J Clin Pharmacol* 1996;42:697–705. 182

Littlejohns P, Hollowell J, Hayward P, *et al.* Comparison of asthmatic patients admitted to hospital from health districts experiencing high and low asthma mortality rates. *Postgrad Med J* 1994;70:92–9.

Neville RG, Clark RC, Hoskins G, et al for the General Practitioners in Asthma Group. National asthma attack audit 1991–2. *BMJ* 1993;306:559–62.

Neville RG, Hoskins G, Smith B, *et al.* How general practitioners manage acute asthma attacks. *Thorax* 1997;52:153–6.

North of England Asthma Guideline Development Group. North of England evidence based guidelines development project: summary version of evidence based guideline for the primary care management of asthma in adults. *BMJ* 1996;312:762–6.

Quadrel M, Lavery RF, Jaker M, *et al.* Prospective, randomized trial of epinephrine, metaproterenol, and both in the pre-hospital treatment of asthma in the adult patient. *Ann Emerg Med* 1995;26:469–73. 183

Richardson DB. The access-block effect: relationship between delay to reaching an inpatient bed and inpatient length of stay. *Med J Aust* 2002;177(9):492-5.

Schneider S, Zwemer F, Doniger A, Dick R, Czapranski T, Davis E. Rochester, New York: a decade of emergency department overcrowding. *Acad Emerg Med* 2001;8(11):1044-50.

Schneider SM, Gallery ME, Schafermeyer R, Zwemer FL. Emergency department crowding: a point in time. *Ann Emerg Med* 2003;42(2):167-72.

Sears MR, Rea HH, Fenwick J, *et al.* 75 deaths in asthmatics prescribed home nebulisers. *Br Med J Res Educ* 1987;294: 477–80.

Sibbald B. Patient self care in acute asthma. *Thorax* 1989;44:97–101.

Snooks H, Hartley-Sharpe C, Booth H, *et al.* Audit of care of acute asthma patients by ambulance crews in London. *Pre-hosp Immed Care* 1999;3:76–80.

Sobie JM, Gaves D, Tringali A. ED "hold" patients: is their care also being held? *J Emerg Nurs* 2000;26(6):549-53.

Sorelle R.A real solution to overcrowding. *Emergency Medicine News* 1993;25(6):1,8-10.

Spaite DW, Bartholomeaux F, Guisto J, *et al.* Rapid process redesign in a university-based emergency department: decreasing waiting time intervals and improving patient satisfaction. *Ann Emerg Med* 2002;39(2):168-77.

Teichtahl H, Buckmaster N, Pertnikovs E. The incidence of respiratory tract infection in adults requiring hospitalization for asthma. *Chest* 1997;112:591–6.

Wathen CG, Crompton GK, Carrington D, *et al.* Treatment for acute asthma in the ambulance. *Br J Gen Pract* 1990;40:388.

Weiss SJ, Anand P, Ernst AA, *et al.* Effect of out-of-hospital albuterol inhalation treatments on patient comfort and morbidity. *Ann Emerg Med* 1994;24:873–8.

Windom HH, Burgess CD, Crane J, *et al.* The self administration of inhaled beta agonist drugs during severe acute asthma. *NZ Med J* 1990;103:205–7.

Wong BJO, Hargreave FE. Bioequivalence of metered-dose inhaled medications. *J Allergy Clin Immunol* 1993;92: 373–9.

5

Management of Hospital Reception

Reception is the first point of contact between the patient/his relatives and the hospital and thus the reputation prestige and image of the hospital depends upon the reception. That is why, there is a great need to ensure the setting up a reception counter managed by receptionists, their number and would depend upon the strength of a hospital. Reception counter must work for all the 24 hours in a day. The hospital must design the reception counter with all the facilities so that patents can get all information promptly. Reception counter must be managed by well trained receptionists round the clock. Since the post of receptionist is most important, therefore, essential training for a month needs to be given to the incumbent. This must be followed by refresher training as and when new electronic gadgets are used. The receptionist has to use a number of electronic instruments, he should be made perfect in all of them. Let us first discuss the essential qualities of receptionists who can serve the patients nicely.

A. QUALITIES OF RECEPTIONISTS

1. Complete Knowledge of the Hospital

The receptionist must be given training about the hospital, i.e. location of different facilities, their functions and the personnel managing them. In addition, there may be a chart hanging on the wall near the reception depicting to whole organizational set-up.

2. Complete Knowledge of the Laboratories and their Procedure

The receptionist must be aware of the location of laboratories and diagnostic facilities including their details, i.e. where the blood sample is to be given, from where the result of the sample obtained, etc.

3. Directory

The receptionist must keep a directory containing all telephone numbers land line and mobile of all the employees so that where about of them can be found in case of need. This is very important as the patients find it difficult to locate the Doctor or Nurse, etc. These directories may be classified in different manner so that the delay in locating them may be minimized.

4. Receipt of Outside Call

It has been generally seen that outside calls at the reception are not attended properly causing great resentment to the callers. Receptionists must be prompt in attending the telephone and providing full information needed by the caller. This would create a good image of the hospital.

5. Excellent Behaviour

Most of the problems today are the result of rude behaviour of majority of employees towards citizens. Their behavior has alienated the people from the functioning. Inspite of 73rd and 74th amendments, people still have not been given their due place and recognition in public governance. How to go about it? We may suggest the following remedies:

(i) Training may be imparted in the art and science of communication.

(ii) Employees using filthy language should be dealt strictly by imposition of fines or recording the demeanor in the confidential reports.

(iii) A column about behavior should be incorporated in ACR.

(iv) Employees should be encouraged to be polite, nice and courteous. Superiors should set a personal example by observing same standards while dealing with their bosses as well as subordinates or members of public.

(v) Supervision should be done strictly and if required dialogues of citizens and employees depicting different situations—very negative, negative, positive, very positive, be recorded for training purposes. To quote Aristotle, "Anyone can become angry—that is easy. But to be angry with the right person, to there right degree, at the right time, for the right purpose and the right way is not easy."

(vi) A new concept called "Equilibrium Thinking" has been tried out with police trainees both with veterans having thirty years experience and freshly recruited officer trainees. Several of the trainees reported remarkable breakthroughs in managing anger and of the emotions. Equilibrium is produced when positive values or vices are balances. The positive values need to be affirmed or reinforced and the negative values need to be denied, weakened and uprooted.

6. Faith in Oneself by receptionist

Faith is a quality of the self. It is a great power of the mind. It can be used beneficially be everyone, at all times. Faith is certain to have a positive effect on our life, health, profession and our mind. Faith is the key with which we can open the secret treasures of this universe. It is the path that leads to the Supreme Being who is the repository of all power and glory that manifests in this world. It is also the means of acquiring tremendous energy. It is faith that given us the steadiness to hold on, with optimism in the midst of gloom and destruction. "With true faith, one can attain enlightenment", says the Gita.

Those who tend to believe that they are culturally, socially and intellectually inferior should, first of all, shake off their inferiority it out. Of course, it is not so easy as throwing away an unwanted article. Our first and foremost need- nay, duty, is to develop confidence in our own immense power, which is latent, in the past, seers and men of limited powers of man are hidden unlimited mysterious powers, if only we had the skill to discover them. Today, psychologist are reaffirming the same fact with the help of their experimental observations. To arouse the powers, nothing more than self-confidence is required. We should strive to rise from the state in which we are right now. We should gradually attain success, scaling each step through efforts.[1]

Swami Vivekananda repeatedly stressed the need for cultivating the faith in one self: "the ideal of faith in ourselves is of the greatest help practiced, I am sure a very large portion of the evils and miseries that we have would have vanished. Throughout the history of mankind if any motive power has been more potent than another in the lives of all great men and women, It is that of faith in themselves. Born with the consciousness that they were to be great, they became great. Let a man go down as low as possible; there must come a time when out of sheer deperation he will take an upward curve and will learn to have faith in himself. But it is bitter experiences in order to gain faith in ourselves? We can see that all the difference between man and man is due to the existence or non-existence of faith in himself. Faith in ourselves will do everything."

Unlimited energy is latent in each one of us. But because of our restricted imagination we act as if we have hypnotized ourselves into inaction. Self-confidence will activate the spirit of enthusiasm and lead us along the pat of achieving great things in life.[2]

Self-confidence and the conviction that virtuous acts lead to one's highest good and success have their source in the power of faith, faith in God. A scientist and a religious person both pay their tribute to faith. Faith is life, William James, remarked: "Faith is one of the forces by which men live and the total absence of it means collapse." Faith is the foundation of spiritual life; it is the means to acquire the grace of the Lord. Everything is possible through faith. Is it possible in one day to have such unflinching, unshakeable trust? Faith begets faith.

7. Love

Love is the elixir of life. It has been found to have power even to cure physical and mental disorders. One who has hatred in his mind not only loses his mind, but also undermines his health and life. On the other hand, love, sympathy, and friendship not only contribute towards building one's peace of mind, but also create a balance outlook. A man who develops these qualities will acquire serenity, joy and peace in spite of all external circumstances.

8. Need of Enthusiasm and Dynamism

To make life worthwhile and fruitful, we must generate enthusiasm within ourselves. Generation of enthusiasm will take place when we discover for ourselves a goal and attach ourselves to the Altar with a spirit of dedication, reverence and love. Once we have surrendered ourselves to it, the ideal itself will provide us with the inspiration and strength. The nothing can hinder the progress of our march towards that Goal and the ideal. The love for the ideal will overcome and vanquish all the hurdles from the ideal, and if it comes to that, life itself will be cast-off with a smile in dedication at that Altar. That was how Bhagat Singh could walk to the gallows with a smile on his face. What is important is that one should choose the right ideal. An ideal worthwhile even if it comes to sacrificing one's own life in the endeavor. The ideal should be inspiring, it should arouse the spring of activity in use. Thus, the discovering of the ideal is the secret of generating in ourselves Dynamism and Vitality in its fullness.[3]

9. Interest in Work

The first factor necessary for success is work. An individual has to work even though he or she would like to have success without work. There is only one place whre success comes before work, and that is in the dictionary. So work is a must for success. We see many people working laboriously. Still, they do no seem to accomplish anything. This is because there is no efficiency in their work. Efficincy is the second factor required for success. The skill of knack of working or performing an action in such a way that it well bear the desired fruit is called efficiency. The third factor required is knowledge, for to perform work knowledge is a must. Knowledge means: (1) knowledge of our desired goal; (2) knowledge of the means to attain the goal; (3) knowledge of the performer who is going to adopt the means and strive for the goal. This knowledge is called proficiency.

A person who has knowledge but no efficiency cannot be successful. The difference can be seen in the material progress of India as compared to other countires such as the United State or Japan. In India, more emphasis is given to theretical knowledge is overlooked, while in America more emphasis is given to the practical aspect and work is done efficiently. Therefore, even though so many students are graduating from universities in India with outstanding degrees, what is the condition of India materially? We are speaking only from the material point of view at the moment. India's prosperity cannot be compared to the prosperity of the United State, Canada or Japan because India has neglected the practical aspect.[4]

When a person works with inspiration, he never gets tired or exhausted. When man works only for himself, there is perspiration; but when he works for a noble goal there is inspiration. In cases where a man cannot dedicates his actions to the Lord, even if he works for some ideal or goal he will derive tremendous strength from his chosen altar of dedication. The nobler the goal, the greater will be the strength he gains. This is the beauty of love and dedication, which brings efficiency in life.[5]

Work ethic embraces work responsibility, work conscience, ethical work conduct. If one has the satisfaction that he is contributing his very best to his organisation and is not just earning the bread, then his would be the true feeling of work ethics. Work ethic demands that one works for attaining organisational objectives in its fullest measures.[6]

Today belongs to us. Success is like oxygen to a person. Every time you ahieve success, enthusiasm in you increases. Your respect gets doubled. When you succeeed, world gives you recognition. All will be with you or following you. Everyone will compete to say that they are acquainted with you. Your relatives will be proud of you. Failure pulls down a person. Success give new strength. No one will hand over to you success in a golden plate. You have to make all efforts to succeed. Your can forget about the efforts made and difficulties undergone after you have achieved victory. But it is not so easy to achieve success. Merely thinking that I want to become a winner is not sufficient. For reputation, constant pursuit, oncentration strength to face defeat, desire to achieve something, personal development, time management, keen observation/examination, patience and expertise to detect a mistake and rectify it, etc., are required. Firm resolve to travel in that direction is most important. Today belongs us, yesterday was; tomorrow will be; but today is with us. Everyday is bursting with opportunities for us to do and to serve, to act and to express, to love and to live.

We must make use of these lush chances and diligently make our life rich, fruitful and useful for others at all times. When we have such a teak of even a few courageous and honest servants of God, the nation is made, the world is saved.[7]

10. Truthfullness and Honesty

"Never complain, about the number of hours you have put in, to do a job. Your nobility must estimate how much of you was put into each hour of your daily work." Cultivate friendliness, charity, concern for others. You are never then alone anywhere, at any time.

"Proficiency in any field, we gain through study and discussion in institutes and colleges. The knowledge we have gathered in our proficiency, when expressed through diligent and planned activities, becomes the play of efficiency in us. Proficiency in an individual is not creative until it transforms into efficiency. The means is to act diligently, with your heart in your work, with a gusto to improve, a spirit to outshine your own present abilities. This spirit of challenging yourself by yourself is the secret of self-improvement and personality-unfoldment."

11. Work Culture: Importance of Work—Work is Worship/Dharma

The first factor necessary for success is work. An indivicual has to work even though he or she would like to have success without work. There is only one place where success comes before work, and that is in the dictionary. So work is a must for success. We see many people working laboriously. Still, they do not seem to accomplish anything. This is because there is no efficiency in their work. Efficiency is the second factor required for success. The skill or knack of working or performing an action in such a way that it will bear the desired fruit is called efficiency. The third factor required is knowledge, for to perform work knowledge is a must. Knowledge means:

(1) knowledge of our desired goal;
(2) knowledge of the means of attain the goal; and
(3) knowledge of the performer who is going to adopt the means and strive for the goal. This knowledge is called proficiency.

A person who has knowledge but no efficiency cannot be successful. The difference can be seen in the material progress of India as compared to other countries such as the United State or Japan. In India, more emphasis is given to theoretical knowledge. India universities impart a lot of information, but practical knowledge is overlooked, while in America more emphasis is given to the practical aspect and work is done efficiently. Therefore even though so many students are graduating from universities in India with outstanding degrees, what is the condition of India materially? We are speaking only from the material point of view at the moment. India's prosperity cannot be compared to the prosperity of the United State, Canada or Japan because India has neglected the practical aspect.[8]

When a person works with inspiration, he never gets tired or exhausted. When man works only for himself, there is perspiration; but when he works for a noble goal there is inspiration. In cases where a man cannot dedicate his actions to the Lord, even if he works for some ideal or goal he will derive tremendous strength from his chosen altar of dedication. The nobler the goal, the greater will be the strength he gains. This is the beauty of love and dedication, which brings efficiency in life.[9]

Work ethic embraces work responsibility, work conscience, ethical work conduct. If one has the satisfaction that he is contributing his very best to his organisation and is not just earning the bread, then this would be the true feeling of work ethics. Work ethic demands that one works for attaining organisational objectives in its fullest measures. Behind every achievement that we see in this world today, is the unseen hand of the human will. The material comforts, scientific achievements are all the products crystallised out of the human will and determination. The human will power has conquered Nature, and made Her a slave for the welfare of making, and in the process has ever created things which were not even available in the world before. Behind all the technological progress are the determined efforts of hundreds of dedicated men and women, who faced all the challenges to make their dreams come true.

Many of what we see today as solid facts of life and proof of man's achievements were only mess ideas yesterday in the minds of a few men of great will power. Those ideas would not have become realities, had they not the will and determination to put their ideas into practice. Our scriptures too have given us examples of men of great will, like Viswamithra who could even create a new world out of his sheer power of willing. All men of achievement had the blessing of tremendous will power in their makeup, and History is full of names of such men of achievements.[10]

Bata K. Dey in his Article, "Work Culture in India—Achievements and Failure" rightly says that culture is not something which can be imported or transplanted; it must grow from within; it grows, and it does, in fertile solid and congenial climate. Gap in capital equipment or technology can be filled by import. You can even buy management, but not dedication, commitment, culture. How to create that is a million dollar question. An inexpensive answer to such a costly question if that, work culture tends to be congruous with and is an extension of, the societal, indeed national culture. And the later, at the moments, is the elusive commodity, despite this country ancient civilization and old culture. The search is on. And we shall succeed.[11]

Murtaza Mithani, Chairman and Managing Director of Wintech Group in his article, "The High Road", in *The Tribune*, dated June 28, 2000 expects his employees to be committed to their work. "As the head of an organization, I, expect my employees to be innovative, competitive and flexible. They should possess total commitment, be actively involved in every day work, and have no hastiness while interacting. He wants his team to be able to work in synergy with various departments. Failure and challenges should be treated as a stepping stone to success. Think big, create your own space and help yourself.

12. Devotion and Dedication

Emotional intelligence can promote Devotion and Dedication. Emotional intelligence is concerned with achieving one's goals through the ability to manage one's own feelings and emotions, to be sensitive to, and influence other key people, and to balance one's motives and drives with conscientious and ethical behaviours. The following are the characteristics of EI:

(a) Inter-personal sensitivity covering competencies like listening and sensitivity.
(b) Motivating, including impact and energy.
(c) Emotional Resilience.
(d) Influence and Adaptability covering both influencing and negotiating ability and being adaptable in various types of situations and cultures.
(e) Decisiveness and assertiveness.
(f) Integrity.
(g) Leadership including motivating other people.

Inner Self Control and Happiness

Happiness that arises from consistent effort and inner self-control can yield a greater beauty and a larger sense of fulfilment. In the beginning its practice may be painful and arduous, but a person who has the necessary courage and heroism, to walk the precipitous path of self-purification, creativity, and inward balance comes to enjoy the subtlest happiness and the all fulfilling absence of inner peace. The flimsy happiness that is gained through sense indulgence and sense gratification is a joy that is fleeting, vanishing as quickly as it comes, and after its drags us into ill-reputed dissipation. This happiness lasts only so long as the sense organs are actually in contact with sense objects.

13. Perfection

Perfection is very important to impart quality to attain success in life and to reach the desired goal one must have a positive attitude. Faith in oneself and in God, courage, strength and fearlessness are the characteristics of a positive intellect. For a man of intense faith nothing is impossible in this world. Perfection has its two aspects in man, which to some extent be separated, the perfection in being and perfection in doing. It can be imagined that through some training or compulsion, good works may possibly be extorted from a man who personally may not be good where the question is not that of utility but of moral perfection, we hold it important that the individual be true to his goodness. His outer good work may continue to produce good results, but the inner perfection of his personality has its immense value, which for him is spiritual freedom and for humanity is an endless asset thought we may not know. For goodness represents the detachment of spirit from the exclusiveness of our egoism, in goodness we identify ourselves with the universal humanity. In order to realize his unity with the universal, the individual man must live his perfect life which alone given the freedom to transcend it.

14. Communication

Communication is an integral part of every function of administration. It is a two way process between people. In communication, a message is transmitted and received.

Transmission Reception

Message transmitted is the first half of the communication and message received and understood is the second half of the communication. Millet rightly describes communication as the "blood stream of administrative organisation." Pfiffner also portrays it as "the heart of management." In the words of Louis A. Allen, "Communications is the sum of all the things one person does when he wants to create understanding in the mind of another. It involves a systematic and continuous process of telling, listening and understaning."[12] According to M.W. Cunning, "The word communications describes the process of conveying messages (facts, ideas, attitudes and opinions) from one person to another so that they are understood."[13] In the words of Millett, communications means "shared understanding of a shared purpose." According to Tead, "the underlying aim of communication is a meeting of minds on common issues."

Communications can be transmitted through audio, visual and audio-visual means. Communications plays the same role as the nervous system in a body. Norbert Wiener has rightly observed, "Communications is the cement that makes an organisation." Communications is central to the exercise of authority in an organisation. In the words of Ordway Tead, "Communication is the touching of mind by mind, of person with person, whether it be one man, or a thousand. It can include conversation, interview, dialogue, visual technique carefully used."[14]

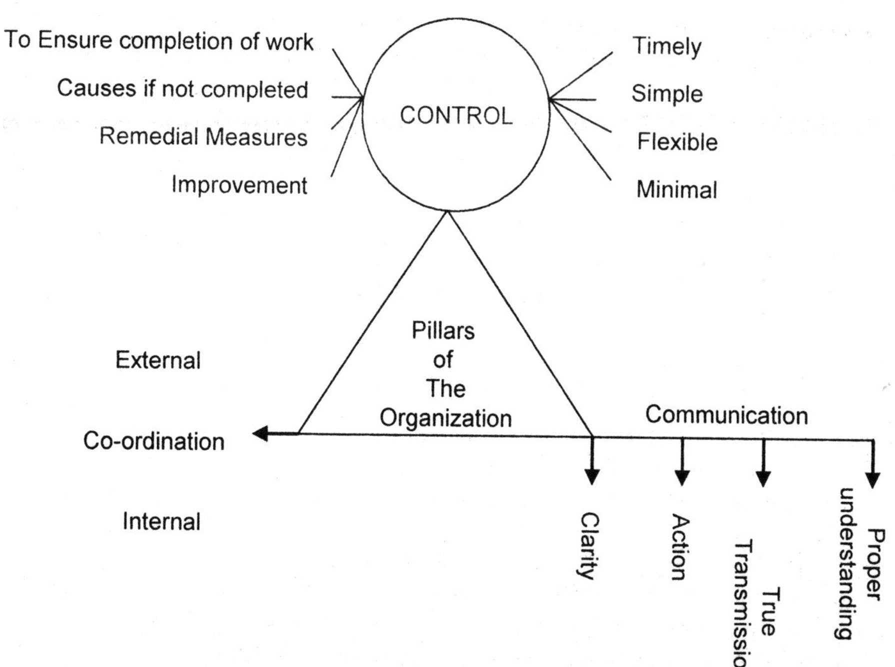

In the context of administration and management, William Scott defined communications as a process which involves the transmission and accurate replication of ideas ensured by feedback for the purpose of eliciting actions which will accomplish organisations goals.[15] To quote Goddard: "Efficient communication is essential to all aspects of effective administration. Staff must be adequately and currently informed about plans, methods, schedules, problems, for practical application to all concerned, and that they are so clearly presented as to make misinterpretation or misunderstanding impossible. Proper and adequate communication is not just in one direction. It requires two-way passage. Administrators must be certain that they know and understand the problems of workers for whom they are responsible. Communications must flow from the bottom upwards, as well as from the top down."[16]

Broadly speaking, communication is the means through which intentions of the programmes are translated to ensure fruitful results. It may even be looked upon as the means by which special information inputs are fed into social systems. It is the means by which behaviour of the personnel engaged in the programme is modified; change is effected, information is made productive and goals are achieved.[17] Barnard has viewed it as the means by which people can be linked together in an organisation to achieve the objectives of the programme.[18] Newman and Summer have viewed communication as an exchange of facts, ideas, opinion, or emotions by two or more persons.[19]

Communication Management

Communication management means the designing of communication strategy, procedures and contents in advance, according to the nature and objectives of the organisation, to smoothen its operations and avoid misunderstanding and other complicated problems, which could be generated out of the communication gap.

Essentials of Communications

The essentials of communications are:

(a) Clarity of Thought

The first sine qua non of good communication is that the idea to be transmitted must be absolutely clear in the mind of the communicator. It must spring out from a clear head. It should be understood by the personnel, so that it may be fully appreciated and acted upon.

(b) Importance to Action Rather than Words

In all communication, actions are more significant than words. Example is better than precept. An officer who is not punctual cannot succeed in enforcing the time-rules on the subordinates.

(c) Participation

In this connection it is essential that both the parties (the communicator and the recipients) should participate in the communication. It is only way to make the communication effective.

(d) Transmission

The communicator must plan carefully what to communicate, with whom to communicate and how to communicate. How can the top personnel communicate with the workers when they themselves do not know or cannot understand all the facts about the new plans? Further, delegation of authority without responsibility breaks down the spirit of communication.

(e) Keep the System Always Alive

The system of communication should be kept open and alive all the year round. It is only by honest attempts that good communicative relations can be developed.

(f) Cordial Employer-employee Relations

Effective communication requires good employer-employee relations, which enable mutual appreciation of different viewpoints.

(g) Examine the Purpose of each Communication

According to Terry, eight factors are essential in making communication effective:

(a) Inform yourself fully;
(b) Establish a mutual trust in other;
(c) Find a common ground of experience;
(d) Use mutually known words;
(e) Have regard for context;
(f) Secure and hold the receiver's attention;
(g) Employ examples and visual aids; and
(h) Practice direct relations.

15. Courteous, polite and smiling

Receptionist should be courteous, polite and smiling. These qualities can impress the patients and they can be feel secure in the hospital.

CONCLUSION

- Understand the environment in which you work. It is better to test the waters before you take a dip.
- Adaptability and flexibility can take you a long way.
- Maintain focus on your priorities in terms of work and the goals you want to achieve.

- Work on the business priorities in terms of work and the goals you want to achieve.
- Work on the business priorities. It is too easy to get caught up in everyday emergencies and other people's requests.
- Learn to delegate and trust that your people will do their job.
- You may be phenomenal at some specific skill, but that talent will do you no good, if it's not a key element to the job you are performing.
- Be more than good at whatever job you accept—be exceptional.
- Learn to be effective with people because, believe it or not, your peers play a big role in your promotion.

Reception is the nerve centre of hospital. If properly organised, it can change the perception of hospital in the minds of people who would willingly co-operate with hospital authorities.

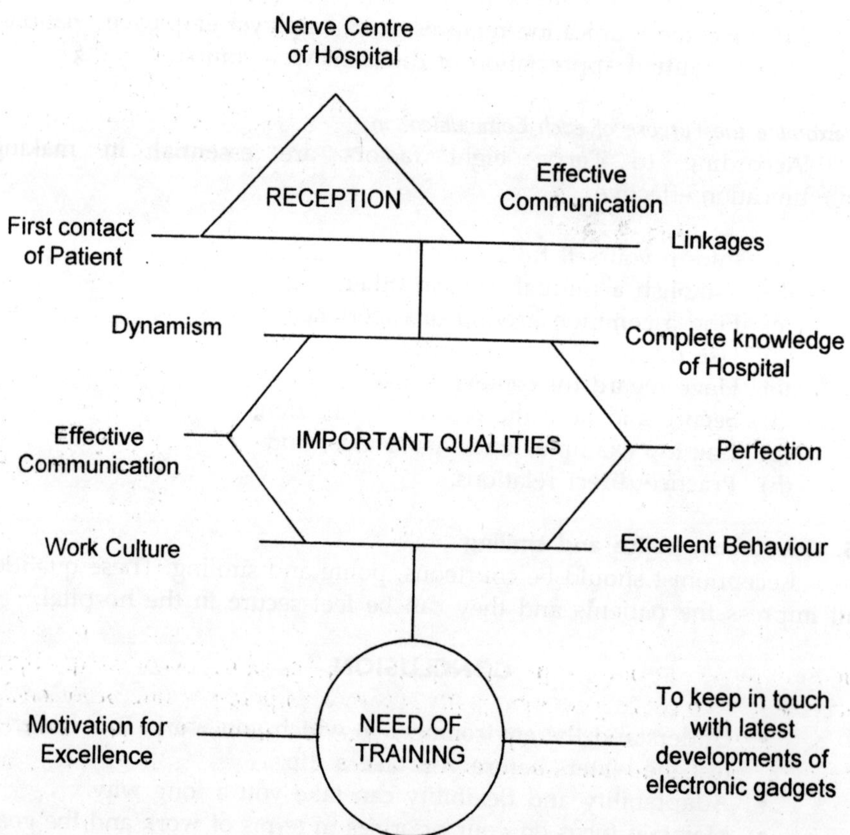

Notes and References

1. Swami Jagadatmananda, Learn tô Live, Vol. 1, *op. cit.*, p. 243.
2. *Ibid.*, p. 251.
3. Swami Chinmayananda, A Manual of Self-Unfoldment, *op. cit.*, p. 42.
4. CCMT, Mumbai, 2002, p. 53.
5. Swami Tejomajananda, Right Thinking, CCMT, Mumbai, 2002, p. 29.
6. S.K. Bhatia, Business Ethics and Management Values, New Delhi, Deep & Deep, 2002, p. 14.
7. Swami Chimayananda, We Must, Central Chinmaya Mission, Mumbai, 2001, p. 30.
8. Chinmayanand Self-Discovery, CCMT, Bombay.
9. Swami Tejomayananda, Right Thinking, CCMT, Bombay, 2002, p. 29.
10. Swami Chinmayananda, A Manual of Self-Unfoldment, *op. cit.*, p. 24.
11. Bata K. Dey, *IJPA*, April-June 1989, p. 175.
12. Louis A. Allen, *Management of Organization*, p. 297.
13. M.W. Cunning, *The Theory and Practice of Personnel Management*, 1972, p. 334.
14. Ordway Tead, *The Art of Administration*, New York, McGraw-Hill, 1951, p. 45.
15. Scott William, G., *Organization Theory*, Richard D. Irwin. Homewood, Ill., 1967, p. 153.
16. Goddard, H.A., *Principles of Administration Allied to Nursing Service*, World Health Organisation, Geneva, 1958, p. 85.
17. Koontz Hand C. O'Donnell, *Principles of Management: An Analysis of Managerial Functions*, London, McGraw Hill, Kogakusa Ltd., 1972, pp. 538-40.
18. Barnard, Chester I., *The Functions of the Executive*, Cambridge: Harward University Press, 1968, pp. 226-27.
19. Newman, H.H., C.E. Summer, The process of Management: Concepts, Behaviour and Practice, Englewood Cliffs, N.J. Prentice Hall, 1961, p. 59.

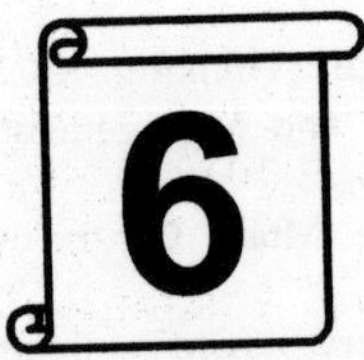

Dietetics and Food Services Development

INTRODUCTION

Dietetics and Food Services Department is an integral part of the hospital supportive services, which provides clinical dietetic services and food services to the patients, visitors and hospital staffs. The patients and other visitors are in need of food that may be hygienic, affordable and healthful. In fact the hospitals should set an example to serve food that may be palatable as well as healthful. This will be an extension service to the community to prevent disease and preserve health. Dietetics service is provided to all patients admitted to the hospital and referred by doctors from specialist clinics, wards, polyclinics, private hospitals and district hospitals. Dietetics and Catering Department will strive for continuous improvement in food services, clinical dietetics and health promotion for the wellness of patients. This department will aim for further innovation, technology and knowledge towards continuous quality improvement. That the food is nutritive and not a junk food, goes without saying. In a study more than 40% of hospital food was found to have been wasted. Energy and protein intakes were low and patients did not, therefore, meet their recommended intakes. This helps to explain continuing weight-loss in hospital patients and represents a large waste of resources.

Despite a wealth of research over the past three decades showing that fresh, well-prepared food is packed with natural disease-fighting nutrients to speed healing and prevent illness, hospital food has hardly been a model of healthy eating.

Hospital feeding policies therefore need reviewing and made more appropriate to the needs of the sick. The routine of a hospital is frequently monotonous and the regular appearance of meals can give some relief from the strangeness and tensions of hospital life. So, apart from the nutritional value of the food itself, well-cooked and pleasantly presented food in hospitals could to some degree relieve the tedium and it may even have therapeutic value. Most hospitals in this country transport hot food from the kitchen to the wards where it is served. The method whereby the food is kept hot can vary but the most common method is to use a heated trolley. The trolley is connected to the electricity supply in the kitchen area and the containers within are preheated before the cooked food is placed inside. After transportation to the ward area, the trolley is reconnected to the electricity supply in order to keep the contents warm until service is completed. This system results in considerable wastage of food, loss of palatability and some loss of nutritional value. Variants on this system which reduce wastage have been developed around the idea of putting the food on the plate in the kitchen. A conveyor belt is an essential part of any 'plated meal system' and a number of methods of keeping the plates hot during transport and service are available. These transport and service methods generally apply to the food destined for patients requiring special dietary treatment as well as to food for patients on a normal diet. Dietetics and Catering Department's missions are:

Providing and preparing quality foods that meet the nutrient requirements, catering procedure, hygiene and food safety principle, using the up-to-date catering technology. Managing department according to the policies, circulars and head instructions Providing professional dietetic services and assisting in medical treatment through medical nutrition therapy and health promotion according to evidence-based practice.

PARTICIPATION AND CONTRIBUTION IN NUTRITION AND DIETETICS RELATED RESEARCH AND STUDY

Specific Objectives

1. To ensure normal diets and therapeutic diets are catered for first, second, third class and pediatric patients according to diet ordering from the wards.
2. To ensure first class diets are served to doctors and sisters on-call, according to their entitlement.
3. To ensure night rations are provided to on-night duty staffs according to their entitlement.
4. To ensure medical nutrition therapy for oral diet and nutrition support are provided to patients referred by doctors.
5. To facilitate in catering practical training and dietetic internship training for students from higher learning institutes.
6. To partake in research and study related to catering services, clinical dietetics and community dietetics for future development and improvement.

Dietetics and Catering Department provides the following services:

a. Receiving, storing and issuing of items;
b. Quality control of goods (foodstuffs);
c. Preparation of patient's meal;
d. Preparation of on call doctors and on call sisters meal;
e. Ordering and issuing of 'on-night' ration for Hospital staff;
f. Clinical dietetics and dietary counseling;
g. Dietary education services;
h. Ordering and issuing of linen material and shoes for Hospital staffs;
i. Monitoring of Hospital Canteen.
j. Refreshment for meeting and in-house training.

Diet tips for a healthy life

- Eat healthy to lead a healthy life.
- As age advances, eat less, exercise more.
- Make breakfast the largest and dinner the lightest meal of the day.
- Be a nibbler, not a gourmet.
- Don't starve yourself and overeat subsequently.
- Include all colors of food in your diet.
- Don't use excess salt or sugar or fat.
- Eat your salad before you eat the meal.
- Eat fresh vegetables and fruits—avoid canned/tinned and preserved food.
- Consume a variety of refined oils.
- Take 2-3 liter of water per day.
- Take exercise and walk half an hour daily.

The delivery of adequate and appropriate food to patients

Intake of nutritious food is crucial for patients who are recovering from the effects of medical or surgical procedures. Patients who receive good nutrition may have shorter hospital stays, fewer post-operative complications and less need for drugs and other interventions. In order to ensure the effective delivery of good nutrition in health care facilities a team-based approach is essential. Caterers, kitchen staff, dieticians, nurses, doctors, ward housekeepers and porters all have an important part to play. A major challenge facing caterers and nutritionists is the number of patients entering health care facilities in a malnourished state. Studies show that up to 40 per cent of hospital patients are malnourished on admission. This means they have not been eating well enough to keep themselves healthy.

In order to address the issue of malnourished hospital patients the Council of Europe has published a major report. The report contains 117 recommendations designed to support health care providers across Europe.

Factors to be Understood before Instructing the Patient

Income is most important; it controls the standard of living to a great extent and must therefore be given full consideration in relation to the diet. Unfortunately, food is usually the first essential to suffer restriction when the income is low or reduced. The nationality, racial habits and religious principles of the patient affect both the choice and preparation of the food and play a large part in deciding the eating habits of the individual. Home conditions influence the management of the diet. Space for storage of food, larder accommodation, cooking facilities and water supply all determine the selection and preparation of the food. The occupation and daily routine affect both calorie intake and the planning of meals. Extra rations of certain foods are allowed for men doing heavy manual labour, the agricultural worker is allowed an extra allowance of cheese. The hours of work may be in shifts. For the patient on a special diet this may mean detailed adjustments each week. Canteen facilities, time allowed for meals, and the distance between the home and the place of work may also determine the type of meal. The dietitian must have a thorough knowledge of the current rations and of the available un-rationed foods and of their cost.

Unpalatable Food Will Not Help

Dieticians must be aware of the fact that serving patients unpalatable food will not help them recover early, said Jyoti Lalwani, Chief Dietician at PD Hinduja Hospital, Mumbai. She was speaking at a conference on Gastroenterology, recently held by PD Hinduja National Hospital and Medical Research Centre, Mumbai. The purpose of the conference was to update dieticians on the latest findings in the field of gastroenterology. The seminar was attended by more than 120 dieticians. It has been a practice since decades to reduce the food intake of the patient suffering from any gastroenterology-related problems. "But, why follow the theoretical knowledge blindly? Reducing food intake only results in malnourishment," said Lalwani, who had organised this conference, adding, "We can be 'slightly' liberal with the patients."

Dr. Philip Abraham, Consultant Gastroenterologist, Hinduja Hospital, said, "Most milk products actually help in digestion, so there is no need to avoid all milk products." He further added, "It is important to include fats and proteins in the diet of patients suffering from malabsorption. Dieticians should use medium chain triglycerides (MCT), which assist in fat absorption. Though MCTs are unpalatable, patients can tolerate 15 ml per day (to be divided in three-four doses). Also, the patient must be given slightly more protein than a normal person, as he is losing protein at a very fast pace."

Dr. Anirudh Phadke, Gastroenterologist at KEM Hospital, Mumbai, observed, "Liver is the workhouse of human body. The most common liver disorders are cirrhosis, acute hepatitis, and fulminant hepatic failure (FHF). Severity of malnutrition correlates with the severity of the liver disease. Also, restriction on water should not be imposed unless the sodium in the body is more than 120 mmol/l."

Priya Palan, Dietician with Hinduja Hospital, stated, "Increase calcium intake while treating the gastro intestinal tract. Also, glutamine is an essential amino acid which helps in curing the disease." Dr. Sudeep Shah, Consultant GI and HPB Surgeon, PD Hinduja Hospital, informed, "Of all the kinds of stones, the cholesterol stones are the only ones that have a direct relation with diets. In the US, 10-15 per cent of population has gallstones and 93 per cent of them are asymptomatic. And, there is no need to operate on asymptomatic stones unless there is calcified GB or sickle cell disease." He also explained the importance of nutrition in post-operative care by citing various case studies. "Enteral and parental feeding, both almost give the same results in post-operative care and hence there is no need to ponder much on them. One should keep in mind to start the food intake slowly, e.g. with 20 Kcal/day and monitor vitamin levels on a regular basis," he added.

The Meal Delivery System

The food when presented to the customer should be:

- Of good quality
- Attractively served
- At the correct temperature
- Acceptable
- Microbiologically safe
- Economically compatible with the goals and standards of the organization.

Considerations for a Tray Delivery System

One major consideration is that the patients may be at some distance from the kitchen. This means that there must be an organized method to transport meals to the point where they will be served. Keeping food at the correct temperature is a big problem when time and distance to transport are considered.

Decentralized Foodservice

In early days of patient foodservice, food was prepared in the main kitchen and then distributed in bulk in a heated cart. Bulk food cart The cart was moved to patient floors and the food was portioned and plated in a galley on the unit. Some foods which required last minute preparation such as eggs and toast could be produced in the galley. Food was placed on trays which were made up in the galley. The tray was delivered to the patient as soon as it was served. The temperature of the food tended to be very good because of rapid service.

This method of tray production had a number of inherent problems. It is a costly way to produce trays because of food, labor and equipment costs. More food than was necessary to serve the patients was likely to be sent to each unit to assure that server would not be short of food. Skilled staff who could prepare short order items and who knew all of the patient modified diets were needed to cover each unit. Complete galleys were placed on each unit. These galleys could have griddles, coffee makers, dish machines, and a variety of other expensive equipment. In addition, the space used by the galley was unavailable to use for other patient requirements.

Centralized foodservice Health care organizations have moved away from decentralized to centralized patient foodservice. In this method food is produced, portioned and plated in the central kitchen and dispatched to the patient units where trays may be served either by foodservice staff, nursing staff, or a patient services aide (PSA). The advantages of this method are lower food, labor and equipment costs because the majority of production occurs in the central kitchen. In addition, there is supervision of tray assembly so that portion sizes and accuracy of the items placed on the tray may be better controlled.

Menus

As with every aspect of a foodservice, menus control the activities of patient tray service. It is crucial to know what each patient is to be served for each meal. Menu delivery process is very complex and every health care organization will have a different method. Diet Order A diet order is generated by the physician and entered into the patient's medical record. This order is communicated to the foodservice department either electronically, by telephone, or by a paper transmission. No food may delivered to any patient without a current diet order. Menus are provided to the patients.

Menu for Patient Foodservice

There are a number of variations on the types of menus which can be used.

Select Vs. Non-select Menu

With a select menu the patient is able to choose from a variety of menu items in each category of foods. There may be from two to about 12 entrees from which to select along with a variety of appetizers, salads, desserts, breads, beverages and breakfast items.

In a limited select menu there may be choices of entrée and beverage, but no choice in other food categories. A non-select menu offers no choices to the patient. Customarily a representative from foodservice will have visited the patient or resident upon admission to determine preferences.

Cycle Vs. Static Menu

A cycle menu is one in which a series of menus is created for a defined period of time and then is repeated. The length of the cycle is determined by the length of patient stay. In an acute care setting with a very short patient stay, a seven or eight day cycle is adequate. For long-term care a much longer cycle is necessary. The cycle menu may be select, limited select or non-select.

A static menu does not change. The same menu is offered each day. Static menus usually have a large number of choices in each menu category to allow the patients an adequate variety so they will not tire of the offerings.

Menu Delivery

Menus must be made available to patients. They must then be retrieved, sorted, assembled, and provided to the central kitchen for tray assembly. Again, there are many variations in this process depending on the type of foodservice organization and which type of menu was developed.

Long-term care

Most long-term care facilities use cycle menus, frequently from three to six weeks. These menus are not usually delivered to the residents. Determinations of what food is provided is through resident preferences and the diet order. With this information menus are generated and the food is served on a tray for in-room service or to the resident seated in a dining room.

Acute care

Hospitals traditionally have used a cycle menu. A menu for one day is delivered to each patient by one of several methods. It may be sent on the breakfast tray, delivered by staff from the foodservice department, or by volunteers. The menu is retrieved and the patient may be helped to complete the menu. The menu is sorted either by hand or electronically by patient unit. It is reviewed by a diet clerk for completeness and to identify if any non-standard menu items have been requested.

Dietetic technician checking menus

These non-standard items will be compiled to give the production staff guidance on what special menu items have been requested. Menus will be divided into meals (breakfast, lunch, dinner) and will be cross-checked with diet orders prior to each meal to assure that each patient who is supposed to have a meal will receive the proper diet based on the most current diet order.

Menu for breakfast, lunch and dinner of the following day

This menu is usually for the next day. This means that, for example, at 10:00 in the morning the patient is choosing meals for tomorrow. There are many problems with this system:

- The patient may choose meals based on how he is feeling on one day which may not be true for the next day. He may over order or under order.

- The patient may think he is choosing meals for today and is disappointed when what he selected does not arrive today.
- The patient may be transferred or discharged and never receive what he ordered.
- New patients may not receive menus for several meals and get food that they would not have chosen.

For these and other reasons, patients are not completely satisfied with this method of choosing what they will eat. Variations on menu delivery systems.

A permanent static menu (restaurant-style) may be kept in the patient room. The patient may fill out a daily disposable menu using the static menu as a guide to what is available. These disposable menus would be delivered and collected in the same way a cycle menu is managed.

A spoken menu is being used by some hospitals to reduce the amount of time between patient ordering and meal delivery. Prior to the meal a foodservice employee or volunteer visits each patient, offers a limited select menu orally, and asks what the patient would like to receive. The spoken menu is usually a cycle menu.

A TV menu uses one of the in-house TV channels to display the non-select cycle menu available for each meal. The patient is instructed to review the menu prior to each meal. If he does not like the offered menu, he calls foodservice and requests another choice. If there is no call, the non-select tray is delivered. The TV menu is usually a cycle menu. Problems with menu delivery

Many acute care hospitals experience significant difficulties with delivery of extra trays due, primarily, to problems with the diet order and menu delivery processes. Menus are assembled by diet clerks prior to the beginning of the tray assembly process using the most current information available and those menus which have been collected. This means, for example, that at about 10:00 A.M. the lunch menus are being assembled by the clerks. These menus will be provided to the central kitchen between 11:00 and 11:30 for lunch. If a diet order is not transmitted to the diet clerk before the menus are provided to the central kitchen, the wrong tray, no tray, or a tray for a discharged patient may be produced. This means that the foodservice department will have to make a correction after tray assembly has begun. The problem is not limited to the lunch meal. In many organizations, dinner orders continue late into the evening, well after the kitchen should have closed for the night.

With current practice of very short patient stays and transfer of patients to new rooms and units, trays may easily be not delivered in the most efficient method. Some hospitals experience the necessity to prepare an additional 25% or more trays for diet changes, transfers, new admissions, and patients who did not like what they received. This additional burden on the foodservice organizations is a severe impediment to managing an efficient organization. Foodservice staff are required to create and deliver additional trays throughout the facility.

Foodservice employee delivering late tray

All foodservice organizations are exploring methods to reduce the number of late trays. Technology holds the promise to expedite the diet order process and provide more timely information about the status of each patient in the hospital.

Another method of tray assembly and delivery which has been introduced recently is Room Service. With this method the patient calls foodservice when he is ready to eat and orders what he wants from a static menu. Patient satisfaction increases and duplicate trays are eliminated with room service.

Tray Assembly

Once the food required for the patients has been prepared and the menus for the meal have been delivered, trays are assembled and sent to the patient units. This process of tray assembly has many variations for consideration.

Tray assembly in a cart

In the simplest method, patient tray delivery carts are used to assemble the food.

A delivery cart used to transport trays to patient units

Trays with tray covers and flatware are placed in the delivery cart. A menu or tray identification card indicating patient name, room number and diet along with any preferences noted is placed on each tray. Cold foods (juice and other cold beverages, salad, dessert, bread, condiments) are placed on the tray. Finally, hot foods are plated, covered, and placed on the tray. A thermal heat retention method such as pellet system should be used to maintain the hot food temperature. The cart is wheeled to the patient unit where the trays are delivered to each patient.

Patient tray line

An assembly line is usually used to produce individual trays for patients. The tray line has multiple stations, each of which has clearly identified items to place on the tray depending on the menu requirements.

Configuration of the patient tray line

Tray lines may be either straight or circular. Circular tray lines, when found, are usually associated with large facilities. They offer the advantage of saving space when many trays with a large number of different menu items need to be provided.

Components of a Patient Tray Line

Tray Conveyor

There will be some method to move the trays from one position to the next. Three options currently exist:

- Non-powered rollers
- Non-powered skatewheels
- Powered belt

With the first two options, employees push the trays to the next station after they have completed all of their activities.

Tray starter

Equipment to hold trays and tray covers, flat ware, condiments. May include heated pellet bases.

Entrée station

Equipment to hold hotel pans of entrees, soups, vegetables, sauces and gravies, heated plates. May include cooking equipment to produce eggs, pancakes, etc.

Salad and dessert stations

Equipment to hold made up (or bulk ingredients to make to order) salads and desserts, sandwiches, breads, juices, milks, frozen desserts. May include toaster.

Beverage stations

Equipment to dispense coffee, hot water, soft drinks, ice, cups.

Checker station

Equipment to store lids. From this station, trays are placed in carts which are delivered to each patient unit for service. On the unit the trays may be served immediately or held for predefined time before service.

Determining the proper number of positions on the tray line

For most small foodservice organizations, four to five are the minimum number of positions. In larger foodservice operations many of these positions may be divided into two or more stations to increase the speed of the tray line. For example: some foodservice organizations divide the hot food station into regular diets, modified diets, soups and purees.

There are suggested methods to decide how many positions are required. These are based on the type of health care organization, the meal, the number of trays to be served, and the amount of time allowed to complete the task. As a general principle, the greater the time allowed to assemble the trays, the fewer positions are required.

For acute care the formula is:

Breakfast—Number of positions = number of trays x 1.4 labor minutes/Allotted time

E.g. = 240 trays x 1.4 labor minutes/60 minutes = 5.6 positions—> 6 positions.

Lunch and Dinner—Number of positions = number of trays x 2 labor minutes/Allotted time

For long-term care the formula is:

Breakfast—Number of positions = number of trays x .8 labor minutes/Allotted time

Lunch and Dinner—Number of positions = number of trays x 1 labor minute/Allotted time

Line balancing

Being certain that every position on the tray line has the same amount of work to accomplish is an important aspect of improving the efficiency of the tray line, controlling labor costs, and getting the meals to the patient units on time. The goal is to have each position perform for the same amount of time for each tray. The position which has the most amount of work on the tray line is the bottleneck position. The line can never move faster than the time that position takes.

Line balancing is a method to determine how much time each position takes and to modify the tasks required in each position to achieve equity. Two excellent resources may be consulted to understand the theoretical framework of line balancing are:

Options in tray assembly temperatures

The type of food production method will determine, in part, what temperature will be used in tray assembly. The two choices are hot tray assembly or cold tray assembly.

In hot tray assembly, food that is to be served hot is held hot on the tray line. All food to be served hot is held in hot food tables which maintain a temperature of at least 140°F. Food is portioned and plated to heated plates and placed in a thermal retention system. Hot tray assembly may be used with any food production system. The food will either be produced immediately prior to service (conventional and commissary) or re-thermalized in bulk immediately prior to service in the central kitchen (ready prepared and assembly serve).

In cold tray assembly, food that is to be served hot is held cold on the tray line. All food is held in cold food tables which maintain a temperature of less than 41°F. Food is portioned, served to chilled plates and placed in refrigerated storage until the time of service. It is then re-thermalized by one of several methods. Cold tray assembly can only be used with ready-serve or assembly serve food production methods.

Meal Distribution Systems

From the tray line, meals are moved to where they will be served. In this process it is crucial to maintain the quality of the food so that the patient receives an aesthetically pleasing product. There are a variety of distribution systems which have been developed to reduce the deterioration of the food as it travels through time and space to get to the patients.

Hot food retention systems

When food is portioned and plated hot there are a variety of methods to retain the heat.

Dome covers

This is a technologically simple method of providing for temperature retention. It is appropriate and adequate for use in restaurant or catering operations when the kitchen is close to the point of service. When paired with a heated plate it could be expected to hold temperature satisfactorily for less than 10 minutes. For most health care organizations this is not sufficient time to deliver meals. This is a passive method of temperature retention.

Unitized pellets

This is the most frequently used method of heat retention. A metal base which is heated to 225°F is placed under the heated plate containing hot food. The metal base may contain either a metal alloy, a gel or melted wax. The pellet base may also be chilled/frozen and used with cold entrées.

Unitized pellet base

Pellet heater cart—used to heat pellet bases to 225°F.

A cover is placed on top of the plate. These unitized pellets can be expected to retain a satisfactory food temperature for from 40 minutes (metal alloy) to one hour (melted wax). This is considered an active method of heat retention.

Hot and Cold Food Retention Systems

Some tray distributions systems have been developed to provide thermal support for both hot and cold foods.

Insulated components

An entire tray can be completed with insulated components which are used to retain the temperature of both hot and cold foods. This is a passive temperature retention system.

Insulated components

Insulated bowls and mugs are frequently used as companions to unitized pellets to retain the temperature of salads, desserts, soups, cereals, and beverages.

Insulated Trays

Fully insulated trays consist of two molded plastic shells with foam insulation. These shells form a top and bottom and fit snugly together. This is a passive temperature retention system.

Match a Tray

Electrically heated and chilled carts are used to maintain food temperatures. Two trays are sent down the tray line. The larger is for cold food and is placed in the cold food section of the cart. Trays with menus, flat ware, and cold items are placed in these sections. The smaller contains hot food and is placed in a pull out drawer in the heated section of the cart. Many of these carts contain heated wells holding hot beverages and soup which can be dispensed at the point of service.

Electrically heated and chilled carts—the left two sections are chilled. The right section is heated. The top right section can contain coffee, hot water and soup.

The carts are heated in the central kitchen. After they are loaded, they are moved to the patient unit where they are plugged in again. Trays are assembled for service by placing the hot entrée, soup and beverage on the cold tray. Food can be held at an appropriate temperature for an extended time period, although hot food will dry out if held too long. This is an active temperature retention system.

Split Tray

Electrically heated and chilled carts are used to maintain food temperatures. Both hot and cold foods are on one tray. This is an active temperature retention system.

Methods to re-thermalize foods assembled in a cold food assembly system

When food is produced using ready prepared or assembly serve methods, one opportunity results. Food may be re-thermalized closer to the point of service. The advantage of this is reducing the time that food is held heated. Many foods deteriorate rapidly when held hot. To improve the quality of the finished foods, many foodservice operators have opted to distribute food chilled and re-thermalize immediately prior to service. There are four technologically different methods to re-thermalize.

Microwave ovens

In a galley on the patient unit, individual plates may be heated using microwave ovens. In some organizations, batteries of these ovens may be used so several plates may be processed simultaneously.

Convection ovens

Plates to be re-thermalized may be loaded in the galley on the patient unit into stacked frames. These structures may be loaded into convection ovens. All plates are re-thermalized quickly and then the trays may be re-assembled.

Convection Oven with Stacked Plates

Infrared ovens

Plates to be re-thermalized may be loaded in the galley on the patient unit into stacked frames. These structures may be loaded into infrared ovens. All plates are re-thermalized quickly and then the trays may be re-assembled.

Contact plate heater carts

A technologically sophisticated method of re-thermalization uses conduction heating.

Comparison of Distribution Methods with Criteria

Whatever method is used to distribute foods, the criteria first suggested must be considered.

The food when presented to the customer should be:

- Of good quality
- Attractively served
- At the correct temperature
- Acceptable
- Microbiologically safe
- Economically compatible with the goals and standards of the organization.

Some of the methods presented fail to maintain correct temperature, or present food which is no longer attractive, or cost too much. Each foodservice operation must select the distribution system which best meets the needs of the organization.

The Quality of Hospital Food; A study

Platt, Eddy and Pellett (1963) have surveyed 152 hospitals in England and Wales and described defects in hospital catering which result in food of poor quality. They concluded that, as the size of hospital increased, the food quality decreased. Up to 45% of the cooked food sent to the wards was wasted owing to defects in communication between kitchen and ward. There was a tendency to overcook vegetables, and in half of the largest hospitals it took more than 1.5 hours to cook and serve potatoes to patients, resulting in complete loss of ascorbic acid from potatoes. The loss of ascorbic acid from green vegetables was 75%. Quality-deterioration also occurred during hot trolley transport between kitchen and ward, which can be a considerable distance in a large hospital. There was a lack of variety and there were low food-quality standards in large, acute hospitals.

Extremely poor (average ascorbic acid content I 1-12 mg/d) level of vitamin C in the food was a major defect. These defects were considered to be due to (I) old-fashioned kitchens and equipment, (2) bad communications, (3) organizational faults and unnecessary division of catering responsibility, 'Too much depends upon administrative routine and too little on direct observation of the patients to discover what they need, what they eat and when they eat', (4) the attention of medical and nursing staff is concentrated on the special dietary requirements of particular diseases to the exclusion of the general requirements of patients.

In this survey the patients were not asked about food quality, but the observations of the team involved in this work are sufficient to conclude that the food in large hospitals is frequently unpalatable, and is produced and distributed in such a way that losses of some nutrients are inevitable. It is possible that there is some disparity between what the patient wants to eat (outside the constraints of special dietary treatment) and what the caterer or hospital administrator thinks he wants to eat. There is also the element of ease of production or cheapness which must also be considered in hospitals. A national survey of hotel and restaurant customers showed that the caterer is not necessarily a good judge of the market for certain dishes (Anonymous, 1966). A survey compiled from the hospital records of a group of hospitals in northern England showed large differences between the choice exercised by the patients in the two hospitals, though both were in the same region with a similar number of patients (E. Washington, personal communication, 1970). Sixty per cent of patients in one hospital chose cereal far breakfast, whereas only 7% in the other hospital made this choice. Breakfast cereal in the latter hospital may be less readily available for financial or other reasons. It is suggested that patients do not necessarily receive what they want to eat even when there is a theoretical choice of dish. It sometimes occurs that, because of the pressure of other duties, nurses are unable to ask patients to choose; the choice is made on behalf of the patients by the nursing staff. These two reports suggest that, both inside and outside hospital, the consumer does not always receive dishes that he prefers to eat even when he is theoretically being offered a choice. In 1968, a survey was performed at a hospital in Harlow (Anonymous, 1968) where seventy-six patients were interviewed shortly before discharge. In this hospital, food is transported to the wards in bulk-heated trolleys and is served by Ward Hostesses under the control of the nursing staff. Table I shows some of the results of this survey. It can be seen that patients were generally satisfied with the quality and variety of the food and were less satisfied with its temperature. A quarter of the patients did not find the food hot enough when it reached them.

Brown, Carden, Stanton and Stock (1969) sent questionnaires to 287 patients in twenty-one hospitals in various parts of the United Kingdom. The object of this survey was to find out what foods were particularly liked. Fish in various forms was liked by more than 70% of the sample; eggs and cheese were liked by 90%. Peas, sprouts and cauliflower were the vegetables most liked. Sweet-corn, marrow and spinach were among the most unpopular vegetables. Fruit was popular, as were tea and coffee as beverages. Roasting of meat mas the most popular cooking method.

It is interesting that 887 of the sample said that hospital meals were served at different times to meals at home, but 92% of these did not mind. These authors concluded that a varied menu with a choice was desirable.

Glew (1968) has studied the attitudes of patients to the food served in the General Infirmary, Leeds (800-bed teaching hospital). Patients requiring treatment for many medical and surgical conditions come from an area within about a 32 km radius of Leeds. Patients requiring special diets were excluded from this study.

The food at this hospital is cooked, then transported to the forty-three wards in heated trolleys. All patients eat simultaneously and, in order to ensure that the trolleys reach the ward area in time for the meal, they must leave the kitchen up to half an hour before service. Service may also be delayed if a consultant is examining a patient in the ward. The meal-pattern in this hospital was that soup, main course and sweet (either hot or cold) were provided both at midday and in the evening. A cooked breakfast was always available and very light afternoon tea was served.

This catering system, with no choice offered to patients, and the same menu throughout the hospital at any one meal, is the most common in hospitals in this country.

The survey method has been described in detail elsewhere, (Glew, 1968) and consisted of a questionnaire sent by post to all patients over 10 years of age within a few days of discharge. During a period of I month (March-April 1967), 839 questionnaires were sent out, of which 84% were returned after one reminder letter. Patients were evenly distributed in terms of age and sex, two-thirds were married and one-quarter were unmarried. Answers to questions were coded as far as possible and transferred to punched cards before automatic processing.

The questionnaire was divided into two parts. Six questions requested opinions on food quality, temperature, appearance, variety, size of portion and whether the patient disliked any dish served. Two questions were concerned with the type of meal preferred by patients in hospital and further questions enquired about the patient's eating habits outside the hospital. In addition to closed-ended questions of the 'Yes/No' type, opportunity was also given for patients to write comments on likes and dislikes and on any other matter shows the degree of satisfaction with the food and it can be seen that males are more satisfied with the food than females. Patients from the two treatment groups, medical or surgical, did not differ in their replies to the six questions on food quality, but analysis of variance indicated a statistically significant difference between the replies of males and females (P<o.oog). The age of patients had a marked effect on their responses to the questionnaire. The difference in response (between the age groups) was significant at the 0.01% level of probability and it was clear that, as age increased, degree of satisfaction with the food increased. Analysis of variance also showed that both the response and the effect of age differed between the sexes.

The length of stay in hospital did not influence the answers to the quality questions.

There was a significant difference (P<o.ooI) between the response of married and single people to these food-quality questions with single females being most dissatisfied.

The preference for two cooked meals each day in hospital differed between both age groups (P<0.005) and sexes (P<o.ooI). Many males

disliked salad, whereas no female listed salad as a dislike. Sausage and fish were also frequently disliked. A very large variety of foods were listed as 'favourite foods' but the only pattern discernible was the frequent mention of high-protein foods.

Patients were asked when they normally ate a cooked meal at home. It was found that males and females normally have cooked meals at different times and that, in general, age does not influence the pattern of when cooked meals are eaten. But it is interesting that for people aged over 65 years the main cooked meal is at midday and also that in this age-group only 19% of the women normally have a cooked breakfast.

The general conclusions from this survey were that hospital patients of different sex, age and marital status had different impressions of the food quality and also had different eating habits outside hospital. It was considered that the provision of a choice of dish could improve the degree of satisfaction with the food. As part of another experiment (an experiment in hospital catering using cooklfreezc system) in the University of Leeds, a choice system was introduced into a part of the United Leeds Hospitals (The Hospital for Women) and surveys were conducted both before and after the introduction of a choice menu (choice between two hot and one cold dish at lunch and supper). The hot trolley distribution system was used during both surveys and a choice of dish was made by each patient during the afternoon of the day before the food was served. Some of the results of these surveys and it is clear that the provision of a choice improved the patient's assessment of the food quality. This result could be due to patients themselves being able partly to avoid being presented with a dish that they do not like.

Nutritional Problems of the Hospitalized Patient

An ill person needs more food than a well one, in order to heal and recover. For example, a patient who has had surgery needs a diet, which has a lot of vitamin C and protein since these help with healing. Also, proteins are especially important to fight off infection because the antibodies that the body uses to fight infection are proteins. Often people use up their protein reserves when they have surgery or are injured or have an illness with fever. An adequate diet is essential. Many illnesses, however, make it difficult for a person to eat, or make it hard for the person to digest food. Conditions making it difficult to get adequate nutrition:

- A person with a very sore throat may find it hard to swallow food.
- A person who has a stomach problem may be nauseated by food.
- A person who has a fever is likely to have no appetite.
- Patients who are in the hospital are almost always at risk of getting insufficient nutrients either because of their illness or because of the treatment for their illness.

- Many patients are already undernourished when they enter the hospital.
- The food served in the hospital may be different from the food the patient is accustomed to eating. Patients may not like the hospital food.
- Meals may be served at times when the patients are not accustomed to eating and when they do not feel hungry.
- Patients are often put on a special diet in the hospital to help treat their disease (for example, a person who has had a heart problem will usually be put on a low-salt diet).
- Patients may not like the change in diet.
- The patient's family may live far away so they cannot bring the foods he or she likes, or the family may not know the right foods to bring, or may not be able to afford the right foods.

How to meet the nutritional needs of the patient

To make sure that the people who are seriously ill or who have just had surgery get enough fluid and at least some calories, they may be fed intravenously until they are able to eat. Intravenous fluids provide enough fluid, but not enough calories. Patients cannot live on intravenous fluids alone. Patients usually go from intravenous feedings to liquids, to a soft diet and then to a regular diet. Sometimes people are able to go straight from liquids to a regular diet.

Liquid diet

Liquids include coffee, soft drinks, fruit juices, coconut water, clear soup or broth and sweetened tea. The person on liquids can also eat gelatin, sugar and hard candies. A liquid diet will give the patient enough fluids and some carbohydrates (from sugar and fruit juices). It will not supply proteins, fats, iron, or enough calories or vitamins. Usually a person should be on a liquid diet for only a short time after surgery or while recovering from acute stomach or intestinal diseases. A patient who has to be on a liquid diet for a long time should be given a nutritional supplement.

Soft diet

A soft diet includes all foods that can be easily chewed and digested. For example, a soft diet might include various cooked, mashed root crops such as taro, kumara, cassava, and yams as well as rice, eggs, very tender lean meat or fish, pasta, tapioca, soft or pureed cooked greens or other vegetables, cooked fruits, bread, and soft desserts. This diet is used for patients who have difficulty chewing and swallowing.

Regular diet

A regular diet is the food the patient normally eats, in particular local foods, which are high in protein, fibre, iron and vitamins.

Help the patient to eat

Make the patient comfortable. To help a patient who is having trouble eating and who is in pain, it is useful to give pain medication 30 minutes before meal times. This will keep the pain from interfering with eating. For a person who has a fever, give paracetamol or other anti-fever medication before meals to keep the fever from interfering with appetite. Also, avoid doing painful or uncomfortable treatments before meals. Explain the importance of good nutrition. Explain the importance of eating properly. Encourage the patient to try to eat at least small portions to help with recovery. Encourage the family to bring foods the patient likes from home. Make sure that the family understands what foods the patient can and cannot eat. Use this opportunity to teach the family about a proper diet. This will help all members of the family as well as the patient. Explain to them the importance of using pasteurized milk, not raw milk, of washing foods such as lettuce which are eaten raw, and of thoroughly cooking meat, poultry and eggs. Tell them to store cooked foods carefully, protect foods from insects and rodents, and keep surfaces clean where food is prepared. Remind them to boil water unless they know it is safe and always wash their hands before preparing food. Position the patient for eating. If the patient is allowed to sit up, help him or her to do so for meals. It is much easier to eat in this position.

Make the surroundings pleasant. Clean the bed table and make sure there is room for all dishes. Food should be served on a clean tray and should look attractive. Make sure there are eating utensils. Keep the surrounding area clean and free of unpleasant smells.

Remove bedpans, urinals and other such objects from the patient's sight. It is important that the patient's room and table offer a pleasant environment for eating. Place the food conveniently for the patient. Give help as needed. Encourage the patient's family to visit at meal times and to help him with eating. Remind them to wash their hands before helping the patient. If necessary, help the patient eat. Some patients require special help with eating. For example, elderly patients are weak and easily tired. The effort of getting food to their mouth may be more than they can manage. You may need to feed such patients if their families are not there to feed them. Wash your hands first. Ask the patient if he or she would like help. If so, ask what he or she would like to eat first. Feed the patient in small bites. Allow time for chewing and swallowing before offering the next bite. Offer the patient something to drink after every three or four bites. Do not rush the patient or show that you are in a hurry. Use the time to get to know the patient. Take away the eating utensils when the patient has finished and see that they are washed.

According to a recent research revolving around the quality and overall acceptance of hospital food, patients find the dishes practically inedible, with a quarter of patients buying their own or ask friends and family to bring in meals for them.

One in three patients was unhappy with the quality of food they were served recently in the hospital while being held there for observation or treatment, a survey for consumer organization found: More than a quarter (27%) found the portions too small, with a third (34%) saying they did not like the type of food provided. Almost two-fifths (38%) said they did not feel meal times matched when they were able or wanted to eat. Around one in five staff in hospitals (21%) said they would be unhappy to eat the food served to patients each day. Researchers said they had heard of a hospital staff member being unaware of egg products in food such as quiche and pasta when caring for a patient with an egg allergy. The organization said it had also heard of a patient with tonsillitis and an abscess who was offered pie and chips when they were struggling to even drink.

Nutritional Support and Critical Care through Food

The Dietetic Department at a tertiary care hospital specializes in a number of clinical areas including Nutrition Support and Critical Care, stroke, gastroenterology, pediatrics, oncology, home enteral feeding and diabetes. Dietitians provide impartial evidence based advice about nutrition and health, and advise about food related problems and treat disease and ill health. Each ward has an allocated dietitian who will provide nutritional support to any patient who is referred to the Dietetic Department during their hospital stay. The dietitian will assess, advise and monitor both adults and children who require particular nutritional advice. This advice may be on:

- Finding ways of treating malnutrition (via oral, enteral or parenteral nutrition)
- Changing food intake due to particular disease or condition such as Diabetes, Coeliac Disease, Renal disease or allergies.
- The dietitians work closely with other Therapists, medical, nursing and catering staff to ensure that patients' nutritional status is maintained and improved during their inpatient stay.

The dietitians also provide an outpatient consultation service, which includes specialist clinics and group sessions to reach the needs of the patient. Specialist outpatient clinics include: gastroenterology, nutrition support, eating disorders, diabetes, home enteral feeding, oncology and paediatric clinics. Specialist daytime and evening group sessions for obesity management (adults and paediatrics) are run on a weekly basis and group sessions for Coeliac disease and healthy eating during pregnancy are run each month. Dietitians are involved in many areas of patient care as part of the Multidisciplinary therapy team which cover inpatient wards.

The main groups of patients seen are very low-birth-weight neonates; infants and children with poor growth; feeding issues; constipation; overweight; type 1 diabetes and inborn errors of metabolism; women with gestational diabetes; type 2 diabetes; hyper-lipidemia and cancer-related complications (e.g. poor appetite, low protein stores).

Apart from patient counseling, the dietitians also provide nutrition education for staff and public as well as nutrition consultancy to external organizations. A balanced diet in terms of calories, proteins, fats, carbohydrates, minerals, electrolytes and vitamins is essential for a healthy life. A proper diet provides daily requirement of nutrients to the body, thus enhancing the immunity of the person.

The department also provides diet counseling for different type of diseases like:

- Diabetes
- Cardiac Disorder
- Cancer
- Migraine
- Kidney Disease
- Liver Disease
- Paediatric Diet
- Diet Related to Pregnancy and Lactation
- Weight Management
- Burn Patient
- Allergic Diet
- Endocrine Disorder Diet
- Organ Transplant
- Diet Information Related Different Surgery
- Others

Instruction to the In-patient

The stay in hospital offers an excellent opportunity for food education. A patient should leave hospital with new ideas on menu planning, on the serving of food and on balancing a diet. The patient on a special diet, provided he is not too ill, commences his dietary instruction at the first interview with the dietitian. The object of this interview is to establish good relations between the patient and the dietitian, who, in the course of conversation, tactfully finds out any food preferences and dislikes, and emphasizes the importance of co-operation. This talk should, if possible, be carried out in an unhurried manner, an ideal difficult to achieve when precious time is slipping away and work is piling up. If a sense of hurry is allowed to creep into this interview many patients will hesitate, both then and later, to ask questions. As a result small but important dietetic problems often remain unsolved. Daily visits by the dietitian give opportunities for further instruction. Co-operation comes with understanding.

We all tend to be conservative in our food habits, which are a product of our upbringing and present circumstances. It is, however, well to realize that a diet that has to be more or less a permanency, as for the diabetic, can be planned to meet these habits to a large extent. One pitfall the dietitian must avoid is underestimation of the intelligence of her patient;

she must also avoid encouraging food fads and fancies by over-emphasizing likes and dislikes for particular foods. It should be suggested that presents of food, such as fruit and eggs, should be sent to the kitchen for inclusion in the diet and not allowed to remain in the locker and eaten as extras.

We have found that an individual menu slip, complete with the name of the patient and the type of diet, placed in a prominent position on the tray, stimulates interest in the meal and gives rise to many questions. It is interesting to note how many patients, particularly men, collect these slips for use when they go home. Here he learns how to plan his own meals using the daily menu, his own diet sheet and the alternative food list. He learns to write his own menu slips. We take this opportunity to demonstrate the use of homely measures and how to use a pair of scales. Simple tips are given, for example an ice cream scoop of mashed potato weighs 2 oz., and a slice of bread from a cut loaf weighs approximately 1 oz. These hints are helpful to those who will have to take meals in canteens or in restaurants. In this way the patient appreciates that his diet is well within his capabilities and his home circumstances.

Instruction to the Patient on Discharge from hospital

With the diabetic it is wise to make sure that the scales, if these are supplied, are satisfactory. The nature of insulin reactions and the importance of carrying sugar or glucose tablets must be emphasized.

In certain conditions a certificate for priority foods is given. The patients must be told then in detail how to obtain the recommended foods. It is often better to give instructions directly to the members of the family upon whom the patient is dependent for the preparation of his food, rather than to the patient. For example, the wife or mother of a patient with a permanent gastrostomy ought to visit the diet kitchen and be told the ingredients of, and the most satisfactory method of mixing, a highprotein, high-calorie mixture. This removes many doubts and fears, and proves that a complete diet can be produced in fluid form. We are proud of one patient who has had a gastrostomy for 4 years and continues to live a full and useful life.

Food Management of a Diabetic

A common enemy of humans, which is as much due to today's sedentary habits and culture, as it is a hereditary phenomenon, diabetes, requires strict and stringent rules for one own lifestyle and eating habits. Diet plays an important role in the treatment of diabetes. The diet may be used alone or in combination with insulin injections or oral hypo-glycaemic drugs.

The diet plan of an individual is based on height, weight, age, sex, physical activity and nature of diabetes. One should consider the following points while planning a diabetic diet:

- Determining energy requirements
- Determining the type of carbohydrates, fibre and food preparations
- Presence of any other complication such as high blood pressure, high cholesterol levels, etc.

In case of insulin dependent diabetes mellitus, the energy intake is based on needs for normal growth and development, physical activity and maintenance of desirable body weight. In case of non insulin dependant diabetes mellitus, the majority of patients are overweight or obese. Therefore, calorie restriction is required to achieve a desired weight.

Type of carbohydrate and amount of fibre: More of carbohydrate must be given as complex starches rather than simple sugars as they breakdown more slowly to release glucose in blood. The presence of fibre in complex carbohydrate like grains, vegetables and other starches slows the glucose absorption. One should emphasize more on the high fibre foods instead of high fibre supplements available in the market.

To remember:

- It is important to control the amount and time of food intake.
- Meals should not be missed.
- Consider the likes and dislikes of the patient.
- Try to substitute the craving for sweet by taking some fruit.

Foods to be avoided

Glucose, sugar, honey, all sweets, chocolates and candies. Foods to be restricted Potatoes, yam, arbi, sweet potatoes, mangoes, grapes, bananas, alcoholic beverages, fried foods, paranthas, poories, pakoras, mathris, deep fried foods, dry fruits, salad oils, cakes and pastries. Foods to be used freely.

Green leafy vegetables, tomatoes, cucumber, radish, soups, buttermilk, tea and coffee without sugar.

High Blood Pressure

Throughout the world a reduction in salt intake is recommended for people who have high blood pressure. Low salt intake is also recommended in many types of kidney diseases and sometimes for pregnant women who have edema (toxemia). High blood pressure increases the risk of stroke and heart attack.

Studies over the years have shown that people have adapted and can remain healthy on sodium intakes of 200 mg. or even less. But with the advent of fast foods, convenience foods and processed foods, there has been an increasing trend in the salt consumption of people. The average consumption of sodium today amounts to about 8-15 gm. of salt (sodium chloride).

Apart from restricting the salt intake, the dietary potassium intake should also be increased as this will help in regulating blood pressure.

Potassium is present mainly in fruits and vegetables. Including more fruits and vegetables helps to reduce the sodium intake and at the same time decreases the amount of saturated fat in the diet as well increases the fibre content.

Some tips to reduce Sodium intake:

- Do not use common salt while cooking and also at the table. Use salt substitutes such as Lo-salt or K-salt.
- Use onions, garlic, chillies, herbs etc to make food tasty.
- Use fresh herbs such as coriander leaves, curry leaves, mint, etc. to add flavor to a salt free dish.
- Avoid use of curry powders, flavor enhancers like monosodium glutamate and processed sauces, chutneys, pickles, preserved foods containing salt, papads, cheese, salted butter.
- Do not use soda while cooking. Limit your intake of baked foods e.g. biscuits, cakes, doughnuts, nankhatai.
- Avoid organ meats like liver, kidney, brain, etc.
- Avoid processed foods, canned foods, salted nuts, etc.

Cholesterol and Heart Disease

There has been a great deal of publicity concerning cholesterol and its relationship to coronary artery disease. A high level of cholesterol in the blood stream is considered a risk factor in the development of coronary artery disease, yet there is an inadequate body of evidence which would suggest that reducing dietary cholesterol alone can lower blood cholesterol levels significantly. Recent evidence supports the fact that decreasing the amount of saturated fat along with cholesterol (i.e. decreasing the consumption of meats) in the diet will decrease blood cholesterol significantly.

Cholesterol is present ONLY in animal products, not in vegetable products. Since Americans on the whole consume a diet high in animal products, they also consume a large amount of cholesterol. Cholesterol and fat are insoluble in water and must be carried in the blood by protein substances known as lipoproteins. Lipoproteins are composed of fat and protein (hence their name) and each lipoprotein carries different amounts of cholesterol. Low density lipoproteins (LDL) carry mostly cholesterol, and very low density lipoproteins (VLDL) carry mostly fats (triglycerides). High levels of these carriers have been linked with the development of coronary artery disease. Another carrier known as high density lipoprotein (HDL) consists of mostly protein. HDL's carry cholesterol away from the body cells, back to the liver to be excreted in the bile. This may be the reason why high levels of HDL have been found to lower the risk of coronary artery disease.

Investigators have not determined what an "ideal" blood cholesterol level should be. In general, the risk of coronary artery disease due to blood cholesterol level alone rises slowly when the level is BELOW 200 milligrams per deciliter (mg/dl). The risk of coronary artery disease begins to increase more rapidly ABOVE 200 mg/dl, especially as levels rise ABOVE 240 mg/dl. In short, many experts recommend a blood cholesterol level BELOW 200 mg/dl. It is interesting to point out that very LOW cholesterol levels (under 110-125) in the elderly population have been associated with malnutrition and a depressed immune response to disease. It is likely that more research will be needed in this area.

Dietary Recommendations for Heart patients

1. Lower the amount of total fat in your diet by eating fewer high fat foods. High fat foods often contain large amounts of saturated fat (most undesirable fat source).
2. Lower the amount of saturated fats while increasing the amount of polyunsaturated fat in the diet.
3. Lower cholesterol intake. Eat more fruit and vegetables and less animal products.
4. Eat more complex carbohydrates (starch and fiber). Foods high in complex carbohydrates are usually low in fat and contain no cholesterol.
5. Lose weight, if overweight, by decreasing the number of calories taken in and increasing the number of calories used.

To Eat Less Total Fat:

1. Within any food category, there are high fat and low fat items. Read labels to learn which foods are low in fat.
2. Sausage and most processed luncheon meats are high in fat and saturated fat.
3. Cream, sour cream, ice cream, butter, and many cheeses are high in fat and saturated fat.

To Eat Less Saturated Fat:

1. Steps you take to reduce total fat will also reduce saturated fat.
2. Most animal fats generally contain high proportions of saturated fat, whereas the fat in chicken and fish contains higher proportions of polyunsaturated fat.
3. The vegetable oils from palm kernel, coconut, and palm, and cocoa fat contain large proportions of saturated fat.
4. Vegetable oils with the highest proportions of polyunsaturated fat are safflower, sunflower, corn, soybean, and cottonseed oils.
5. Many margarine's are lower in saturated fat and higher in unsaturated fats than butter.

To Eat Less Cholesterol:

1. Cholesterol is found in high amounts of red meats, organ meats (liver, kidney, sweetbread, brain), and egg yolks. Shrimp is also high in cholesterol.

To Eat More Complex Carbohydrates:

1. Vegetables, fruits, cereal grains, dried peas and beans, rice, and pasta contain complex carbohydrates, little or no saturated fat, and no cholesterol.

To Help Lose Weight, If Overweight:

1. Fats are high in calories. Fat and oils supply 9 calories per gram as compared to protein, and carbohydrates, which supply only 4 calories per gram.

Which People need to adhere to the above advice?

1. Everyone, the younger you start healthy eating habits the better.
2. Patients with a history for hypertension, congestive heart failure, coronary artery disease, stroke, peripheral vascular disease, or diabetes MUST make an extra effort to watch what they eat to lower their risk of atherosclerosis.

Nutrition for Cancer PATIENTS

A good nutrition is very important for Cancer Patients under treatment. It helps them—

- Maintain well-being and improve the body's ability to fight infection. In short, helps build body's immune system.
- Helps them to cope better with the effects of treatment and recover sooner.
- Maintain their weight, and helps them feel better in themselves.
- It also helps wounds and damaged tissues to heal better. This is the most important reason, whether after surgery, radiotherapy, chemotherapy or any other medical treatment.

WHAT DOES EATING WELL MEAN?

Eating well means giving your body the food it needs to keep working properly.

The best way to 'eat well' is to eat a variety of foods from the following five food groups everyday.

1. Cereals and Breads 5 to 6 serves (like chapatti, etc.).
2. Vegetables and fruits 5 to 6 serves.
3. Milk and milk products 2 to 3 serves.
4. Meats or legumes 2 serves.
5. Fat 1 tablespoon.
6. Fluids. This is an essential part of any diet. Aim for at least 6 to 8 glasses of fluids per day. These may include: Water, milk, lassi, butter milk, soups, green tea, milk shakes, juices, coconut water. Tea and Coffee may be taken in moderation as they have little nutritive value and so also, soft drinks, as they contain extra calories and can also increase acidity. Complan and Resource are high in protein and energy and may be included. Alcohol in moderation may be taken to stimulate appetite but should be avoided in case of sore mouth and throat, heartburns (acidity) or diarrhea.
   - If the patient is not eating enough, and is losing weight, he will need more proteins and calories in his diet, to help stop weight loss.
   - If the weight is within normal range, efforts must be made to maintain his weight.
   - If he is overweight, then also, he must aim at maintaining that weight during treatment. His nutrition will suffer if he loses weight. Weight loss should be considered only after completion of treatment, and that also after discussing with the doctor.

There is no known diet, food, vitamin, or mineral supplement that will cure cancer. Therefore, patients should be advised not to follow any other diet, which may be promoted as 'natural remedies.' These diets are often found to be lacking in essential nutrients, due to elimination of some types of food; often require use of supplements which may be harmful to the body; are often rigid and monotonous, and could cause further loss of weight; apart from them being expensive, they could interfere with the treatment.

HOW CANCER TREATMENT CAN AFFECT EATING?

All methods of treating cancer, namely, surgery, radiation, or chemotherapy, are very powerful. Although these treatments target the cancer cells in the body, they can sometimes damage the normal cells, as well. This may produce unpleasant side effects that cause eating problems. Side effects vary from patient to patient; the part of the body being treated; length of treatment; or the dose of treatment. Patients may also experience loss of appetite when they are upset, worried or afraid.

1. *Surgery:* Surgery increases the need for good nutrition because it puts stress on the body. Surgery may slow down digestion, or

lessen the ability of the mouth, throat and stomach to work properly, or make them sore. During this time, the patient may receive nutrients through a tube in their nose or stomach, and be put on a liquid diet.

2. *Radiation*: Radiation to the head and neck or chest area may cause 'dry mouth', 'sore mouth', 'sore throat', 'difficulty in swallowing', 'change in taste of food', and or 'dental problems'. Treatment in the stomach area may cause nausea, vomiting diarrhea.
3. *Chemotherapy*: chemotherapy may cause any of the following—nausea and vomiting, loss of appetite, diarrhea, constipation, sore mouth or throat, weight gain, change in taste of food.

COPING WITH/OVERCOMING COMMON PROBLEMS

(A) Loss of Appetite/poor Appetite

This is caused by a lot of factors, such as worry, stress, treatment, treatment schedule, medication, etc. The patient will not feel hungry, but the body needs nourishment. So try the following:

- Try and keep a regular eating pattern,
- Eat small nourishing meals, but more frequently (ie have something every 2-3 hours),
- Avoid fluids at meal times, but drink nourishing drinks in between meals,
- Gentle exercise can stimulate appetite,
- A small glass of alcohol half hour before meals may stimulate appetite,
- Make a meal, a social occasion, a family occasion, and
- Try your favorite foods.

(B) Loss of Weight

If the patient is underweight, or is losing weight, he needs to include more protein and calories in his diet:

- For extra protein, include foods such as 'cheese', 'milk and milk powder', 'complan and resource', 'yogurt', 'eggs', 'nuts', 'wheat germ', 'meat and fish', 'beans and legumes', 'soya products', etc.
- For extra calories, incorporate foods high in fats and sugar, such as 'butter'.
- 'Cream', 'salad dressing such as mayonnaise', 'honey', 'jam', 'dried fruits', 'eggs', etc.

(C) Nausea and Vomiting

This could be caused by the cancer itself or by its treatment. The patient should be advised to—

- Ask the doctor for medicine to control nausea/vomiting Eat small meals often, because NOT EATING WORSENS THE NAUSEA.
- Try foods like dry toast, crackers, yogurt, and biscuits. Drink fewer liquids, with meals.
- Eat slowly.
- Avoid food with strong odors and cooking smells.
- Try cold foods, or eat at room temperature.
- Avoid eating in a room that is too stuffy or warm.
- Avoid fatty, rich and spicy food.
- Take cold clear fluids.
- Wear loose clothes.
- Avoid eating one or two hours before treatment.
- Rest after meals, but try and avoid lying flat on your back.

(D) Chewing and Swallowing Problems: or sore mouth: sore throat

Some of the treatments can cause mouth or throat sores, or ulcers. The treatment may change the amount of saliva in your mouth, or cause dryness in the mouth. This could make the mouth feel hot; and make swallowing painful. The patient experiences dryness of the lips, and tooth and gum problems may occur. In all of the above cases, try the following:

- It is essential to ensure good oral hygiene. Keep the mouth clean with frequent mouthwash and gargle (one teaspoon of salt+one teaspoon of baking soda, mixed in four cups of water makes for a good mouth wash).
- Avoid foods of extreme temperatures.
- Avoid spicy food.
- Avoid foods that may sting the mouth, such as alcohol, salty foods, vinegar, lime, pickles, etc.
- Avoid dry, rough and crunchy food, like wafers, biscuits, etc.
- Eat soft foods, overcooked, blended, or pureed.
- Add extra milk, cream, sauces, custard, butter to moisten the food.
- In extreme cases, try using a straw for drinking.

(E) Dry and Coated Mouth

The following are recommended for this—

- Use mouthwash regularly, specially after every meal.
- Eat moist foods only, totally avoiding all dry and crunchy foods
- Suck on ice, sweets, or sorbets in between meals.
- Drink fluids, with meals.
- Ask doctor to prescribe for artificial saliva.

(F) Loss of Alteration of Taste or Change in Smell

Some of the treatments can raise complaints like—'all foods taste the same', 'food tastes like card board', 'food has a metallic taste', 'all my favorite foods are not my favorite foods anymore', 'I cannot stand the sight of food', 'I lose my appetite when I smell the food cooking at home', etc. Try some of these tips—

- Keep your mouth clean and moist
- Unpleasant flavors could be improved by adding extra seasoning or herbs such as (i) if the food has no flavor, add salt, garlic, cheese, herbs, sugar, chocolate, etc. (ii) if the food tastes too sweet, add extra salt, lemon juice, coffee powder, etc. (iii) if the food tastes metallic, add extra salt, sugar, honey.
- Eat foods with an extra tart in them, such as orange, lemon, etc.
- Serve food at room temperature.
- Drinking through a straw could bypass the taste buds.

(G) Indegestion and Heartburns

This may be a result of radiotherapy to the stomach area, or could also be due to chemotherapy. Try the following:

- The patient is recommended to eat his meals slowly, and have frequent small meals (smal amounts, every 2 hours).
- Avoid spicy, fried and fatty food.
- Caffeine, alcohol, tobacco worsens the condition.
- Avoid fluids with meals.
- Avoid lying down directly after a meal.
- Avoid bending over, directly after a meal.
- Avoid tight, restrictive clothing like belts, etc.

(H) Diarrhoea

This may have several causes. It could be due to chemotherapy, radiation, infection, or due to food sensitivity, or emotional upset. During diarrhoea food passes quickly through the bowel, before the body can absorb the vitamins, minerals and water. So, severe or long-term diarrhea could cause dehydration. Therefore, patients should be advised to—

- Drink plenty of liquids.
- Eat small amount of food throughout the day.
- Eat more food containing sodium (salt) and potassium, such as bananas, peaches, apricots and potatoes.
- Eat low fibre food, such as yogurt, rice, eggs, white bread, cottage cheese, etc.
- Eliminate fatty, greasy foods, raw fruits and vegetables, all high fibre vegetables such as corn, beans, cabbage, peas, etc.

- Limit caffeine intake, including chocolates.
- Sometimes, diarrhea can cause temporary lactose intolerance, so avoid milk and milk products and shift to soya milk, instead.

(l) Constipation

Some anticancer drugs and pain killer medicines may cause constipation. Constipation may also be caused because of reduced food intake by the patients, as well as insufficient fluid intake, inadequate exercise, or reluctance to go to the toilet due to discomfort. Some suggestions for reducing constipation are—

- Drink plenty of liquids.
- Eat high fibre foods, like whole meal breads, cereals, pasta, fresh fruits and vegetables, legumes, pulses, and nuts.
- Get some exercise. A walk for 30 minutes a day is recommended.
- Check with your doctor for some laxatives, or stool softeners.

Tooth Decay

Cancer and its treatment can cause tooth decay and gum problems. Change in eating habits may also add to the problem. The patient is advised to do the following:

- Brush his teeth after each meal or snack.
- See the dentist regularly.
- Use a soft toothbrush. Ask the dentist for special tooth paste if the gums are sensitive.
- Rinse mouth often.
- Limit the amount of sugar in one's diet.
- Avoid eating food that sticks to the teeth.

Cramping and bloating

Few people suffer from cramping or bloating in their gut. They are advised to avoid the following:

- Foods that create gas in the stomach, e.g. cabbage, cauliflower, onion, beans, lentil.
- Carbonated drinks.
- Drinks at extreme temperatures.

Sometimes patients gain excess weight during treatment without eating extra calories. For example, certain anticancerous drugs (such as prednisone) can cause body to retain fluids (edema), causing weight gain. It is important not to go on a diet during treatment, instead, discuss the weight gain with the doctor.

Diet during Chemotherapy

Chemotherapy refers to the delivery of anticancer medications into the body to destroy the cancer causing cells. Chemotherapy, in most cases, has the additional side effect of suppressing the patient's immune system, making them more vulnerable to infection. Patients receiving chemotherapy require proper nutrition to maintain their immune system, strength, and vitality.

- *Improves Tolerance of Therapy*: A well nourished body is stronger and more resilient than a poorly nourished one. Studies have shown that nutrition can decrease the severity and duration of chemotherapy side effects such as vomiting, nausea, weakness, lowered immunity, and susceptibility to infection. There may be other specific side effects, but in general, people who eat well while on chemotherapy tend to feel better and stay more physically active and alert mentally.
- *Increases the Effectiveness of Therapy*: When patients feed themselves they also feed their cancer cells. Studies have shown that "well fed" cancer cells multiply more readily and are more susceptible to anticancer drugs than are slow growing undernourished cells. A good nutritional status may allow patients to withstand higher doses of drugs and increase the effectiveness of the therapy.
- *Speeds Recovery from Treatment*: Nutrients are the building blocks the body uses to rebuild the normal tissues that have been affected by the chemotherapy. If the proper nutrients in the adequate amounts are available, this recovery process takes place much more quickly and efficiently than when deficiencies are present.
- *Regulates Your Weight*: Many patients lose weight on chemotherapy, but some gain weight. Underweight and overweight are both undesirable for the chemotherapy patient. Both of these conditions can lead to weakness, lethargy, depression, embarrassment, and a lack of self-esteem.

Goals of Nutritional Management in the Case of Cancer

- Achievement and maintenance of reasonable weight.
- Prevention or correction of nutritional imbalances and deficiencies.

Adequate calories to meet energy requirements, sufficient protein to permit tissue growth, fats, minerals, vitamins, and fluids all must be supplied in appropriate amounts to meet the patient's requirements. Careful attention to nutrition is important because malnutrition induced by cancer and its treatment adversely affects the patient and complicates further treatment of the disease.

Appetite loss in cancer is apparently a varied symptom, with diverse causes. Attention must be paid to the individual causes. The following steps are recommended:

- Determine symptoms that might be related to appetite loss.
- Probe for specific food likes and dislikes.
- Patients should be given nutritional and dietary counseling.

Practical Guidelines for Eating

When you feel well, take advantage of it by eating well and by preparing meals that you can freeze for the down days. On the good days, eat when you feel hungry, even if it isn't mealtime. It is important to eat foods with good nutritional value; many nutrients can be stored in your body for later use.

Before you try home remedies, be sure you problems are not symptoms needing medical attention, or unwanted side effects associated with the chemotherapeutic agent. DO NOT hesitate to ask your physician questions and to tell the doctor what seems to be bothering you.

Take advantage of time saving and effort saving foods and appliances. These include foods that can be prepared as a meal in a dish with little preparation and cooking. Frozen dinners, when served with a fruit, milk, and canned foods, such as soups, spaghetti sauce, or gravies, can be mixed easily with fresh cooked meat for a good dinner.

An attractively set table with flowers or other such items can take your mind off a slumping appetite. Good odors also help such as baking bread and cakes. A glass of wine or beer with your doctor's approval prior to meals is helpful in generating an appetite.

Stay away from raw eggs and raw meats: This is particularly important if your chemotherapy makes you more susceptible to infection.

End-stage Kidney Disease and the Diet for Patients

The diet for patients with end-stage kidney disease who are on dialysis is usually high in protein and low in sodium, potassium, and phosphorus. Fluid intake is also restricted. The purpose of this diet is to maintain a balance of electrolytes, minerals, and fluid inpatients who are on dialysis. The special diet is important because dialysis alone does not effectively remove ALL waste products. These waste products can also build up between dialysis treatments. Most dialysis patients urinate very little or not at all, and therefore fluid restriction between treatments is very important. Without urination, fluid will build up in the body and cause excess fluid in the heart, lungs, and ankles. Patients on dialysis need to get enough protein and adequate nutrition because they can become malnourished.

The dialysis diet controls the intake of fluid, protein, sodium, potassium, and phosphorus. The amounts of these nutrients in the diet are based on your blood levels of sodium, potassium, phosphorus, calcium, albumin, and urea. These levels are measured before and immediately after a dialysis treatment. Fluid restriction is based on the amount of urine output and weight gain between dialysis treatments.

RECOMMENDATIONS

PROTEIN

Before dialysis, you may be asked to limit protein to slow the progression of kidney disease. At the start of dialysis, you will need much more protein. Patients on peritoneal dialysis need even more protein, because a large amount of protein can be lost in the peritoneal fluid that is discarded. However, dialysis patients still need to limit salt, potassium, and phosphorous, which makes it a little challenging to get enough protein. Also many dialysis patients have a poor appetite, especially after they just start dialysis. Every dialysis center has a dietitian who can explain dietary modifications, suggest foods, and prescribe supplements if you need them.

SODIUM

Most patients need to control the sodium (salt) content in their diet. This helps maintain fluid balance in the body to avoid fluid retention and high blood pressure.

POTASSIUM

The daily intake of potassium is also controlled. This helps prevent high potassium levels in the blood (hyperkalemia), a common problem for people on dialysis.

PHOSPHORUS

The mineral phosphorus is also controlled in this diet. Phosphorus is not effectively removed by dialysis treatments, so you need to reduce your intake of dairy products and other foods high in phosphorus. Your doctor may prescribe calcium supplements, which bind to phosphorus in food. It is important to take calcium tablets with meals. Or, you may be given a non-calcium phosphorus binder. How much of the binders you need to take is determined by your blood levels of phosphorus and how many phosphorus-containing foods you eat.

FLUIDS

During kidney failure, the amount of urine produced drops. The urine output usually stops completely once patients have been on dialysis for more than 6 months. Patients on peritoneal dialysis usually continue releasing urine for a longer time and have less restricted fluid intake. The recommended daily amount of fluid is based on the amount of urine produced in a 24-hour period and the amount of weight gained between dialysis treatments. Other considerations are:

- Amount of fluid retention
- Level of dietary sodium
- Whether you have congestive heart failure

Patients on peritoneal dialysis usually have fewer restrictions on fluid, sodium, and potassium intake because they have dialysis treatments every day. The intake of these substances needs to be individualized in these patients.

OTHER FACTORS

People with kidney disease are more prone to heart disease and often need to follow a low-fat diet. The daily calorie intake needs to maintain proper nutrition and prevent the breakdown of body tissue. Your health care provider should regularly monitor your weight and protein status. Many patients need to take vitamin supplements. Diet alone can usually meet the requirements for the fat-soluble vitamins (A, D, E, and K). Vitamin D may be supplemented, depending on your calcium, phosphorus, and parathyroid hormone levels. Vitamin D is usually given through a vein during the dialysis treatment.

The intake of water-soluble vitamins is often not enough, because this diet restricts several good food sources of water-soluble vitamins. Water-soluble vitamins are also lost during dialysis treatments. All dialysis patients should receive water-soluble vitamin supplements. The doctor will monitor your calcium and iron levels. Whether you get a daily calcium supplement depends on your blood calcium levels. Calcium is also given in the dialysis solution and is adjusted according to the blood calcium levels. Iron supplementation is based on iron studies, which are usually monitored every 3 months. Most dialysis patients do not get enough iron, and must receive iron through a vein during dialysis treatments.

Diets for the Obese

The overweight patient on a low-calorie diet attends the clinic at frequent intervals.

Good results are obtained by careful explanation of a diet planned to show the patient what he may eat. Merely giving a list of forbidden and of permissible foods has not proved nearly so satisfactory. It is important to discuss the reason for dieting and the loss in weight to be expected in a given time. From the commencement of the treatment the patient should know that, once the weight reaches a satisfactory level, instruction will be given on how to keep it there.

Praise and encouragement for progress, or even a little mild bullying, are used in turn. The dietitian must have imagination as well as a wide knowledge of people if she is going to find a point of contact and be able to stimulate the patient to continue over a period of time. Weight cards, and weight graphs, with the target plainly marked, keep the interest alive. Demonstrations of portions of different foods with the same calorie value are both interesting and instructive. The diet is reviewed at each visit and, if weight loss is unsatisfactory, search must be made for ' hidden calories.' How many of the audience does one see consuming potato crisps, peanuts and ice-cream?

Diet counseling in Antenatal clinics The therapeutic approach to dietetics is not applicable to work in the antenatal clinic, where the accent is on a balanced normal diet. A dietary history is taken to supply information on the quantity and kind of food usually eaten and on the amount of cooking that is done. It is useful to know if any of the meals are taken in a canteen or cafC. A simple form, with a list of relevant questions, serves as a guide. The patient's interest is aroused when she sees her intake of food written down. When faults are pointed out and reasoned improvements are suggested she is almost always ready to co-operate. Reasons should be given for the extra food allowances and for the vitamin supplements. On her first visit to the antenatal clinic each patient is seen by a dietitian. If the diet is not satisfactory the expectant mother attends regularly until it has improved. Food Intolerance inpatients with Ulcerative Colitis; Indian study.

'One man's meat is another's poison' was well said by Lucretius Carus (96-55 BC). This describes food sensitivity as a reproducible unpleasant reaction to a specific food or ingredient which one person experiences but others do not. Other types of food intolerance could be due to pseudo-allergy, lack of some specific metabolic enzyme, local irritation, or some other unexplained reasons (Ajit Sood *et al.*). Inpatients with inflammatory bowel disease (IBD), the effect of dietary factors may be primary or modulatory. Various food sensitivities described by patients with inflammatory bowel disease may be the cause of aggravation of symptoms, though not convincingly of pathogenetic importance. Foods commonly identified by patients as causing symptoms on re-introduction, re-challenge, and double-blind challenge include milk, peanuts, citrus fruits, wheat, eggs, fish, and even salicylate rich food:

1. These have been well-studied in Crohn's disease, but attitudes among patients with ulcerative colitis towards diet have not been well elucidated.
2. Food intolerance has not been incriminated as a risk factor in ulcerative colitis but many patients may relate their symptoms to specific ingested food items and they may restrict their diet accordingly. These particular food or food groups may be avoided routinely and that avoidance may be increased during flare-ups. This arbitrary discontinuation or avoidance could lead to decreased intake of specific nutrients, thus raising the question of nutritional adequacy. The present study was undertaken to assess attitudes of patients with ulcerative colitis towards various food groups, how often they considered themselves intolerant to one or more food items, and if any specific offender could be identified.

Amongst patients with ulcerative colitis, maximum intolerance was to milk and milk products followed by legumes (28%), rice (22%), tea (20%), spicy food (20%), and vegetables (18%) in descending order of frequency at the initial stage. A statistically significant difference was seen with milk and its products, alcohol, fruits, and legumes amongst patients with ulcerative colitis and controls ($p<0.01^{**}$). Amongst fruits, mangoes, watermelon, and melon were troublesome. A significantly higher number of controls complained of intolerance to meat/fish ($p<0.01^{**}$). There was no significant difference in the two groups for other food items. Intolerance reported to vegetables, tea, legumes, and spicy foods caused significantly less complaints ($p<0.01^{**}$). However, after dietary manipulation, a significantly higher number of patients were actually intolerant to milk and milk products as compared to controls ($p<0.01^{**}$, $Z = 2.79$). Most patients (84%) were initially intolerant to two or more food items but after dietary manipulations the majority (90%) were intolerant to a single food item ($p<0.01^{**}$, $Z = 5.84$). Food intolerance was not related to the activity of disease. The commonest symptom reported was abdominal pain (55%) followed by regurgitation (50%), nausea (47%), diarrhea (45%), constipation (22%), and flatulence (14%). The majority of patients (81%) had 3 or more symptoms initially and only 1 symptom (84%) after dietary manipulation. The symptom of diarrhea did not show any statistical difference after dietary manipulation; all other symptoms showed a significant decrease after dietary manipulation ($p<0.01^{**}$). Lactose intolerance, Intolerance to the long chain triacylglycerol content of milk, allergy to milk proteins, psychological factors, and various misconceptions are some of the many factors related to patients dairy product sensitivity:

1. In Asians, a high prevalence of lactose mal-absorption has been seen with no specific increase in the number of patients of ulcerative colitis.
2. breath test was not different from that of controls (42% *vs.* 40%), though a significant difference in the incidence of lactose intolerance inpatients with active and quiescent disease was observed (59% *vs.* 32%).

Food Poisoning in Hospital Patients; A Study in South Africa Hospital

A number of food poisoning outbreaks in hospitals have been recorded in South Africa: In order to prevent such outbreaks in the Tygerberg Hospital a comprehensive investigation into all possible sources of food poisoning has been carried out. The investigation covered the bacteriological testing of all raw food supplied to the hospital, the same food after normal cooking, and after subsequent freezing and 'reconstitution' by reheating. In addition, tests were carried out on abattoir, food factory and kitchen personnel. Bacteriological testing was confined to identifying the pathogenic bacteria present in each sample. Only those organisms recognized as being the cause of food poisoning are referred to.

Beef portions: These showed a high degree of infection with food poisoning organisms. (B.M. HORWITZ, *et al.*). The possibility of the meat becoming infected with these organisms during transport from the abattoir, subsequent handling, and cutting up in the butcher's shop must be considered. A single inspection of the premises of one of this hospital's meat contractors, where swabs were taken from equipment, etc., showed the presence of Cl. welchii and pathogenic E. coli on the butcher's block, band-saws, and the overalls and hands; Cl. welchii on the scale. And Staph. ai/reus and pathogenic E. coli on the knife. In addition, a survey of the corned beef pickling barries in the Divisional Council area of the Cape revealed that of 119 samples taken, 3 were positive for Salmonella; 10 for Cl. welchii; and 3 for Sraph. aureus.

Food Handlers in the Hospital Kitchens

Thorough heating for a sufficient length of time should destroy all vegetative forms of bacteria even in heavily infected food. Samples of food cultured immediately after cooking showed, in some instances, that either the temperature reached, or the length of time the food was heated, was insufficient to destroy all pathogenic organisms present. Alternatively, the cooked food may have become infected by a handler in the kitchen directly or indirectly through infected utensils. The presence of pathogenic bacteria or their toxins has been borne out by a number of small outbreaks of food poisoning among this hospital's staff during the period 1970-73. Three of these outbreaks were due to Staph. aureus and three possibly to Cl. welchii.

PREVENTION

In 1972 an experimental kitchen for the preparation of frozen foods was introduced at Conradie Hospital, Pinelands, to investigate its operation under South African conditions. The bacteriological investigations of both the raw and cooked foods were carried out. The frozen food was held long enough for these investigations to be completed before the food was issued. Basically, the system employed is that immediately after cooking the food is placed in disposable covered aluminum trays, and when cool, frozen in liquid nitrogen to approximately –25°C and then stored in a freezer.

After freezing, sample trays of the food are heated in infra-red ray ovens to 80°C for from 20 minutes to 1 hour. depending on the type of food and the size of the container. Samples are then taken for bacteriological culture. If satisfactory, the batch of food is marked as being suitable for issue to the hospital wards. If pathogenic organisms are found, further bacteriological tests are carried out. It still unsatisfactory, the batch is condemned. Food for the wards is issued frozen in trays (4-10 portions per tray) from the central kitchen to accessory ward kitchens. Here food is heated in infra-red ray ovens to 80°C and then served onto plates. All left-overs are discarded.

The following precautions are taken:

1. All food handlers (kitchen staff, and ward-kitchen staff) are tested regularly every 3 months—both throat swabs and faeces samples are taken.

2. The staff are lectured on food hygiene and the absolute necessity for the clean handling of food.

3. The central kitchen used for the production of frozen foods and the ward kitchens for the feeding of patients are supervised by qualified dietitians who are responsible for the enforcement of hygienic handling of all food.

4. Use is made of the agar syringe modification' of the Ten Cate agar sausage technique, to check on the efficacy of cleaning of all utensils and working surfaces and as a means of demonstrating to the staff the absolute necessity of good hygiene.

5. Random samples of raw foods and of all cooked foods are taken daily for bacteriological control. In those sections of the hospital using food prepared by conventional methods of cooking and direct feeding after cooking, a number of small food-poisoning outbreaks have occurred. In the two kitchens supplying conventional food, the precautions taken are the same as those described for the central kitchen, except that the food is not frozen and then reheated before use. The possibility of infection of food by the human carrier, either directly or indirectly, and the multiplication of the contaminating organisms while the food is kept warm during serving, is thus not eliminated. Unlike the wards, where each container holds only 4-10 portions, the containers here are large and hold approximately 20-40 portions. When there is a delay some of the food may be held for more than an hour. No containers are re-used until thoroughly cleansed, but with the type of labour available this system could break down. Every attempt is made while serving to keep the food at a high temperature (approximately 800C), but constant supervision is necessary to enforce this. The major objection to the use of the frozen food system is that it is more expensive due to the costs added by rapid freezing, freezing rooms, reheating, and disposable containers. The cost of hospitalization of a patient in this hospital is estimated at ± R30jday.

Dietetic Course at K.K. Women's and Children Hospital, Singapore

Entry Criteria to teaching course in dietetics

- *Students*: Completed 3 years of BSc course leading to Degree in Nutrition and Dietetics or Dietetics, or completed 1 year of MSc course leading to Masters in Nutrition and Dietetics or Dietetics.
- *Professionals*: Degree in Nutrition and Dietetics or Dietetics.

Expected learning/learning objectives on completion, the trainee will:

- Understand the range of dietetics services offered in a women's and children's hospital.

- Understand the roles of the dietitian in a multidisciplinary team approach to patient management.
- Observe and obtain hands-on experience on the various roles of the dietitian, so as to gain knowledge of the skills required in the profession.

Teaching Programme

Observation of dietitians in:

- Group counseling
- Individual counseling
- Combined clinics (feeding clinic, weight management clinic, diabetic clinic)
- Nutrition talks (antenatal)
- Multi-disciplinary team meetings (catering support committee, gynaecological oncology)

Observation of food service:

- Catering department
- Milk room

Participate in:

- Combined journal clubs
- Departmental journal clubs and case study discussions

Project work:

- Clinical audits of dietitians' compliance to standards of care
- Statistical support (data entry, data analysis) for patient outcome reviews
- Development of patient education materials

APPLICATION PROCEDURE

Interested candidates are required to send a request in writing to:

The Dietetic Internship at Brigham and Women's Hospital

The dietetic internship is an 11-month generalist program of post-baccalaureate study accredited by the Commission on Accreditation for Dietetics Education of the American Dietetic Association (CADE). The address and telephone number of CADE are 120 South Riverside Plaza, Suite 2000, Chicago, IL 60606-6995, 312-899-4876. The program is designed to give theoretical and practical experience in medical nutrition therapy, community nutrition, nutrition research, and food service management.

Candidates must possess the ability to participate in a multifaceted program. This includes strong personal motivation for library and seminar work; initiative to become involved and contribute to all aspects of patient care; willingness to teach; and an interest in research.

Brigham and Women's Hospital firmly advocates that the graduate who successfully completes the accredited dietetic internship can face his/her future with justifiable confidence and self-assurance. Leadership comes to those who achieve professional competence, are adaptable, and who have a perceptive mind. Classes, seminars and field trips are combined with the supervised practice experience to provide greater depth and learning in all areas of dietetics. Joint classes with other Boston internships are held monthly to provide insight into the specialties of the other hospitals and expose interns to the rich medical education and health care experience that Boston offers. The geographic location of Brigham and Women's Hospital—across the street from the Harvard Medical School and Harvard School of Public Health; adjoining Boston Children's Hospital Medical Center and the Dana Farber Cancer Center; and within walking distance of the Beth Israel Deaconess Medical Center—provides interns with opportunities to attend lectures, rounds, clinics, and conferences conducted by leaders in their fields. Harvard University's Francis S. Countway Library of Medicine also adjoins the hospital and is available for study and reference work.

Mission Statement for the Dietetic Internship

The Brigham and Women's Hospital Dietetic Internship is committed to providing the highest quality training in order to prepare interns who will function competently, creatively, compassionately, and collaboratively in a dynamic health care environment.

To further define the BWH internship's mission, goals have been established that reflect the ends toward which the Program's resources will be directed. The Program will:

Goal I—The program will prepare graduates to be competent entry-level dietitians.

Outcome measure-I

Over 5 years, graduates achieve at least 95% pass rate on the Registration Exam.

Outcome measure-2

Within 12 months of program completion 80% of graduates will have passed the registration exam and obtained employment relating to dietetics.

Outcome measure-3

All interns will complete the program requirements and achieve a satisfactory rating for the clinical, community, and food service competencies on the Intern Evaluation Forms.

Outcome measure-4

Employer surveys will provide feedback that rates 90% of graduate work performance as good or excellent.

Goal 2—Through encouragement, motivation, and support, internship director and staff will ensure that Dietetic Interns will complete the internship within 100% of the time planned for completion.

Outcome measure-1

90% of dietetic interns will complete the dietetic internship within a 11 month period of time.

Outcome measure-2

Dietetic interns indicate on Rotation Evaluations, 90% satisfactory or better scores with respect to motivation and support by preceptors.

Outcome measure-3

100% of all at risk students are identified after an unsatisfactory rotation evaluation.

Goal 3—The program will inspire graduates to utilize their nutrition knowledge to help their communities.

Outcome measure-1

The Dietetic Interns will be involved in nutrition education/ counseling in the community.

Outcome measure-2

At least 20% of graduates will be involved with nutrition education/ counseling in the community.

Outcome measure-3

Dietetic Interns will indicate on Alumni Survey that 20% participate in one or more community activities.

Goal 4—The program will provide qualified entry-level dietitians to practice at Brigham and Women's Hospital who will support the education of the next class of dietetic interns.

Outcome measure-1

20% of graduates will be selected for positions at BWH.

Outcome measure-2

Within 6 months of being hired the BWH graduate RD's will precept interns.

Dietetic Intern Rotations

- Orientation—2 weeks
- Clinical Rotations—16 weeks
- General Medicine or General Surgery—3 weeks
- Metabolic Support Service—2 weeks
- Hematology/Oncology—3 weeks
- Cardiac Surgery/Transplant or Cardiac Medicine—3 weeks
- Renal/Dialysis/Transplant—2 weeks
- Medical or Surgical Intensive Care—3 weeks
- Neonatal Intensive Care Unit (optional)

Specialty Rotations (12 weeks)

- Dana Farber Cancer Institute—5 weeks
- Children's Hospital—2 weeks
- General Clinical Research Center—3 weeks
- Special Rotation of Your Choice—2 weeks
- Food Service Management—5 weeks
- Purchasing
- Tower Room Service
- Food Service Production and Distribution
- Catering/Cafeteria
- Ambulatory Service/Community Rotation—7 weeks
- Obstetrics—3 weeks
- Nutrition Consult Service—4 weeks
- Ambulatory Diabetes Center
- Brookside Family Health Center
- Administration—1 week
- Staff Relief—3 weeks
- Vacation—1 week

Dietetic Intern Class Days

- Class days are held every Monday from mid-October through May.
- 2 Mondays/month classes are held at Brigham and Women's Hospital, which include attending lectures at Harvard School of Public Health and speakers from the Department of Nutrition, Medicine, and Allied Health Fields.
- 1-2 Mondays/month classes are held at other Boston Internships, including Massachusetts General Hospital, Beth Israel Deaconess Medical Center, Mount Auburn Hospital, Simmons College, Boston University, Frances Stern Nutrition Center at Tufts Medical Center.

Minimum Admission Requirements

- o Verification Statement from a DPD Program and at least a bachelor's degree from a regionally accredited school.
- o Enrollment fee of $200.00 payable upon acceptance.
- o GPA 3.0 or above.

Application Procedure

Application materials should be sent to:

Robin H. Abourizk, MA, MS, RD, LDN
Associate Director of the Dietetic Internship
Department of Nutrition
Brigham and Women's Hospital
75 Francis Street
Boston, MA 02115

The completed application packet must include:

- Completed application form. The Brigham and Women's Dietetic Internship uses the Dietetic Internship Program Application and Reference forms found at http://www.depdpg.org. (Dietetic Educators of Practitioners—DEP website).
- Official Transcripts and records of courses and grades at all colleges attended.
- Verification Statement by faculty advisor of completion (or intent to complete) the academic requirements of an accredited Didactic Program in Dietetics.
- A two-page maximum typed letter of application, which highlights your achievements, interests and goals.
- Three letters of recommendation (at least one from a faculty member in dietetics or nutrition).
- Application fee of $70.00. Make check payable to Brigham and Women's Hospital, Department of Nutrition.
- All applicants to Dietetic Internships must participate in computer matching. Applicants should request instructions and a mark/sense card to prioritize their DI preferences. Applicants should request this material from an ADA-approved Didactic Program in Dietetics or from D & D Digital Systems. This request should be made to allow turn-around time for submitting by February 15th postmark deadline. There is no charge for this material; however, there is a $50.00 charge for computer matching that is due with the applicant's prioritized ranking.

Address requests to: General Information

- o 11 month program
  - 2 starting dates
  - 1st week of August
  - 1st week of October
  - 12 dietetic interns selected each year
  - On program completion, graduate is eligible to take the Registration Exam for dietitians
  - 9 holidays per year
  - 1 week vacation
  - Meals provided by hospital
  - Housing information is provided by the Internship Associate Director, who will aid interns in making their own housing arrangements
  - Work hours vary with requirements and activity of the unit to which the intern is assigned. The intern hours will be similar to those of the preceptor to whom she/he is assigned. Due to the professional nature of the internship, extra time may be required to complete assignments and projects
  - Intern stipend of $4500.00 per year
- o Cost of program:
  - Housing and parking are very expensive. We recommend not bringing a car.
  - Housing costs vary but an estimate for a 4 bedroom apartment is between $2500-$3000/month.
  - Public transportation is recommended and with the hospital subsidy of 50% the average transportation cost is $30.00/ month for travel using the MBTA system within Boston.

Health insurance is supplemented by the hospital and can vary from $10-$15/week. If you are under 25 and can be covered by your parents' insurance the hospital reimburses you $75.00 monthly. The service aims to:

- Provide high-quality dietetic services to help to fulfil Addenbrooke's role as a provider of comprehensive health services to the residents of Cambridge and the surrounding area.
- Increase specialist work and develop specialist dietetic teams within the department.
- Improve the links between these specialist teams and other dietitians in the region.
- Ensure quality is amongst the best, and adopt an approach to constant quality improvement.
- Employ high-calibre staff and invest in their education and training.

- Use evidence-based practice to develop effective therapies and new treatments.
- Work to the highest professional standards.
- Work with others to ensure nutrition is included as a priority inpatient care.

What Dietitians do?

- They are qualified to translate the science of nutrition in health and disease into practical information about food.
- Work as members of a multidisciplinary team to look after patients who are under the care of a consultant at Addenbrooke's. They visit patients receiving hospital care (or their carers) to check on their health and ensure their diet meets their requirements. They can also be involved in treating disease by diet, for example people who have diabetes or coeliac disease.
- Work to promote good health by teaching the public and other health professionals about diet and nutrition.
- Act as advisors to the Trust on the nutritional standards and specifications for the patient food service to ensure that the needs of all patients can be met.

They provide:

- *Nutritional support*: This means feeding patients who are unable to feed themselves. Examples of this type of patient include patients who have had a stroke, or a patient who is very weak following an operation at the hospital. If we ensure a patient is fed properly, it can improve recovery rates, reduce the chance of further difficulties and reduce the time the patient needs to stay in hospital.
- *Therapeutic diets*: Patients receive medical or surgical help with their conditions, but some have conditions that can also benefit from special diets. Eating more of certain foods, and/or avoiding certain things can help to control a patient's symptoms. In some cases, by carefully monitoring what a sick patient eats and drinks, the dietitian can reduce the chance that patient will have problems in the long-term, and can establish and/or help maintain the patient's quality of life.
- *Advice to the Trust on nutritional issues*: Members of the department work with Trust staff on the following groups and committees: Nutrition Steering Committee, Essence of Care Project Team, Corporate Nutrition Standards and Better Hospital Food Project Team.

- *Education*: The department has a substantial commitment to educating other health professionals through English National Board (ENB) courses and National Vocational Qualifications (NVQ). The Dietitians' Board of the Health Professions Council (HPC) has approved the Department as a base trainer for student dietitians.

FAQs ABOUT FOOD SERVICE

Q. Which departments and wards of the Hospital have nutrition and dietetics services? All inpatients and outpatients are under the care of the Addenbrooke's dietitians.

Q. What information about nutrition and dietetics is available for patients? The Department publishes a number of useful leaflets and sheets, which will be offered to you or can be requested from your dietitian. It also has access to information published by other organizations. If you have other communication requirements, please let our staff know.

Q. Which wards of the hospital receive dietetic services? Every ward has an allocated dietitian responsible for all dietetic services to that area.

Q. If I am referred to a dietitian, how long will I have to wait to be seen? Once referred to a dietitian by a member of the ward staff, we aim to see you within one working day of the referral being made.

Q. What if I need dietary advice at the weekend? An inpatient emergency on-call advisory service is available at weekends.

Q. How will I recognize my dietitian when they arrive on the ward? All of the qualified Addenbrooke's dietitians wear black or navy trousers or skirts and a purple collared short or long-sleeved shirt. An Addenbrooke's ID badge is worn at all times and the dietitian will introduce themselves.

References

Adam E., Ebert R., Production and Operations Management. Englewood Cliffs, NJ: Prentice-Hall; 1982.

Anonymous (1966), The British Eating Out, Thames Uitton, Surrey: Smethursts Foods Ltd.

Brown, A.M., Carden, P.T., Stanton, B.R. and Stock, A.L. (1969), Nutrition, Lond, 23, 217.

Cooper, E.D. (1959): *Ibid.*, 33, 542.

Croom, J.H. (1950). *Edinburgh med.* J. 57, 185.

Finlayson, M.H. (1943): *Ibid.*, 17, 173.

Glew, G. (1968), Nutrition, Lond, 22, 195.

Grady, G.F. and Keusch, G.T. (1971): *New Engl. J. Med.*, 285, 831.

Horwitz, B.M. (1974): *S. Afr. Med. J.*, 48, 271.

Instruction of the Patient Attending the Dietetic Department of a Hospital By ELLA SCOTT, Senior Dietitian, The London Hospital, Whitechapel.

Jones V.A., Workman E., Freeman A.H., *et al.* Crohn's disease: maintenance of remission by diet. *Lancet* 1985; 22: 177-80.

Journal of Indian Academy of Clinical Medicine, Vol. 4, No. 1, January-March 2003 33.

Kochhar R., Mehta S.K., Goenka M.K., *et al.,* Lactase intolerance in idiopathic ulcerative colitis in north Indians. *Indian Journal of Medical Research* 1993; 98:79-82.

Lawrence, R.D. (1951), *Lancet,* 260, 1318.

Le Riche, H. and Dunsian, T. (1953): *S. Afr. Med.* J., 27, 102.

Millcross, I. (1973): *Royal Society of Health Journal,* 93. 133. 464

Mishkin S. Controversies regarding the role of diary products in inflammatory bowel disease. *Can J Gastroenterol* 1994; 8:205-12.

Mishkin S. Dairy sensitivity,lactase malabsorption and elimination diets in inflammatory disease. *Am J Clin Nutr* 1997; 65: 564-7.

Mitch W.E., Chronic kidney disease. In: Goldman L., Ausiello D., eds. Cecil Medicine. 23rd ed. Philadelphia, Pa: Saunders Elsevier; 2007: chap. 131.

Pearson M., Teahon K., Leir A.J., Bjarnason I. Food intolerance and Crohn's disease.Gut 1993; 34:783-7.

Platt, B.S., Eddy, T.P. and Pellett, P.L. (1963), Food in Hospitals. London: Oxford University Press.

Thomas E.C., Management engineering in the food service department. In Rose, J.C., 1984. Handbook for Health Care Foodservice Management, Aspen Publications. pp. 221-234.

Tolkoff-Rubin N. Treatment of irreversible renal failure. In: Goldman L., Ausiello D., eds. Cecil Medicine. 23rd ed. Philadelphia, Pa: Saunders Elsevier; 2007:chap. 133.

Wilkerson, H.L.C. and Krall, L.P. (1947), J. Amev. med. Ass. 135, 209.

Wright R., Truelove S.C. A controlled therapeutic trial of various diets in ulcerative colitis. *Br Med J* 1965; 22: 138-41.

IT and Health—Telemedicine Services: Need and Scope in a Hospital

With the area of 32,87,268 sq.km, population of 1.1 billion, urban-rural divide, inaccessible hilly regions, islands and many tribal areas, India is an ideal setting for telemedicine assisted health care delivery. Growing number of medical, paramedical colleges and schools with lack of adequate infrastructure, learning materials and teachers needs is a matter of grave concern. E health technology has the potential to create a national level GRID which can form the backbone to be shared by health care providers, trainers and beneficiaries. A strong fiber backbone and indigenous satellite communication technology in place with large mass of human potential trained in IT and local presence of telepathy industry, E health application and implementation should not be a problem technically. Further a number of pilot projects over last five years with successful outcome stand to its testimony. A ground work on telemedicine in the country has already been laid with the efforts of ISRO and Information Technology department partnering with many State Government and specialty Institute/hospitals. Policy standardization and infrastructural issues have already been researched. However, a country level plan is long due to steer the Telepathy ship by the Captain (M/o Health and Family Welfare/Government of India) with its crew (technology and health care providers/educators) and passengers (citizen) in right direction (policy, implementation, application, security, social and legal issues) to reach at the destination (Quality health care and wellness).

Health Telematics is defined as a composite term for health-related activities services and systems carried out over a distance by means of information and communications technologies for the purpose of global health promotion, disease control and health care, as well as education, management and research for health. Telemedicine, the practice of transferring medical data using interactive audio, visual, and data communication systems, is quickly becoming indispensable in modern medicine, health care delivery, and education. Telemedicine has been defined as the use of telecommunications to provide medical information, services, and care to people located at any place. At the University of Kansas telemedicine Program, telemedicine technology has been used for several years for oncology, mental health care to patients in rural jails, hospice care, and most recently, to augment school health services by allowing school nurses to consult with physicians.

Cyber medicine, defined as 'the science of applying Internet and global networking technologies to medicine and public health? adds a new dimension to telemedicine. The global coverage of networks extends the scope of information available to patients. In this evolution, physician-physician and patient-physician communications are enhanced by patient-patient relationships (e.g., through e-mail exchanges or formalized discussion groups). Curative and palliative care are complemented by predictive and preventive medicine in which the active patients, not only the health care providers, are at the center of the health network. For example, health assessment tools can directly provide the individual with a personalized analysis of his or her lifestyle habits and risk profiles for common diseases, as well as orientations for changing behaviour (e.g., stress management, body weight reduction, smoking cessation, etc.). Self-medication and self-care become part of a global health care process in which the gatekeeper role of the general practitioner (primary care) is bypassed by the creation of direct links between patients and specialists (secondary care) from one side, and patients and non-physicians (e.g., nurses, community pharmacists, patients' groups) from the other side. It also paves the way for a new business, the e-health business, for which providers are looking for future clients in the promising market of citizen-oriented health products (e.g., dietetic and pharmaceutical products, fitness programs, behavioural programs, etc.).

Although a variety of telecommunication media can be employed for telemedicine systems, in general these systems link clinicians and patients together synchronously or asynchronously. Systems that provide a synthconous or 'serial' link allow one clinician to interact with one patient at a time. This often necessitates a predetermined appointment for the interaction to occur so that both parties are available. Although this approach lessens patients' travel burden, it is still labor-intensive. In general, 'serial' systems are video-based, either with direct video links or streaming video through the Internet.

Telemedicine systems that operate asynchronously or 'in parallel' allow one clinician to monitor multiple patients simultaneously. These systems are partially or fully automated and usually have a computer system interacting with the patients. Using predetermined algorithms, these automated systems supplant the routine monitoring of patients and notify appropriate personnel when problems are detected. Although the degree of personal clinician inter-action varies with these systems, by necessity it is limited compared to face-to-face interactions. Personnel costs are decreased with these systems, and patient monitoring, albeit automated, can be increased. These systems often employ store-and-forward technology.

Telemedicine in its true sense is the transmission of medical information in the form of audio, video, text and images of patients from one location to another, using telecommunication channels. The main communication is between two or more clinics, hospitals, institutions and health centres, within a country or outside, for consultation, advice and opinion. Telemedicine also means transfer of expertise from one point to another and it is the fastest means of communication for consultation for improvement and efficiency in diagnosis and treatment. In addition, high quality medical services of specialists and super-specialists can be readily available using telecommunication and computer technology.

The Telemedicine system can improve rural health care especially primary and secondary care of patients attending community and district hospitals. The technology can improve professional interaction between rural health professionals and their colleagues with urban medical specialists. We must understand that the quality of interaction between distant physicians becomes significantly improved when they communicate via telemedicine networks because it conveys more than just their voices through telephone conversation and discussion. The Store and Forward architecture in Telemedicine system allows consultants and specialists to share images, sound clips and graphical data of the patients, not confined to verbal discussion. The interactive and synchronous video conferencing allows physicians and distant specialists to interact with each other along with their patients and not just voices on telephone. We must realize that in Telemedicine technology the whole nature of interaction between the physicians along with the information (patient's record) conveyed to them is greatly enhanced. In fact, this is a face-to-face discussion or advice and opinion between the patients and their physicians located at different and distant places.

Dr. Prakron Vuthipongse, permanent Secretary, Ministry of Public Health, Thailand, in Inter-country Workshop on Tele-Medicine for Health Development in 21st century from 30th March-3 April, 1998 at Bangkok said that as a decision-maker he was aware of the advancement in today's technology, especially in its applications which will help to bring letter quality of health care to people in remote and rural areas in a cost-effective manner. He also said that the initiation of Tele-Medicine in the Ministry of Public Health has emerged from the fact that, in remote and rural areas, there has been mal-distribution of medical specialties, resulting in poor health care services. He expected the workshop to come up with fruitful recommendations on regional and national plans of action as well as on inter-country cooperation.

However, this very conference cautioned about the use of Tele-medicine: Health Telematics raises certain ethical issues, such as the acceptability of transmitting personal information across cultural boundaries; young doctors getting professionally affected, and the confidentiality of the relationship between the patient and the treating doctor. Full cooperation of the medical and paramedical staff involved, as well as patients is essential. Even in the most advanced form, Health Telematics might not provide a blanket solution for each situation. There would be cases where human intervention is needed. It also raises concern on widening the gap between the poor and the privileged. Thus, in the new millennium the use of tele-medicine offers a potential source of latest knowledge, however, we must use it with great caution and thought.

Dr. R.A. Mashelkar, Director General, Council of Scientific and Industrial Research, delivered the convocation address at the 30th Convocation of Indian Institute of Technology, New Delhi. He said, "Knowledge without innovation is of no value. It is through the process of innovation that knowledge is converted into wealth and social good. Innovative nations lead the world today. When one looks at India, one feels that centuries of subjugation have perhaps undermined our capacity for innovation and creativity, which has got to be revived. We cannot Allow the "T" in India to stand for imitation and inhibition, it must stand for innovation. This requires an all pervasive attitudinal change towards life and work-a shift from a culture of drift to a culture of dynamism, from a culture of idle prattle to a culture of thought and work, from difference to confidence, from despair to hope. Revival of creativity and the innovative spirit needs to be made into a national movement today, in the same spirit and on the same scale as marked our freedom struggle.

Dr. R. Chidambaram, Chairman, Atomic Energy Commission and Secretary to the Government of India, Department of Atomic Energy, delivered the Convocation Address at the Third Annual Convocation of Shivaji University, Kolhapur, he said, "For a nation to grow and advance rapidly, it has to strive for excellence in all its spheres of activity.

Dr. Shivayogi P. Hiremath, Vice-Chancellor, Kuvempu University, Shimoga (Karnataka) delivered the Convocation Address at the Graduation Day- 1999 of JJM Medical College, Davanagere. He said, Doctors on the net is a common caption in most of the Western Countries. Why are so many people turning online for medical information? Experts suggest that there is something inherent in the quick turnover medical office visits that it leaves patients wanting more and more connection, more personal interest, more explanation and more help."

A doctor has to be a constant student and should always work hard to keep abreast of the field by regularly attending the Continuing Medical Education (CME) programmes.

ADVANTAGES OF TELE-MEDICINE

1. Accessibility

Providing health care services via telemedicine offers many

advantages. It can make specialty care more accessible to underserved rural and urban populations at a low cost with high quality. Video consultations from a rural clinic to a specialist can alleviate prohibitive travel and associated costs for patients. Videoconferencing also opens up new possibilities for continuing education or training for isolated or rural health practitioners, who may not be able to leave a rural practice to take part professional meetings or educational opportunities. Continuing Medical Education is essential as the technology is changing fast.

2. Useful for Low Income and Underserved Children

"A TCP Press Release, September 13, 2007 observes "Telemedicine is a powerful tool that helps overcome major obstacles low-income and underserved children and families face in obtaining the health care they need", said Wendy Lazarus, Founder and Company-President of The Children's Partnership. "For children living in medically undeserved areas—both rural and parts of urban areas—telemedicine can address health care provider shortages, transportation costs, and lost time from work and school, by using technology to bring the care to where the children are."

3. Useful in Emergencies and Disasters

It is not too much of a stretch of the imagination to realize that telemedicine will soon be just another way to see a health professional, just as seeing friends and family while talking to them on the phone is becoming commonplace. Farther down the road, it has been theorized that we each could have a 'personal Diagnosis System' as part of our home entertainment centers. This system would monitor our daily health status and automatically notify a health professional if we become ill.

4. Outreach to Remote Areas

Telemedicine in clinical practice is a new concept to India while it has been in practice in the developed world for quite sometime where it is also culturally accepted. We have a situation where a patient irrespective of the distance he/she is located, can get almost instant specialist/ superspecialist advice for his/her ailment which facility hitherto was available only to those living in metropolitan cities. In the absence of availability of proper guidance from a specialist, we have lost many precious lives. The importance of Telemedicine will be appreciated only when its benefits trickle down to our remote rural and semi-urban areas where 80 percent of our population lives. It is doubtful whether there is any other single development, which will allow social justice in our Health Care programme, if the technology is implemented properly. The technology helps us make full use of the specialist/superspecialist services available for bringing solace to millions of people living in semi-urban and rural areas.

5. Consultative Services to Individual Patients

The FDA (The Food and Drug Administration, USA) an authority which regulates the medical field as well, define Telemedicine as the delivery and provision of health care and consultative services to individual patients and the transmission of information related to care, over distance, using telecommunication technologies and incorporating:

1. Direct clinical, preventive, diagnostic and therapeutic services and treatment,
2. Consultative and following-up services,
3. Remote monitoring of patients.
4. Rehabilitative services, or
5. Patient education.

6. Helps in Continuous Medical Education through Distance Education

While considering the educational paradigm shift, the Report of the Task Force of International Council on Distance Education (1996) identifies four major factors as drivers of educational change:

1. The Explosion of Information.
2. Emergence of Information Technology.
3. The Changing Nature of Work.
4. Changing Student Population.

All the developed countries are now moving from the industrial to the post-industrial or information societies. Some of the changes in fields such as computer applications are so fast that the packages become out-dated within 2 to 3 years and new technologies/applications offer more economical, generalized and integrative solutions to current issues. In fact, the speed of changes is making any long-term visualization very difficult. Our vision of the 21st century, therefore, cannot go far beyond and, therefore, we may restrict ourselves to the first quarter of the 21st century that networking with broad band communication with integrated multimedia can afford.

7. Patient Empowerment and Professional Education

To enter into a win-win mode of cooperation with proactive patients. Health care professionals should be prepared for in-depth revision of their education and training programme and accept deep change in their attitude with patients. Appropriation communication and Internet technique is a technical prerequisite for all physicians who need to collaborate with other professionals and patients through health information networks. Physicians' background on the principle of evidence-based medicine is another prerequisite to be able to respond to the checklists und to the structured questions that might arise from their patients. Knowledge on the general aspects of prediction (e.g., genetic counseling), prevention and environmental disease relationships should complement highly specialized knowledge on disease prevention and treatment strategies. Physicians should be ready to direct patients to sources of high-quality Health-related Web sites including bibliographic databases, evidence-based Knowledge sources such as the Cochrane Library or dedicated interest groups. Physicians also should share their favorite sources of information with other Professionals and Patients, providing information on the Internet is no longer.

8. Potentialities of the Holistic View of Media

With the integration of a variety of communication media into the education system, distance education has come to play a major role in universalizing medical education. The technological environment of distance education has changed more significantly with the introduction of live, interactive media. These media are markedly different from other distance education media, in the sense that they are directed towards group interaction rather than individual interaction. With the explosion of technology, distance education is increasingly being defined not by the technology used for delivery but by the nature of interaction involved in the educational process (Garry E. Miller, 1994).

Teleconferencing, because of its interactive nature is also referred to as 'virtual conference'. Virtual conference creates an analogue of communication forms that typically occur in a face-to-face conference, including paper presentation, discussion, moderation, questioning and answering, etc. IGNOU has been using Interactive ETV for its students and counselors. Many experiments have been conducted to experiment the utility of these technologies like CEC-ISRO-UGC-IGNOU Teleconference (December 15-24, 1994), NOS, DECU-ISRO Talk back Experiment, (December, 1996), etc. Based upon these experiments D.R. Goel and D. Sarang made the following observations which need analysis. To quote them:

- (i) The technical, instructional, economic feasibility, legal viability and social acceptability was established and it proved the operational possibilities of an interactive Distance Education system.
- (ii) Potency of teleconferencing as an instructional tool in direct classroom, enrichment education and professional training was realized through the experiments.
- (iii) In most cases technical coordination among the technologists and pedagogists was very successful.
- (iv) Except in few cases of improper use of media-materials due to technology unfamiliarity on part of the academicians and learners, occasional technological shortcomings and personnel management, the experiments were successful in preparing for the operational level.

However, it may be added that its large scale use needs caution, advance preparation and financial resources availability, pooling of resources, understanding the environment of the country, and the needs of the learners.

9. Training in Latest Medical Technology

Conventional classroom training is considered to be too slow and inefficient to keep pace with change. Moreover, administrative hurdles, which include setting up infrastructure and finding tutors, have stymied the growth further. Traditional distance education modes like postal coaching have also failed, as these are non-interactive. Special packages can be developed for different specializations and given to special category.

Limitation

There are many limitations to use telemedicine:

(a) Medical personnel who have neither high qualifications nor experience can cheat the public to make money.
(b) Facilities of telecommunication are the essential feature of telemedicine. It is non existent in many areas of developed countries and more so in developing countries.
(c) Funding for telemedicine is limited. Funds are being allocated mostly for direct hospital services.
(d) Efforts are being made but still not very effective by pooling the resources from health, education, government and business to make use of the facilities. It means pooling of resources.
(e) All the medical personnel are not competent in handling health care through telemedicine.
(f) There have been many frauds in telemedicine. There is a need of law and policy for medicine.

Recommendations of Eleventh Five Year Plan

Information Technology is now one of the major components of the technological infrastructure for health management. All sub–sectors dealing with the generation, transmission and utilization of demographic and epidemiological data such as bio–informatics, bio–statistics, HMIS and the decision support systems (DSS) are finding increasing use in health planning and management. The nationwide network of NICNET provides rapid reporting mechanism for health information; MEDLARS Biomedical Informatics Programmes provides ready access to medical databases to post-graduates and research workers as well as practicing physicians. Planning Commission has provided additional central assistance to the UHSs in Karnataka, Andhra Pradesh, Tamil Naidu, Punjab and Maharashtra for strengthening of libraries and networking them through IT. This effort has to be augmented and all medical colleges need to be brought into the network.

Indian Space Research Organization (ISRO)

ISRO has been actively engaged in applying space technology for health care and education through specific initiatives which include *inter–alia*:

(a) Providing telemedicine technology and connectivity between remote/rural hospitals and super–specialty hospital for tele–consultation, treatment and training of doctors and para–medics.
(b) Providing technology and connectivity for continuing medical education between medical colleges and post–medical institutions/hospitals.
(c) Providing technology and connectivity for mobile tele–medicine units for rural health camps in the areas of opthalmology and community health.

A number of initiatives in tele–medicine have been made in the private sector, SGPIMS, Apollo Hospitals, Asia Heart Foundation, Escorts and others are presently engaged in extending consultations through tele–medicine and are conducting regular tele–education, tele–consultation and tele follow–up sessions with patients.

Need for strengthening telemedicine/e–health initiatives in India

Despite the massive public health infrastructure, health care in rural areas remains a critical challenge. The magnitude of health care services required in the context of the existing shortage of medical officers and trained para–medics clearly demonstrate the need for strengthening tele–medicine and other e–health initiatives over the next Plan. The National Rural Health Mission provides an opportunity for taking tele–medicine to the health care facilities at the primary, secondary and tertiary levels of care. Computerization of health related data would be an essential first step. With the establishment of about 300 Telemedicine nodes by Government/Private/Trust agencies of which 175 nodes by ISRO all over the country and the experiences gained by each of the implementation agencies have brought to bear some of the important issues that needs to be addressed for future implementation strategies for the development of telemedicine and e-health for augmenting the present health care delivery system in the country.

Major thrust areas for 11th Five Year Plan

- Establishment of e–Health department in M/o H&FW in states D/o H&FW with support of state IT Department.
- Computerisation of health care delivery system and health records at state, institutions, district and taluk/block level for the flow of information over the network.
- Computerisation of three tier health care system: CHC/PHC and SC.

- To acquire and implement IT equipments like servers and client systems, multicast video conferencing facilities, data storage and archival facilities in all the specialty hospitals, medical institutions and other centres of excellence who will be providing teaching and training facility.
- To identify agencies within the medical institutions/speciality hospitals/research institutions to develop content for medical education/CME/training modules.
- To acquire and implement terrestrial/wireless/satcom technologies required for various connectivities from taluk/block to district to the state capital.
- To plan for one dedicated medium weight class Communication satellite (HEALTHSAT) for satcom based connectivity which will have the capability to meet the broadband connectivity requirements for various applications of the National Grid.
- The cost of HEALTHSAT with launch, operations and maintenance of the satellite is around Rs. 400 crores. Apart from this, the various connectivity charges by other technologies have to be incorporated. The present cost of a standard telemedicine node including computer hardware/software and video conferencing system is around Rs. 4.0 lakhs at the district hospital level. Whereas at the CHC/PHC level the cost will be around Rs. 1 to 1.5 lakhs. Hence number of nodes which will come up during the 11th Five Year Plan upto the block level may have to be worked out.
- All tele–medicine network should evolve around a National tele–medicine grid. Ultimately, every individual would need to have a unique ID.
- Formal specific training programmes in tele–health for all levels (grass–root to policy makers depending on requirements) and facilitate a support system to provide current information to doctors in the management of patients through new data bases, software packages, etc.
- Medical Council of India to include Information Technology in health care in the curriculum of all medical and para–medical degree courses. Information Technology to be also included in all IT and MBA courses.
- Introduce at least one mobile van in each district.
- Trauma care, ambulance on National Highways to be provided with technology for transmitting audio–video images using EDGE, GPRS, MMS, etc. Pilot studies using tele–medicine and ambulances would be required.
- Setting up of a Tele–health Corporation of India. Given the highly specialized and technical natural of tele–medicine, a Tele–medicine Board of India needs to be established under the aegis of the Ministry, which will include a set of technical

experts with representatives from major health care organizations and NGOs working for tele–medicine. The basic objective of this Board would be to oversee the growth of tele–medicine, develop R&D tools, provide software, manage the National tele–medicine grid and interact with international organizations.

- E-prescriptions at all levels by the end of XIIth Plan but to cover atleast PHCs and above during the XIth Plan. This will necessitate availability of computers and net facility at all health care facility.
- Minimum standards of treatment to be documented and made available on the Ministry of Health website. Details should be available regarding new drugs, banned drugs, new identifications, list of essential drugs, adverse effects, standard treatment protocol, drugs of choice, etc. Skill, knowledge and care should be the corner stone of what we strive for.
- Magnitude of care may vary at different levels but the standard of care to remain the same. This will be possible once the standard treatment protocols are available and will help in identifying the kind and nature of drugs to be placed at each level and the financial requirements for making available these drugs at different health facilities.
- Synergy amongst all existing initiatives and programmes between different Departments/Ministries in the area of health.
- TCI network being created under Department of IT.
- North–Eastern Council initiatives with support from ISRO.
- E–governance initiatives like common service centres under Department of IT.
- Integration of existing infrastructure like CBHI, IDSP, NICD, etc. in the Ministry of Health and F.W. to have proper synergy between them and avoid duplicity in data collection, compilation and transmission.
- Proposed Tele–medicine project by Delhi Government.
- Any other State initiative/Central project which will cater to health needs and requirements.

10. Role of Telemedicine in Disasters

The United Nations telecommunications agency recently deployed 50 satellite terminals, which are capable of providing telemedicine services, in remote areas of southern Peru as part of its efforts to restore vital emergency communication links to the region in the wake of last month's deadly earthquake. The 50 'plug and play' terminals, which are portable devices the size of a small suitcase, allow users to make calls to telephones, access the internet and provide other voice, data and video services, such as telemedicine.

The Geneva-based International Telecommunication Union (ITU) said in a statement that the terminals are being deployed to areas where telecommunications were served because of the damage caused by the quake. Rescue operations in Peru have been hampered by the often mountainous terrain. "We take very seriously the role of telecommunications in mitigating disasters", said Sami Al Basheer Al Morshid, Director of ITUs Telecommunication Development Bureau. "Whenever a country is affected by a disaster, we quickly mobilize and dispatch transportable telecommunications resources that can be used for general communications by government authorities and to provide e-services such as telemedicine that are crucial for saving human lives", he added, voicing hope that the contribution would help Peru cope with the recent massive earthquake. So far, the ITU has allocated more than $ 500,000 to cover the costs of deploying the terminals and paying for their use, but officials said this figure may rise. Cosmas Zavazava, head of the Emergency Telecommunications Division of the ITU, told the UN News Service that the agency is planning to launch in December a framework for cooperation in emergencies that will include a fund to pay for the deployment and use of equipment. The 15th August quake, which measured 7.9 on the Richter scale and struck 161 kilometers south of the capital, Lima, has resulted in the death of over 500 people and injured more than 1000 others, according to the UN office for the Coordination of Humanitarian Affairs (OCHA). In addition, preliminary assessments indicate that over 37,000 houses and four hospitals were destroyed, while 16 hospitals were damaged. *Source*: United Nations Press Release, September, 7, 2000)

11. Role of Telemedicine in Travel especially International Travel

We often see people in the airport preparing for foreign travel who seem far removed from the robust young people featured in travel ads. They are in wheelchairs, supported by oxygen, and many require considerable physical assistance. Yet they are traveling long distances and may be entering a truly alien landscape of medical response, relative to the one that has cared for them thus far. These intrepid travelers are not rare. This chapter does not address the issues of the medical traveler coming to the United States seeking health care. That broad topic is related but is not the subject of this section. The medical evacuation and medical assistance programs available for repatriation will be given only short coverage. The focus of this chapter is the emerging resources of electronic information and telecommunications to support the traveler with regard to health needs. Electronic information and telecommunications applied to health care define telemedicine. No matter where you are, you should be in an electronic continuum with familiar, competent, and interactive health care. In this brief chapter, the scope of medical issues in travel will be considered along with the comparative anatomy of health services in the United States and abroad. Most important, the excellent resources in telecommunications and electronic information will be reviewed along with those services that the public demands and the steadily improving technology may bring to bear in the near future. Ideally, our medical care should be as portable as our medical conditions.

CONCLUSION

With the integration of a variety of communication media into the health and medical system, telemedicine has come to play a major role in improving the health and medical care system. The environment of health and medical system has changed more significantly with the introduction of hire and interactive media, i.e. Telemedicine. Teleconferencing because of its interactive, nature is also referred to as virtual conference. The Telemedicine if properly planned and implement can change the health and medical system in India. It's not too much of a stretch of the imagination to realize that telemedicine will soon be just another way to see a health professional, just as seeing friends and family while talking to them on the phone is becoming commonplace. Farther down the road, it has been theorized that we each could have a 'Personal Diagnosis System' as part of our home entertainment centers. This system would monitor our daily health status and automatically notify a health professional if we become ill.

Appendix I

GOVERNMENT MEDICAL COLLEGE AND HOSPITAL, CHANDIGARH

In view of the ever increasing population of the city of Chandigarh, a second 500-bedded General Hospital had become a necessity not only for catering to the needs of patients in the southern sectors of the city but also to cater for patients from the satellite townships of Panchkula and SAS Nagar. The first 500-bedded General Hospital in sector 16 remains choked with the flow of patients from the first phase sectors of the city and the surrounding states of Punjab, Haryana, Himachal Pradesh and western parts of Uttar Pradesh. The Postgraduate Institute of Medical Education and Research, located in sector 12, Chandigarh was conceived as a premier referral centre for the northern states of India. This is also overcrowded and overburdened.

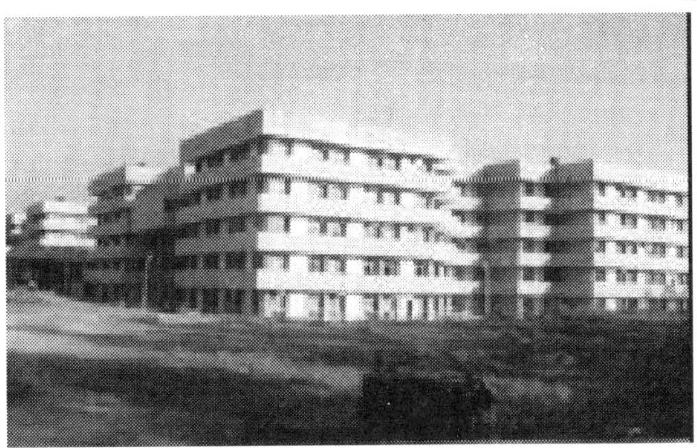

The second General Hospital in Sector 32 had been planned to serve the second phase sectors, thereby relieving pressure on General Hospital, Sector 16 and Post Graduate Institute of Medical Education and Research (PGIMER), so that the latter could serve as a first rate referral hospital.

CHANDIGARH, BEST EDUCATIONAL FACILITIES IN THE COUNTRY

Besides the Panjab University and the Postgraduate Institute of Medical Education and Research, it has an Engineering College, College of Arts, College of Architecture, a number of Government and Private Degree Colleges and other prestigious and important research institutions. Somehow, the city had lacked a Medical College for graduate studies, i.e. MBBS. The deficiency was most glaring. GMC provides opportunity of a career in medicine to many promising students who were denied of this opportunity because of 'domicile' restrictions imposed by the states in which these colleges are located.

BROAD OBJECTIVES OF THE PROJECT

The hospital, intending to meet the medico-social needs of various communities of different economic status, has been obliged to adjust its various services/facilities of general nature and teaching to the present requirements of the society in North India. The broad objectives of the 500 bedded multi-disciplinary teaching hospital are cited below:

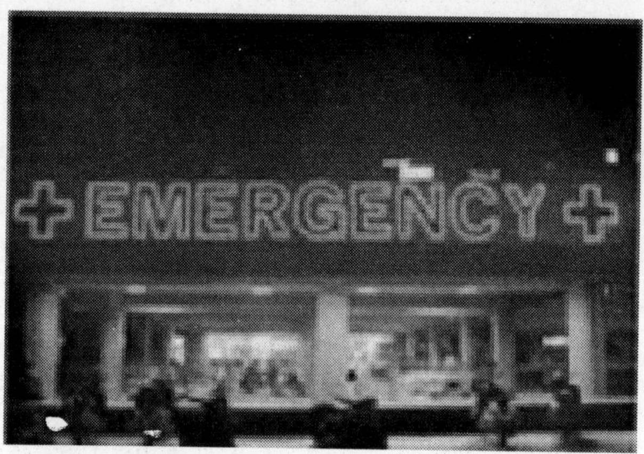

I. To provide comprehensive health care, encompassing preventive, promotive, curative and rehabilitative health care to the residents of North India drawn from the urban/semi-urban and rural areas.
II. To provide out-patient, in-patient and round the clock maternity and emergency care services of all basic and supportive general specialties. These services would be provided free to the poor whereas the more affluent component of the society will add gradually to the government revenue.
III. To provide round the clock facilities of intensive care unit, coronary care unit, burns unit and neonatal intensive care unit.
IV. To provide round the clock state of the art diagnostic services/facilities in clinical pathology, including blood bank, clinical biochemistry, microbiology and radiology, including ultrasound and CT scan.
V. To provide few specialized services in clinical, diagnostic and therapeutic fields like in cardiology, pulmonology, nephrology, neonatology, neurosurgery, urology, plastic surgery and burns, etc.
VI. To act as a free medical institution for direct/first level contact for patients and also as a secondary level referral centre for the referred cases from nearby smaller/large hospitals (Government/private), health centres, polyclinics and dispensaries situated in North India.

VII. To act, specifically, as a regional overflow multi-disciplinary institution (north region) for the referred cases by linking horizontally with other peripheral 100 bedded and 500 bedded general hospitals in the north, with other major teaching institutions and larger multi-disciplinary hospital situated in other parts of Chandigarh.

VIII. To reduce considerably the present workload of other hospitals, especially the Postgraduate Institute of Medical Education and Research, Chandigarh and thereby offer maximum relief to the economically weaker section and middle section of the people residing in rural and semi-urban areas of Chandigarh.

IX. To participate in various national health programmes, including National Family Welfare Programme, by linking with various Government/private hospitals and health centres (horizontally and vertically) and providing necessary infrastructure and facilities as per their demands.

X. To fulfil the glaring deficiency of an undergraduate Medical College in the Union Territory of Chandigarh which offers the best educational facilities in all other fields. The Government Medical College will be attached to the teaching hospital.

XI. To act as a centre for Continuing Medical Education Programmes for various categories of technical and non-technical personnel of different disciplines working within and from other various sized hospitals.

XII. To render facilities for conducting research activities relating to different specialties, as and when required.

XIII. Last but not the least the hospital, as a measure for future expansion, in response to the changing trend in hospital services, would also provide facilities/services (clinical, diagnostic, therapeutic) of various other specialties in future depending upon the real needs of the population.

HOSPITAL AND MEDICAL COLLEGE WINGS

The Government Medical College, Chandigarh was started during the year 1991 in pursuance of the No Objection Certificate issued by the Government of India, Ministry of Health and Family Welfare, vide their U.O.No. 12013/31-90ME(P) dated 15-01-91. The de facto Government Medical College was started in the Prayaas building, Sector 38, Chandigarh after the foundation stone laying ceremony was performed by the former Hon'ble Prime Minister of India, Shri Chandra Shekhar on 20 January, 1991 in Sector 32 on the quilt of 36.09 acre of land allotted by the Chandigarh Administration. In the first instance, the construction for this College and Hospital was started with the outlay of Rs. 100.00 Lac earmarked in the annual plan for 1991-92.

HOSPITAL PLANNING

The hospital building is being constructed with the highest specifications available in the country so that it can be kept hygienically clean and relatively infection free, in the patient's interests. Crevices, projections and other designs, which can collect dust and cobwebs, have been avoided in the construction. Such infection harboring designs have been eliminated.

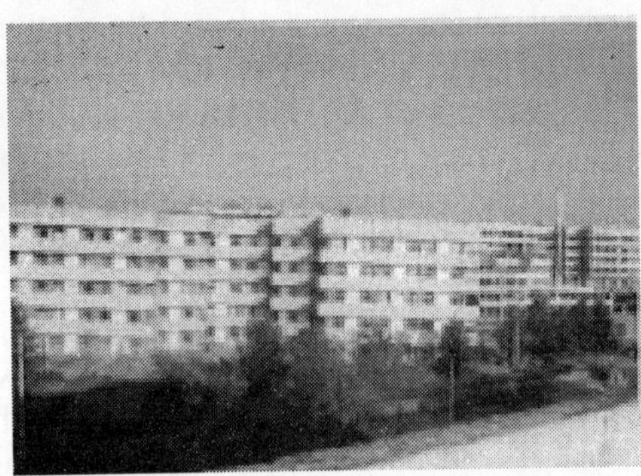

BED DISTRIBUTION AND ARCHITECTURAL DESIGN

Based upon modern technology and the utilization of the modern approach for the building of any complex, especially a large hospital, the Chief Architect, Chandigarh Administration, had evolved a new concept based on the modular system. He proposed the system with self-contained modules for different functions with vertical requirements and a central core which will take away the use of unending corridors of the traditional hospital buildings constructed in the past. The following wings/modules have been proposed and the architectural designs proposed by the Architecture Department of Chandigarh Administration.

Details of each module are as follows:

1. BLOCK-A	Five Floors (45,000 sq. ft. on each floor) Total Area: 2,25,000 sq. ft.
Level-I (OB/GYNAE)	Obst. and Gynae., Antenatal Ward, Neonatal Ward, Labour rooms, Premature Nursery, one Operation Theatre.
Level-II (EMERGENCY)	Medical area, Surgical Area, Paediatrics Area, Emergency Labs, including X-rays, three Emergency Operation Theatres.
Level-III (TRAUMA)	Craniospinal Ward, Orthopaedics Ward, Cardiothoracic and Abdominal Ward, Burns Unit Ward, I.C.U. Ward, three Operation Theatres .

Level-IV (PAEDIATRICS)	Paediatric Medicine Ward, Paediatric Surgery Ward.
Level-V	Private Wards, Kitchen, Canteen.
2. BLOCK-B	5+1 Floors (43,000 sq. ft. on each floor) Total Area: 2,58,000 sq. ft.
Basement	Central Registration Records, Dispensary Stores, Computer Centre.
Level-I	Reception Hall, Registration counters, Canteen, Sample Collection Centre, General OPD (about 12 cabins, screening area),. Information Technology Centre, CT Scan.
Level-II	Obst/Gynae outpatients and MOT, Family Planning Clinic, Antenatal Clinic, Postpartum Clinic.
Level-III	General Surgery OPD, Orthopaedic Surgery OPD, ENT, OPD, Radiodiagnosis Facilities, Day care surgery centre and MOT
Level-IV	Eye OPD, Chest OPD, Skin and VD OPD, Psychiatry OPD and MOT.
Level-V	Medical OPD, Paediatric OPD.
3. BLOCK-C	7+2 Floors (43,000 sq. ft. on each floor) Total Area: 3,87,000 sq. ft.
Level-00	Hospital Laundary, Engg. Services, AC Plant, Electricity Sub-Station, Pump Room, Generator Room, Boiler Room.
Level-0	Stores.
Level-1	Main Kitchen,Canteen, Central Sterlization, Hospital Mortuary.
Level-2	Seven Operation Theatres, Pre and Postoperative Ward.
Level-3	Seven Operation Theatres, Intensive Care Unit.
Level-4	Male and Female Eye, ENT and Orthopaedics Ward, Investigative Labs.
Level-5	Male and Female Medical and Surgical Ward, Cardiac Care Unit, HDU.
Level-6	Skin/VD, TB and Chest and male and female General Medical Ward.
Level-7	Private Wards.
4. BLOCK-D	5+1 floors—Total Area: 2,78,000 sq. ft.
Level-0	Stores, Records and Incinerator—Garbage Collection and disposal.
Level-1	Deptt. of Radiogonisis, Radiothearpy and Dentistry.
Level-2	Blood Bank, Dental Wing.
Level-3	Depts. of Obst. and Gynae., Orthopaedics and Surgery.

	Level-4	Deptts. of Anaesthesiology, Paediatrics and Medicine.
	Level-5	Deptts. of Chest and TB, Dermatology, Psychiatry, Eye and ENT.
5.	BLOCK-E	7+2 FLOORS (43000 sq. ft. on each floor) Total Area: 3,87,000 sq. ft.
	Level-00	Parking.
	Level- 0	Stores and Records.
	Level-1	Central Stores, Hospital and College, Workshop, Tailoring Wing, Lecture Theatre, Staff Canteen.
	Level-2	a. Deptt. of Anatomy. b. Lecture Theatre.
	Level-3	a. Department of Physiology. b. Department of Biochemistry. c. Lecture Theatre.
	Level-4	a. Department of Pathology and Haematology/Transfusion Medicine b. Lecture Theatre.
	Level-5	a. Department of Microbiology. b. Department of Forensic Medicine. c. Lecture Theatre.
	Level-6	a. Department of Pharmacology. b. Department of Community Medicine. c. Lecture Theatre.
	Level-7	a. College and School of Nursing. b. Department of Audio Visual/ Photography/Medical Illustration c. Lecture Theatre.
6.	BLOCK-F	7+2 floor (43,000 sq. ft. on each floor) Presently only 4 floors to be completed.
	Level-00	Parking.
	Level-0	Stores and Records.
	Level-1	Central Library.
	Level-2	College Administration.
7.	BLOCK-J	Animal House.
8.	BLOCK-L	Services Block.
9.	BLOCK-M	Public Parking.
10.	Block-N	Power Sub-Station.

Note: The hospital is striving to offer patient friendly services under the leadership of Prof.. Raj Bahadur, Director Principal. There is a need to abolish the queues at the registration counters and to introduce pre-registration for all patients and to schedule appointments with waiting time to access the first service not exceeding 10 minutes.

APPENDIX 2

A. SINGAPORE NATIONAL CANCER CENTRE

MANAGING CANCER

Singapore is a cosmopolitan and multicultural city with a warm and humid climate all year round. It is also the culinary capital of Asia offering a wide variety of food. With an efficient public transport network of taxis, buses and Mass Rapid Transit (MRT) rail system, traveling around Singapore is hassle free and affordable.

The National Cancer Centre, Singapore (NCCS) is a national and regional centre directed at the prevention and treatment of different cancers, including thoracic, hepatobiliary, pancreatic, head and neck cancers. About 70 per cent of patients with cancers in public hospitals and about half of all cancer patients in Singapore receive treatment from the centre.

As a one-stop specialist centre housing Singapore's largest pool of oncologists, it has state-of-the-art equipment and employs the largest therapies including mini transplants and targeted therapies that maximize outcomes and minimize undesirable side effects.

Physically and operationally designed to provide multidisciplinary services in one location, it allows cross-consultation among oncologists of different specialties. This enables patients to receive customized treatment from a team of radiation, surgical and medical oncologists in one visit. Evidence has shown that a multidisciplinary approach significantly improves prognosis and long-term survival of cancer patients.

NCCS also undertakes cancer research and educates health care professionals as well as the public on cancer.

FOREIGN PATIENT SERVICE

The Foreign Patient Service (FPS) provides keen assistance to patients from other countries and their family members in the following areas:

- General Enquiries
- Medical Referrals and Appointments
- Comprehensive Cancer Screening
- Accommodation Arrangement
- Travel-related Services
- Visa Extension
- Ambulance Services
- Interpreters/Translators
- Visitor Information

CANCER SCREENING PROGRAM

To nip cancer in the bud through screening gives the best chance for cure. Hence, "Nip" (Neoplasm Interception Program)—the name of program. It is unique for its thorough cancer risk evaluation prior to recommendation of a screening program specifically tailored to the individual's risk profile.

A detailed medical and family history will be asked for and analyzed during the initial check-up. A through physical examination will also be done. Risk for major cancers will then be determined. High-risk individuals may require additional special screening tests and/or standard test at screening frequency compared to those with average risk for cancer.

We believe that there is no "standard" package of tests that will be appropriate for everyone. Each individual is unique. Only screening tests that the individual needs, based on risk profile, will be recommended.

The screening tests will include, but are not limited to, blood tests, x-rays, mammogram, ultrasound, CT scans, MRI, and endoscopy. These tests will be done over one and a half days within National Cancer Centre, Singapore as a one-stop service. A detailed explanation of all the test results and discussion for subsequent screening schedule or follow-up action for abnormal tests will take place at the second visit.

We are hopeful that the end of cancer will truly begin with "Nip."

The "Nip" hotline is 6436, 8383 for appointment bookings and general enquires.

HEAD AND NECK CANCER

Head and neck cancer is a term used to describe a range of malignant tumors that appear in or around the throat, larynx, nose, sinuses, and moth. Over the recent years, the management of these tumors has involved increasingly complex, combined-modality programs requiring specialists from various disciplines, including medical oncologists, radiologists otolaryngologist (ear, nose and throat doctors), plastic surgeons, maxillofacial prosthodontists, dentists, physical therapists, speech therapists, nurses, dieticians and social workers. Together, they form a multidisciplinary team to care for each patient before and after treatment begins.

In this issue of Cancer Update, we will review some of the new exciting advances in the evaluation and treatment of these cancers, including the use of functional imaging to improve staging, high precision radiation techniques to reduce therapy-induced side effects, combined modality approaches to improve treatment outcomes and novel molecular targeted therapies such as cetuximab. Often, curative treatment of these cancers also involves radical surgical resection that leaves behind significant anatomical defect. The role of plastic surgeons and speech therapists in restoring anatomy, function and cosmesis will also be addressed in this issue.

While the use of aggressive therapy such as combined chemoradiation has resulted in superior outcomes in the management of patients with head and neck cancers, these improved outcomes are at the cost of increased acute and late toxicities. These include acute local effects such as mucositis, dysphagia, odynophagia, and xerostomia as well as long-term endocrine disturbances such as hypothyrodism and hypopitutarism. Thus, supportive care is also an important area of focus for clinicians who care for head and neck cancer patients and some of these issues will also be discussed. With these improvements in imaging, surgical procedures, radiation techniques and novel therapies, "state-of-art" in head and neck treatment is now being redefined.

ADVANCES IN RADIOTHERAPY

Radiation therapy remains one of the most effective and important treatment modalities for cancer. 60% of all cancer patients will require radiotherapy treatment in the course of their illness. Radiotherapy is the primary curative treatment for many cancer sites and is especially important in head and neck cancer.

In early stage head and neck cancer, radiotherapy is as effective as surgery for control and cure of cancer with better organ preservation and comesis. For patients at high risk of relapse, radiotherapy is often used after surgrey for better local control. The role of post-operative radiotherapy has recently been confirmed by several landmark studies.

Improvement in computer technology and innovation has contributed to many of the recent advances in the field of radiotherapy. For instance, the availability of faster computers has made intensity-modulated radiotherapy (IMRT) possible. With multiple field IMRT, radiation oncologists can now "dose paint" areas, manipulate and visualize in three-dimensions the planned dose distributions before treatment starts. Dose painting allows different doses to be delivered to different parts of the treated volume. This has enabled better tumour control of head and neck cancer while sparing late radiation effects. This is especially important because the head and neck tumours are invariably close to important soft tissue, blood vessels, cranial nerves, exocrine and endocrine glands. With IMRT, tumours that wrap around the brainstem and spinal cord can be treated as the high doses can be 'curved' to avoid these structures. Previously, with parallel opposing fields, the whole volume through the cord is treated.

At National Cancer Centre, Singapore (NCCS), nasopharyngeal cancer (NPC) patients are treated using IMRT as a standard radiotherapy treatment. In addition, patients who are fit also receive concurrent chemotherapy to enhance the effectiveness of radiotherapy. NCCS has recently conducted and published a large randomized control trial on NPC patients that confirmed the superior local control rate and improved survival outcome. We have also established ourselves as one of the main treatment centres in the world contributing to good trial data on NPC.

Another huge recent advancement is image-guided radiotherapy (IGRT) which will minimize uncertainty of target irradiation due to normal body movements like respiration. Before treatment, the exact location of the tumour is ascertained by imaging (by X-rays or with CT). IGRT incorporates time as a fourth dimension in theplannign process. Instead of only a single snap shot in time, with IGRT, the patient is imaged continuously at all paints in a complete respiratory cycle so that the full extent of all body and organ movements are captured for planning in the computer. Using sophisticated techniques like respiratory gating and fiduciary markers, these machines are 'smart' enough to only shoot when the tumour moves into the parameter coordinates within the treatment filed. This enables the radiation oncologist to minimize toxicity, and increase precision without sacrificing tumour control. Stereotactic fractionated radisurgery (SRT) offers yet another option in better precision and conformity in treating certain types of brain cancer. The treatment beams are shaped to match the exact contour of the tumour so that even irregularly shaped tumours can be treated well with good dose conformity. Some of the patients can even be treated without a head shell because the sophisticated software that controls the machine can track with markers, adjust and shoot to a remarkable pinpoint precision. NCCS has recently with industry partners cooperated and commissioned a new Navalis. Brainlabs machine offering SRT.

In October 2007, NCCS will be the first centre in Singapore to use the latest Varian Trilogy machine that has the capability of doing IMRT, IGRT and SRT. Possible new developments in NCCS in the future may involve offering intra-operative radiotherapy, tomotherapy, cyber knife and proton treatment. With all these recent exciting developments in technology, we can continue to offer patients more options to obtain the best possible radiotherapy treatment today and in the future.

Positron emission tomography (PET) is a nuclear medicine functioning imaging modality with direct applications to oncology, cardiology and neurology. At our facility in SGH, we currently perform many oncologic PET/CT imaging which combines PET with CT within a single scanner. PET imaging exploits the glucose metabolic commonly used PET radio-tracer (F-18) fluoro-deoxyglucose (FDG). Various molecular derangements in malignant cells, including increased glycolytic rates and upregulated glucose transporters, result in increased cellular uptake of FDG. A FDG-PET scan can detect and localize such abnormal concentrations of FDG. This short account can only provide a very brief overview of some current indications of PET imaging in head and neck cancers (excluding CNS, NPC and thyroid cancers).

PRIMARY TUMOUR

Apart from nasopharyngeal carcinoma (NPC), squamous cell carcinomas (SCC) account for about 90% of head and neck tumours. Staging is critical in the management of such tumours and provides prognostic information. Cellular cell types such as squamous cell carcinomas are highly FDG avid, several studies have indicated that FDG-PET has good sensitivity in excess of 90% for detecting primary tumour, with failures in very small lesions. However, it should be noted that the clinical information it provides is complementary to that of structural imaging such as MRI. The standardized uptake value (SUV, a semi quantitative index of glucose uptake) obtained may also have prognostic significance.

EVALUATION OF NODES AND DISTANT METASTASES

PET compares with CT or MRI in terms of sensitivity for detecting nodal involvement, although the reported sensitivities can be as low as 50% and as high as 94%. The use of PET in staging lymph nodes of primary head and neck tumours shows that it can detect disease in a segment of patients with NO neck although its exact role is still evolving.[1] In cases of advanced primary tumours, PET imaging allows the concomitant detection of distant metastates, which may alter the plan of management, which may alter the plan of management. Patients with head and neck cancer also have an increased risk of developing secondary cancers in the head and neck, esophagus or lung. One report suggested that PET is able to detect distant metatases or a synchronous secondary cancer in about 10% of patients at initial staging.[2]

POST-CHEMO-RADIATION NECK

PET is useful for assessing residual disease or tumour recurrence in the post-chemo-radiation neck, which may be difficult to assess by structural imaging. A post-therapy PET scan should be performed at 8-12 weeks. A negative scan has high negative predictive value. Nonetheless, it is important to recognize that post-treatment changes such as inflammation can mimic tumour uptake.

DETECTION OF UNKNOWN PRIMARY

Patients with neck metastases of squamous cell cancer are very likely to have the primary lesion within the head and neck region. PET is often useful in detecting some of these tumours when no obvious tumour has been found by other imaging modalities or panendoscopy.

Some limitations for PET imaging in the head and neck include the relative low uptake by some well-differentiated thyroid carcinomas. Certain benign lesions such as parotid Warthin's tumours may give rise to rather high uptake. PET is not optimal for evaluating intra-cranial abnormalities as the physiological uptake of glucose by the normal gray matter precludes a proper delineation of tumours that occur at the base of skull or in the cavernous sinus.

CONCLUSION

In conjunction with structural imaging, PET and PET/CT provide clinical information on status of the primary tumour, nodal and distant metastases and the presence of unsuspected synchronous second cancer. It is useful in the evaluation of post-treatment neck and the detection of occult primary tumours.

POST-RADIATION HYPOPITUITARISM

Hypopituitarism is the inability of the pituitary gland to provide sufficient hormones adapted to the needs of organism.[3] It can be caused by either an inability of the pituitary gland itself or an insufficient supply of hypothalamic releasing hormone.

Pituitary irradiation is a well known cause of hypopituitarism. Hypopituitarism has been found inpatients treated with cranial irradiation for a number of intracranial pathologies, including pituitary adenomas, suprasellar tumours, primay tumours, nasopharyngeal carcinomas, head and neck tumours and bone tumours affetcting the skull. It can also occur inpatients who have received prophylactic cranial irradiatin as part of the treatment scheduled for acute lymphoblastic leukemia in childhood.[4]

Radiation induced toxicity depends on the total radiation dose. The fraction size and the time allowed between fractions for tissue repair.[5] The physical soe of radiation delivered to hypothalamus and pituitary during conventional external beam depends on whether they are included in the radiation filed or whether they are located near the filed, in which the radiation dose delivered will be less.[5] The severity of the hypopituitarism depends on the dose of radiation. Low radiation dose (<50 Gy) usually result in isolated growth hormone deficiency,[2,3] while higher doses (>60 Gy) for nasopharyngeal carcinoma lead to panhypopituitarism.

Irradiation of the hypothalamic-pituitary axis cause a characteristic pattern of hormone loss; growth hormone (GH) is usually affected first, followed by gonadotrophins, corticotrophin (ACTH) and thyroid-stimulating hormone (TSH).[6,7] The hypothaloamic-pituitary dysfunction is progressive and evolves dysfunctinis progressive and evolved over many years. Studies have demonstrated that the number of pituitary hormone deficiencies increase with the length of time from irradiation.[6,7] The rate of which the hormone deficiency develops depends on the dose of radiation used.[3]

Age is another factor that has impact on development of hypopituitarism. Younger individuals are more vulnerable to radiation damage.[5] The progression of the hypopituitarism is also influenced by prior compromise of hypothalamic-pituitary neuronal integrity such as underlying pituitary tumor or previous surgery.[4,5] Lam *et al.* studied 28 patients undergoing radiotherapy for nasophyryngeal carcinoma with normal prior pituitary function.[7] At five years, GH, ganadotrophins ACTH and TSH axes remained normal in 36.5%, 69%, 73% an d85% respectively.

CLINICAL FEATURES

The clinical manifestations of hypopituitarims are variable and often insidious in onset. They are also dependent on the degree of hormonal deficiency. It can be subclinical, indicated only by measurement of hormones, or its clinical onset might be acute or severe.

DIAGNOSTIC TEST

In principle, a combination of low peripheral and inappropriately low pituitary hormones indictes hypopituitarism Thus, as an initial investigation, basal serum hormones should be measured. However, basal concentrations alone might not be distinctive owing to pulsatile, circadian or situational secretion of some hormones. Dynamic stimulation test are indicated in equivocal basal hormone levels or to diagnose partial hormonal deficiencies. Every dynamic test has its specific limitations and the test of choice depends on the local experience and practical considerations.

ACTH DEFICIENCY

ACTH and cortisol secretion follow a diurnal rhythm, with highest levels in the early morning an lowest concentration around midnight. A morning cortisol value below 100 nmol/I is indicative of hypothalamic-pituitary-adrenal (HPA) asix insufficiency, whereas HPA insufficiency can be excluded if the morning serum cortisol is above 500nmol/I.[6]

Between 100 and 500 nmol/I, ACTH deficiency is not unequivocally excluded and a dynamic test is required. Hypoglycemia (blood glucose <2.2 mmol/I) induced by insulin tolerance test is a strong stressor and regarded as a gold standard for assessment of the hypothalamic-pituitary-adrenal axis.[3] A maximum response of 500 nmol/I generally excludes HPA insufficiency although some advocate a higher cut-off level of 550 nmol/I.[8] However, this test has some unpleasant side effects, such as sesating, trembling, fatigue and hunger. It is potentially dangerous and thus requires the supervision of a physician. It is also contraindicated inpatients with heart disease and epilepsy.

As sustained ACTH deficiency leads to adrenal atrophy and ACTH receptor down regulations, standard ACTH stimulation rest (synacthen test) can be used to establish secondary adrenal insufficiency at least 4 weeks after the onset of the ACTH deficiency. Stimulated cortisol level below 500 nmol/I is indicative of adrenal insufficiency. However, there are some patients who pass the synacthen test but not the insulin tolerance test (ITT). There is also a debate as to whether a low dose 1 mcg synacthen stimulation test would represent a more physiological stimulus for maximal adrenal stimulation. A recent met analysis reported similar operating characteristic between the 2 doses.

TSH DEFICIENCY

The diagnosis of TSH deficiency can be made by serial free T4 measurement. Concentrations of free thyroxine are decreased with TSH being low or normal.[1,7] Dynamic testing is generally not necessary, as it does not add to diagnostic reliability. In some cases, TSH can be slightly raised due to secretion of biologically inactive TSH.

LUTENISING HORMONE (LH) AND FOLLICLE-STIMULATING HORMONE (FSH) DEFICIENCY

Hypogonadism in premenopausal women is easy to diagnose because of the menstrual disturbance. Presence of menstrual disturbance and an inappropriately low LH and FSH indicate secondary hypogonadism. Absence of typical post-menopausal rise in LH an dFSH also indicates central hypogonadism. Similarly, in men, the presence of low testosterone and low or normal LH and FSH is indicative of central hypogonadism. Dynamic tests are of limited value and are seldom used.

GROWTH HORMONE DEFICIENCY

The diagnosis of growth hormone deficiency is established by clinical and biochemical criteria. Normal insulin-like growth factor I (IGF-I) concentration does not exclude the diagnosis of GH deficiency have IGF-I in the normal range. Thus proacative tests are usually indicated. Hartman *et al.* however, suggested that inpatients with an appropriate clinical background of pituitary pathology or irradiation, GH provocative test may not be required. The presence of more than 2 pituitary hormones deficiencies or low IGF-I level is sufficient for diagnosis.

Insulin tolerance test (ITT) is still the diagnostic test of choice[9] with peak of growth hormone below 9 mU/I suggesting severe deficiency.

Other alternatives included glucagons stimulation test, growth hormone-releasing hormone (GHRH) plus arginine test and more recently GHRH plus growth hormone releasing peptide 6 test, are easier to do but unfortunately not available at our Center. A point to note is that tests that stimulate the pituitary directly, as in GHRH plus arginine, may produce response that do not reflect the GH status[2,11] as the hypothalamus is the immediate site of damage following irradiation. No test for assessment of growth axis is 100% reliable.

PROLACTIN

Prolactin can be mildly elevated after radiation due to hypothalamic dysfunction. This may not require treatment unless the level is very high and possibly contributing to central hypogonadism.

CONCLUSION

With more patients receiving cranial irradiation having a better chance of survival, more are now left with the prospect of pituitary dysfunction. The frequency and severity of developing hypopituitarism is both dose- and time-dependent. The onset of hypopituitarism is insidious and symptoms are often subtle and non-specific. Hence, an index of suspicion should be present when reviewing patients with cranial irradiation. Periodic screening for signs and symptoms of hypopituitarism and basal hormonal tests should be considered when appropriate.

PLASTIC RECONSTRUCTION METHODS

Plastic surgery may not come to mind intuitively when thinking of cancer patient. However, plastic surgery plays an important ole in restoration of anatomy, function and cosmesis for many of our patients who have lost them due to cancer invasion or, more frequently, the radical treatment require for the cancer. The defect may be as simple as a small skin and subcutaneous defect after excision of a basal cell carcinoma, to something as complex as total maxillectomy-mandibulectomy defect after resection of an extensive buccal carcinoma.

Before discussing reconstruction, resection defects can be optimized by respecting skin tension lines and aesthetic units wherever possible, with the caveat that surgical clearance must not be compromised. Where there is a conflict of resection versus sease of reconstruction, resection must take precedence.

The Principles of plastic reconstruction are:

1. Restoration of function,
2. restoration of anatomy with similar tissue wherever possible, e.g. bone with bone, skin with skin,
3. Simple preferred to complex, and
4. low donor site morbidity.

To achieve these aims, there is a hierarchy of methods, from simple to complex, beginning with primary closure, local flaps, free graft, regional flaps, distant flaps and free flaps.

Primary closure is the technique of choice in small wounds, where closure may be achieved with no tension. This results in the best outcome. Undermining of surrounding subcutaneous tissue may be necessary to relieve tension. Closure may be facilitated by modification of the wound be facilitated by modification of the wound with Z-plasty, W-plasty, V-Y plasty, etc. These allow re-orientation of the whole wound or segments of the wound to allow tension free closure and to break the line of the scar for a better cosmetic outcome.

Where primary closure cannot be achieved, the next best option is local flaps. These include simple advancement flaps, transposition flaps and rotation flaps. Tissue match is usually good as these flaps are typically from adjacent tissue. Donor site morbidity is minimal, although a long incision may be necessary in tissues with little compliance, e.g. the scalp. An example of a transposition flap is the nasolabial flap for reconstruction of a nasal defect after excision of basal cell carcinoma.

Free graft may be sued in areas where cosmesis is not critical or if there is insufficient local tissue for local flaps. They range from thin split skin grafts, full thickness skin graft to complex composite grafts including cartilage, etc. As grafts including cartilage, etc. As graft are not vascularised, survival of grafts are dependent on the vascularity of the recipient, bed, thickness of graft (thinner better) and stability (shearing leads to devasularisation).

Consideration should also be given to the donor site, for tissue match and donor site morbidity. Split skin grafts tend to result in poorer cosmesis, especially if meshed to increase area. However, they take more easily as they are thin and can be used for extensive skin defects. The donor site typically heals with hyper or hypopigmentation. Full thickness skin grafts result in better cosmesis, but their thickness limits their size and decreases take rate. The donor site is closed primarily, usually with good results. Composite grafts have an even poorer survival rate due to complexity and poor vascularity. An example is a full thickness conchal (ear) graft for nasal alar reconstruction.

A large of complex defect after resection typically requires either a sizeable regional flap or free flap reconstruction. The choice is dictated by the patients's fitness to tolerate prolonged surgery, the nature of the defect, whether it requires distant tissue egg bone for the mandible. Occasionally, compromises have to be made in an unfit patient. For instance, when reconstructing a commando defect, a pectoralis major flap may be chosen to reduce surgical time and to ensure greater flap survival instead of a free fibular flap which is ideal in a fitter patient.

Regional flaps may be composed of a combination of different tissues. Foreheaded flaps and deltopectoral flaps are examples of fasciocutaneous flaps. Pectoralis major and latissinus dorsi flaps are myocutaneous flaps. These are transferred base don their blood supply, with the pedicle still attached after the transfer. The advantage is shorter surgical time and a lower risk of flap failure, as the native vascular pedicle is less prone to problems like thrombosis, compared to free flaps, which require microvascular anastomosis. The flap side of having an attached pedicle is limitation of range. Thus a pectoralis major flap is unable to reach a defect over the forehead or scalp.

Before the advent of the operating microscope and expertise for microvascular anatomosis, flaps were sequentially "walked" to from the donor site to the recipient site, or if it came from a mobile appendage like the forearm, the limb had to be kept close to the recipient site until the flap had revascularised form the bed before the pedicle could be detached. This era of microvascular free flap has revolutionized our ability to reconstruct complex defects with like for like. An example is the use of a free fibular flap after commando resection, where the fibula respalces the resected mandible and skin is used to cover the mucosal defect.

With our current reqportoire of plastic reconstructive techniques, almost any defect can be covered. However, a well-designed prosthesis may accasionally yield better cosmetic and functional outcomes than the most technically floawless flap. It takes wisdom and experience not to views everything as a nail when you have a hammer in hand.

MANAGEMENT OF PAIN IN HEAD AND NECK CANCERS

Pain is a common symptom in cancer of the head and neck. Pain may be caused by direct tissue damage due to the disease, or as a result of treatment, both as an immediate side effect of chemotherapy or radiotherapy, or as late sequelae, such as from fibrosis and neovascularization post-radiotherapy. These must be distinguished from other common causes of head and neck pain, such as tension headache, migraine, toothache and trigeminal neuralgia. Accurate assessment of the cause and pathophysiology of the pain is the first step to good pain management.

Pain due to direct tumour damage includes ulcerative lesions of the mouth and palate, tumour destroying bandy structures and tumour destroying boney structures and tumour affecting the cervical spine causing radicular pain of the head and neck. Often the pain is exacerbated by muscle spasm, which is usually reactive and often protective. NSAIDs and COX-2 inhibitors are often useful in ulcer or bone pain, with addition of opioids if pain is more severe. Muscle relaxant, such as baclofen, may help with muscle spasm, though they have to be used judiciously if there is facet joint or spinal instability. Neuropathic pain needs to be treated with adjuvant drugs such as amitriptyline, sodium valproate, gabapeintin or pregabalin, in addition to analgesics.

The commonest cause of pain due to cancer treatment is muscositis. Transcription factors, such as NF-kB, activated by chemotherapy, radiation, therapy or reactive oxygen species paly a major role in triggering a biological cascade that leads to mucosal injury. Mucositis may range in severity from generalized mucosa erythema to widespread ulceration, which may be life threating, depending on the agent and dosing regimen. Treatment is directed towards control of pain and risk of infection.

A common infection causing pain in immunosuppressed patients is oral candidiasis. This may extend into the oropharynx and oesophagus giving rise to odynophagia and compromising oral intake of food and fluids. Management is by removal of Candida plaques with bicarbonate solution and treatment with oral nystatin suspension, 500,000 Units four times daily, or in severe cases, with systemic antigunfal agents, such as fluconazole. Other infections causing pain include Herpes simplex and zoster reactivation. The latter may also cause post-herpetic neuralgia.

Other oral complications of cancer treatment of the head and neck include osteonecrosis of the mandible and radiation tooth caries. It is important before the start of cancer treatment to have dental clearance of tooth and gum disease. Osteoradionecrosis of the mandible is a known complication of radiation treatment, and may be precipitated by a tooth extraction or other trauma to the irradiated bone. It is often very troublesome to treat, as dead bone sequestrate may have to be removed and sometimes the mandible replaced. Hyperbaric oxygen has also been tried. A more recently reported cause of osteonecrosis is that associated with the use of intravenous bisphosphonates.

ROLE OF MOLECULAR TARGETED AGENTS

Cancers arising from the head and neck region are a diverse group of malignancies that include paranasal sinus tumours, salivary gland tumours and malignancies of the lip, oral, cavity, oropharynx, hypopharyns, larynx and nasopharynx. Head and neck cancer has an annual global incidence of over half a million cases and remains the fifth most common cancer worldwide. Of these cases, the majority are head and neck squamous cell carcinomas (HNSCC).

Traditional therapy of HNSCC has involved a multimodality approach employing surgery, radiotherapy and chemotherapy. This last decade has seen the integration of chemoradiotherapy with improvements in quality of life, organ preservation and survival. Nevertheless, most patients with Stage III or IV disease, and nearly all patients with recurrent or metastatic disease will succumb of their illness.

The benefits of conventional therapy are beginning to plateau such that ongoing improvement in outcome for these patients will depend on advances in surgical techniques, radiotherapeutic techniques and molecularly targeted therapies.

ROLE OF MOLECULAR TARGETED THERAPY

Cancer results from aberrations in genetic and epigenetic processes, both of which are paramount for cellular function, differentiation, survival and proliferation. Molecularly targeted agents offer attractive therapeutic options by restoring normal control of oncogenic process.

The epidermal growth factor receptor (EGFR) and its ligands (epidermal growth factor (EGF) and tumour growth factor (TGF-) are fundamental for cel proliferation, motility, adhesion, invasion and angiogenesis. By dysregulating the EGFR signal transduction pathways, the process of tumour formation, growth and metatasis occurs. Both biochemical and immunhistochemical studies have demonstrated expression of EGFR in a number of solid tumours, including 80-90% of HNSC, 1-3 and elevated levels of EGFR protein have been shown to be a poor prognostic factor 2-4.

EFGR inhibition has proved to be an important strategy in the treatment of HNSCC as well as other cancers of the head and neck. Although EFGR is the best understood and studied target in HNSCC, other molecular targets such as vascular endothelial growth factor (VEGF) and ErbB2 are also undergoing further evaluation.

TARGETING EGFR

The use of anti-EGFR therapies is the most employed molecular-trageted stragety studied in HNSCC. The rationale for their use stems from EFGR biology in HNSCC. Preclinical work has shown the importance of EGFR in the pathogenesis of HNSCC. Messenger RNA for both eGFR and its ligand EGF are found to be elevated and over expression of EGFR protein is seen in up to 47% of HNSCC.

Levels of EGFT are also increased based on stage and grade of the tumour. Upregulation of EGFR is further observed as cells change from dyplasia to squamous cell carcinoma. Based on these observations, several phase II studies have sought to establish response to targeting the EGFR (Table 1).

Cohen *et al.* reported on the single agent activity of gefitinib at both 500mg/day and 250 mg/day, the observed response rate was 10.6% and the disease control rate was 34%.

Wheeler et a;, evaluated gefitinib inpatients with recurrent HNSCC and stratified them into two groups; group 1 included patients disease and group 2 included patients who had received only one treatment regimen. Only patients who did not receive prior therapy for their recurrent disease responded to treatment (15% response rate) and theoverall survival for all 32 patients was 6 months.

Soulieres *et al.* evaluated erlotinib in 115 patients with recurrent or metastatic disease and reported an overall objective response rate of 4.3% and disease stablilization rat of 38%.

Cetuximab, a human-murine chimeric lgG monoclonal antibody that binds to the extracellular domain of EGFR has been used in Pase II trails inpatients with recurrent or metastatic HNSCC as a single agent or in combination with chemotherapy. Phase I studies showed no overlapping toxicities when combined with full dose cytotoxic agents. A Phase II study of cetuximab alone inpatients who progressed on platinum-based therapy, documented a response rate of 13%; however, overall survival was still <6 months. Table 2 summarizes some of the phase II studies evaluating the use of cetuximab inpatients with recurrent or metastatic HNSCC.

So far, only two published phase III randomized clinical trials have incorporated a targeted therapy into the treatment of HNSCC. In one of these studies, patients with loco-regionally advanced HNSCC were randomly assigned to radiotherapy alone or radiotherapy plus cetuximab.

Patients were ineligible if they had previously undergone surgery or had previously undergone surgery or had previously received radiotherapy for head and neck cancer. Between the two arms of the study, 424 treatment-naïve patients were enrolled and results showed a median duration of loco-regional control of 24.4 months versus. 14.9 months (p=0.005), favoring the addition of cetuximab.

Of importance, the median duration of overall survival was 49.0 months (p=0.03), again significantly favoring the additional use of cetuximab. The Eastern Cooperative Oncology Group (ECOG) has also recently completed a phase III trial comparing the use of cisplatin plus placebo *versus* cisplatin plus cetuximab inpatients with recurrent or metastatic disease.

These patients were not previously treated for their recurrent of metastatic disease. Based on 117 analyzable patients, those treated with cetuximab plus cisplatin ad statistically superior objective response rates (26% versus 10%, p=0.03) but not median progression-free survival (4.2 months versus 2.7 months, p=0.09) or overall survival (9.2 versus 8.0 months, p=0.21)

OTHER STRATEGIES UNDER EVALUATION

Beyond just targeting EGFR, two studies have recently evaluated the role of lapatinib, a selective and potent dual competitive inhibitor of EGFR and ErbB2.

Harrington *et al.* report on a Phase I study of lapatinib plus chmoradiation inpatients with locally advanced HNSCC and Abidoye *et al.* report on a Phase II trial of lapatinib in recurrent or metastatic HNSCC.

The Phase I study confirms the safety of the combination of lapatinib, cisplatin and standard radiotherapy; however the Phase II tiral showed the drug to have no activity. Other preliminary trials have evaluated antiangiogenic drugs.

A Phase II study of sorafenib, a potent inhibitor multiple receptor tyrosine kinases and serine-threonine kinases including Raf isoforms. VEGFR-2 and PDGFR, inpatients with recurrent or metastatic HNSCC and nasopharyngeal cancer has shown a partial response in 1 out of 23 and stable disease in 9 out of 23 patients.

Finally, Vokes et al recently presented a Phase I/II study of bevacizumab and erlotinib in 55 patients. Overall response rate was 14.6%, with two complete responses observed. Survival data from this study is in keeping with prior studies and the median survival was 6.8 months.

CONCLUSION

The increased knowledge of the molecular alterations present in HNSCC has led to efforts to develop compounds that target these molecular pathways. As EFGR is overexpressed in HnSCC, different strategies to target this activated receptor have reached the clinic. Among them, a monoclonal antibody termed cetuximad and two low-weight tyrosine kinase inhibitors (gefitinib and erlotinib) have shown promising results.

For instance in the treatment of locally advanced HNSCC, cetuximab increases the activity of radiotherapy. In the metastatic setting, cetuximab increases the activity of chemotherapy compounds. Other drugs against the EGFR and other molecular pathways are in preclinical and clinical development. From all of these, anti-VEGF therapies are promising agents especially in combinations with other chemotherapy or targeted agents.

Although these are exciting new advances, important questions remain. Criteria for adequate patient selection for these targeted therapies remain unanswered as well as the best way to increase the activity of these agents.

In conclusion, several compounds have now reached the clinic with successful results. In the future, these therapies and others to come will need to be integrated in a rational way with standard treatments. This will hopefully improve the prognosis of HNSCC.

TUBE FEEDING

Head and Neck cancer patients often present to their physicians in poor nutritional state. Malnutrition is reported to affect up to 50% of this

TABLE I

EFGR tyrosine kinase inhibitor trials in HNSCSS patients

Drug	*Phase*	*N*	*Stage*	*Overall response rate*	*Overall survival (months)*	*Reference*
EGFR TKIs given as monotherapy or in combination chemotherapy						
Gefitinib	II	52	Rec./Met.	10.6%	8.1	Cohen *et al.* (2003)[5]
Gefitinib	II	32	Rec.	9.4%	6	Wheeler *et al.* (2005)[6]
Gefitinib	II	70	Rec./Met.	1.4%	5.5	Cohen *et al.* (2005)[7]
Erlotinib	II	115	Rec./Met.	4.3%	6.0	Soulieres *et. al.* (2004)[8]
EGFR TKIs incombination with radiotherapy						
Gefitinib+ induction chemotherapy followed by radiochemotherapy	II	45	Locally advanced unresectable	85%	5.5	Doss *et al.* (2006)[10] Savvides
Erlotinib + radiochemotherapy (docetaxel)	I	23	Locally advanced			Savvides *et al.* (2006)[11]
Lapitinib + radiochemotheraphy	I	17	Locally advanced			Harrington (2006)[12]

Rec. = recurrent, Met = metastatic

group of patients and it can be a result of a few contributing factors including cancer cachexia, tumour, growth, inability to consume adequate nutrients from chewing and/or swallowing difficulties which may arise from the cancer treatments.

Dysphagio following head and neck cancer therapy or from the tumour growth itself can significantly reduced the patients oral intake. In this circumstance, tube feeding is indicated for those with fully or partially gastrointestinal (GI) tract. Placement of feeding tubes has been shown to be effectively delvivering nutrients into the GI system.

TABLE 2

Trials using anti-ENGFR antibodie in HNSCC patients

Drug	*Phase*	*N*	*Stage*	*Response rate*	*Reference:*
Anti-EGFR antibodies in combination with chemotherapy or as monotherapy					
Cetuximab+cisplatin	II	132	Recurernt, P-refractory	OR 13%, DCR 64%	Herbst *et al.* (2005)[13]
Cetuximab+ cisplatin/carboplatin	II	96	Recurernt, P-refractory	OR 13%, DCR 53%	Baselga *et al.* (2005)[14]
Cetuximab	II	103	Recurrent P-refractory	OR 16.5% DCR 53%	Trigo *et al.* (2004)[15]
A: Cetuximab+cisplatin B: Placebo+Cisplatin	III	117	Rec./Met	OR: A=26% B=10%(p=0.03) OS:A=9.2mo, B=8mo (p=ns)	Burtness *et al.* (2005)[16]
Xalutumumab	I/II	24	Rec.	OR 12.5%	Basthalt *et al.* (2005)[17]
Anti-EGFR antibodies in combination with radiotherapy					
Cetuximab	I	16	Advanced	OR 100%	Robert *et al.* (2001)[18]
Cetuximab	II	22	Locoregionally advanced	OR 15/16 OS(3 yr)76%	Pfister *et al.* (2006)[19]
Cetuximab A: radiotherapy B: radiotherapy+ cetuximab	III	424	Locogregionally advanced	OS: A=29.3 mo, B=49 mo (p=0.03)	Bonner *et al.* (2006)[20]

OR=overall response rate, DCR=disease control rate, mo=months, OS=median survival

There are various tube feeding modalitites. Access to the GI tract through the nose is classified as a nasoenteric tube and access through the skin is termed as enterostomy tube. The decision on the type of feeding tube depends on the patients medical condition and the anticipated duration of tube feeding. Table below shows the comparison of various tube feedings.

Enteral Access	*Indications*	*Advantages*	*Disadvantges*
Nasoenteric			
Nasogastric	• Unable to take adequate/safe oral intake • Requires normal gastric motility and gastric outlet function	• Ease of placement/ easy to remove • Low cost • Allows administration of medications	• Greater risk of aspiration *vs.* nasointestinal feeds • Requires monitoring of gastric emptying
Nasoduodenal/ Nasojejunal	• Preferred route for patients with high risk of aspiration, delayed gastric emptying, gastroparesis, gastro-oesophageal reflux disease	• Decreased risk of aspiration *vs.* nasogastric feedings • Beneficial in patients with gastgroparesis	• Requires endoscopy for placement. • Unable to monitor gastric motility.
Enterostomy			
Gastrostomy (can be surgically or percutaneouly placed)	• Long-term eternal feeding • Indicated in patients with normal gastric function • When transnasal/ transoral route is not available	• Bolus feeding possible • Paticnt comfort • Large bore tube allows medication administration/ gastric decompression	• Increased risk of aspiration in high risk individuals • Stoma care required • Potential for tube dislodgement
Jejunostomy	• Enteral access in upper GI tract unobtainable or contraindicated • Impaired gastric motility • High aspiration risk	• Jejunum functional for early post-operative feeding • Decreased aspiration risk • Can be placed via laproscopy	• Tube patency, smaller bore tubes may clog • Potential for intraperitoneal leakage • Potential for volvulus
Combined gastrostomy/ jejunstomy	• Useful in patients requiring gastric suction or decom-pression with otherwise intact intestinal tract	• May be weaned to gastric feedings over time.	• Potential gastrointestinal intolerance • Smaller bore tubes prohibit medication delivery and may clog

Adapted from American Dietetic Manual for Clinical Dietetics

SELECTION OF ENTERAL FORMULAS

When selecting an appropriate enteral formulation both formula characteristics and patient's specific factors should be considered. Formula variables include digestibility/availability of the nutrients, nutritional adequacy, viscosity, osmolality and cost. Patients variables include nutritional status and requirements, electrolyte balance, digestive and absorptive capacity, disease state, renal function, medical or drug therapy, and possible routes available for administration.

Adult enteral formula products fall into one of the following categories:

Polymeric feeds

Nutritionally complete formulas with macronutrients, vitamins, minerals and trace elements. Some examples are Ensure, Ensure Plus, Resource Standard, Resource Plus, Resource 2.0, Nutren Optimum, Isocal and Enercal Plus.

Disease specific feeds

These formulas have modified nutrient compositions designed to meet specific needs such as:

- Glucose intolerance e.g. Glucerna, Nutren Diabetes, Resource Diabtetic
- Renal failure e.g. Nepro, Suplena, Navasource Renal.
- Type 2 respiratory failure e.g. Pulmocare

Disease-specific feeds are often more costly than standard polymeric feeds.

Predigested or semi-elemental feeds

Formula contain nutrients which are readily absorbed (monoand disaccharides, amino acids, peptides, medium-chain triglycerides and long chain triglycerides). An example of a semi-elemental feed is Peptamen.

Modular feeds

Modular feeds contain single nutrient to enhance polymeric/disease-specific formulas to meet individual patient needs. An example of a modular feed is one with protein. Commonly used protein supplements are Propass, Beneprotien and NutriComp Protein.

MONITROING TUBE FEEDING

Below is a guide for causes, prevention and treatments for common tube feeding complications.

Complication	Courses	Prevention/Treatments
Mechanical Complications		
Aspiration pneumona	Delayed gastric emptying	• Consider post-pyloric feeding • Reduce administration rate • Regularly check gastric residuals and tube placement • Keep patient elevated 30-45° during and after feeding
Gastrooesophageal reflux		• Use small-bore feeding tube to minimize compromise of lower oesphageal sphincter • Keep patient elevated 30-45° during and after feeding. • Regularly check tube placement.
Irritation/erosion at the nasal, oesophageal and mucosal region	Prolonged intubation with large bore feeding tubes	• Use of plastic/rubber tubes • Use small-bore feeding tubes made from bio-compatible materials • Secure feeding tube using tape to avoid placing pressure on the nostrils. • Consider enterostomy sites for long-term feeding.
Tube obstruction	Formula residue	• Flush tube with warm water before and after each feed, medication or gastric aspiration.
	Formula-medication insoluble complexes	• Use liquid form of medication where available. • Vigorously instill and withdraw small amount of warm water or carbonated beverage.
GI Complications		
Diarrhea	Rapid formula administration Hyperosmolar formula Microbial contamination Drug-induced	• Decrease feeding rate temporarily • Select isotonic formula or dilute formula and increase strength gradually • Hygienic handling and administration techniques • Review medications.
Nausea and vomiting	Rapid formula administration Delayed gastric emptying	• Decrease feeding rate temporarily • Consider post-pyloric feeding • Reduce administration rate • Regularly check gastric residuals and tube placement • Keep patient elevated 30-45° during and after feeding.

Constipation	Inadequate fluid intake Insufficient bulk Inactivity	• Ensure well-hydrated • Select fibre-supplemented formula and ensure well-hydrated • Encourage ambulation, if possible.
Metabolic Complications		
Dehydration	Increased fluid requirements or loss of fluid and electrolytes	• Ensure adequate hydration
Overhydration	Fluid overload	• Restrict fluid intake • Change to a hypercaloric formula • Administer diuretics • Replace sodium losses
Hyperglycaemia	Metabolic stress Diabetes Mellitus	• Select low-carbohydrate formula • Monitor blood glucose • Administer insulin if necessary.

Adapted from Enternal Nutritiion Handbook, Abbott Laboratories.

SUPPORTIVE CARE FOR PATIENTS

Head and neck cancer includes cancers of the mouth, nose, sinuses, salivary glands, throat and lymph nodes in the neck. Those who survive and become disease free frequently have altered appearances and/or disabilities associated with treatment[9], and that results in significant medical and psychosocial consequences.

Patients at the National Cancer Centre are counseled before surgery. The patients who undergo head and neck surgery are followed up by a trained staff nurse who identifies new issues that arise, provides counseling, and ensures that the patients are followed up by appropriate health professionals. She refers patients to the medical social worker for counseling, support and financial aid. The patient is introduced to a support group that meets monthly.

After a laryngectomy, the speech therapist helps in voice restoration. The options include the electrolarynx, oesophageal speech and trocheo-esophcqeol speech. The patients are taught effective communication in terms of phrase groups and coordination for the first two groups. Patients using trachea-esophageal speech are assisted in the management of the prosthesis and in using it for communication. The most common form of voice rehabilitation after total laryngectomy is the artificial larynx. Although the tracheoesophageal puncture is a technique deemed as superior to other options of voice restoration, only a relatively small number of patients are successfully rehabilitated long-term.[10]

Aspiration rate following chemotherapy and radiotherapy for the treatment of head and neck cancer is an underreported occurrence.[11] Dysphagia is a significant morbidity of head and neck cancer treatment, and the severity of dysphagia correlated with a compromised quality of life, anxiety and depression.[12] The speech therapist plays a big role in the rehabilitation and supportive care of these patients. They teach the patients compensatory techniques for swallowing and swallowing therapy has been shown to improve dysphagia severity and reduce the need for tube feedings.[13] The patients are also advised on the long-term side effects of radiotherapy, including xerostomia, fibrosis and trismus. Exercises for the oral and neck muscles are taught to prevent further fibrosis.

The prosthodontist is another health professional involved in the care of this group of patients. The patient may be rendered edentulous by cancer treatment or dentures may no longer fit due to gum atrophy or change of the anatomy of the jaw. They may need implants or prosthesis such as a palatal obturator (Fig. 1).

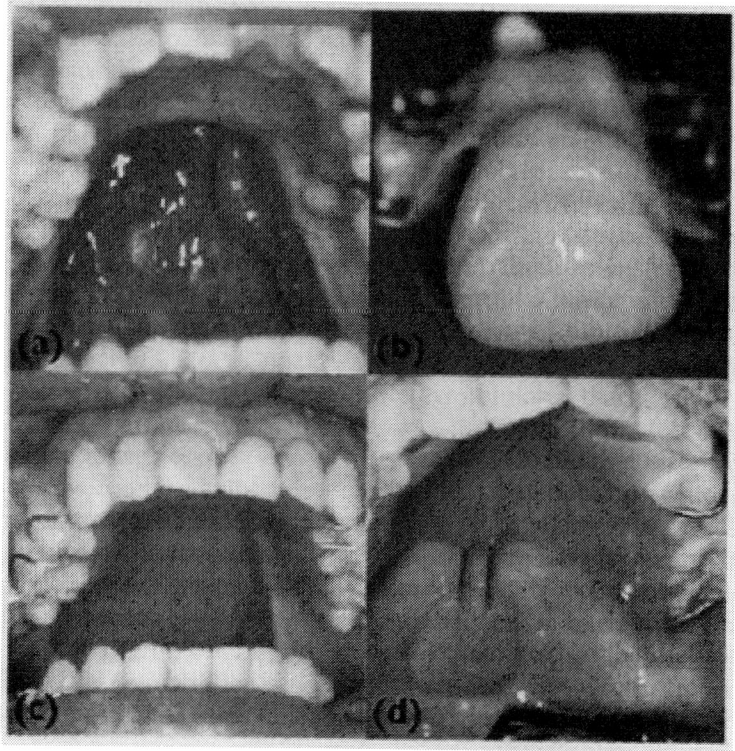

Fig. 1: (a) to (c) before and after insertion of palatal obturator, (d) palatal lift appliance

Having cancer and dealing with the residual effects of treatment can be time consuming, energy and emotionally draining. The patient needs to make adjustments in many ways, including adopting a healthier lifestyle. Smoking and drinking are risk factors for head and neck cancers and these patients may return to these habits in times of distress. Patients need help with smoking cessation, and the avoidance of alcohol. They need support from their families and significant others in eating more healthily, exercising and coping more healthily with stress. Their closed ones need education, in order to support the patient in various ways needed.

Cancer-related fatigue is a late medical effect of cancer, and occurs in those who have been cured. It is easily overlooked. A cancer rehabilitation physician screens for and treats cancer-related fatigue. The contributing causes are identified and reversible factors are treated, for example anaemia, sleep disorders, depression and endocrine disorders such as hypopituitarism. Sleep apnoea often occurs after upper airway surgery, and should be investigated and addressed. Treatment of cancer-related fatigue includes starting an exercise program, teaching the patient to prioritise and pace his daily activities as well as sleep restoration. Methylphenidate is used in the treatment of cancer-related fatigue. There is evidence that it can improve fatigue scores and it has an effect on overall well-being and quality of life scales.[14] It improves one's functional status.

Quality of life includes dimensions such as physical, functional, psychologic and social wellbeing. Other dimensions include spirituality, sexuality and so on. In a study on head and neck cancer survivors, despite some improvements in physical changes and activities of daily living eventually, patients report a decline in certain quality of life domains. They report declines specifically in areas of marital and sexual functioning.[9]

An involvement of the rehabilitation physician is essential for a multidisciplinary approach to the management and supportive care of cured head and neck patients. The rehabilitation physician assesses and coordinates the multidisciplinary care amongst various health professionals and continues to follow up the patient when the patient no longer has surgical issues nor require follow-up for cancer treatment. He deals with the residual effects of cancer and its treatment, including cancer-related fatigue, depression, neuropathic pain, and helps to reintegrate the patient back into family/society, looking into issues such as sexuality, employment and other dimensions in life that is meaningful to the patient.

Data from National Cancer Registry Publication, 2002

Type of Cancer	*Absolute numbers, between 1998-2002*	*Male*	*Female*
Tongue	214	142	72
Major salivary glands	114	64	50
Mouth	188	122	66
Nasopharynx	1465	1079	386
Oesophagus	503	393	110
Nasal cavities and sinuses	96	72	24
Larynx	371	343	28

VOICE RESTORATION

Talking is a basic form of communication. Therefore, losing the ability to talk can be frustrating for a patient who has had a total laryngectomy, i.e. the removal of the larynx. This procedure is done for patients who have cancer of the larynx or voice box. In doing so, the patient loses his or her ability to produce voice as the vocal cords are also removed in the process. The trachea or airway is then diverted to a permanent breathing hole in the neck called a stoma.

After surgery, the patient communicates through alternative ways such as writing, using picture boards, gesturing or mouthing words. These methods are limited in vocabulary and are time consuming, as thoughts are not expressed immediately. Relatives and friends also take some time to get used to these modalities of communication. There are, however, three alternative ways of restoring 'voice' after a total laryngectomy. These methods are:

(1) Oesophageal Speech
(2) Artificial Larynx
(3) Trachea-Esophageal Speech

Oesophageal Speech

This type of speech requires the speaker to learn how to "swallow" air into the oesophagus and create a sound by releasing the air and articulating words at the same time. This method is quite like burping. Sound is created when the air vibrates in the oesophagus and words are produced when this sound is shaped by the articulators, for example, lips, tongue and cheeks, into meaningful words and sentences. This method requires the speaker to learn to sustain the air that is released and involves a substantial amount of coordination and practice.

Artificial Larynx

This method involves the use of a handheld electronic device that translates vibrations into sounds. This device is held on the neck and under the chin. The vibrations produced by this device are converted into speech through slow and deliberate articulation. The voice produced using this method is robotic but the pitch can be altered to suit the speaker. The speaker and the listener will need some time to get used to this type of voice and speech produced.

Tracheo-oesophageal Speech

This mode of speech requires a surgical procedure to create a connection between the trachea and the oesophagus. A voice prosthesis, which has a one-way valve, is then fitted through this fistula. Voice is produced when the speaker occludes his or her stoma to divert all the air from the lungs through the prosthesis and up the pharyngo-oesophageal segment to the mouth. The segment vibrates to produce a sound and this sound is then shaped by the articulators to produce meaningful speech.

As the voice prosthesis is made of silicone, it may be damaged by *Candida*. If the candida grows at the valve and damages it, leakage of fluids will occur resulting in coughing and possible aspiration of fluids. Voice quality may also be affected. When this happens, the patient will need to visit his or her speech therapist to get the voice prosthesis replaced. One way of reducing the growth of *Candido* is to take Nystalin regularly. This helps to prevent the growth of *Candido* and increase the lifespan of the prosthesis.

The Rehabilitation Process

Speech therapists work very closely with post-laryngectomy patients right from the beginning. They meet the patient before the surgery to tell them more about it and the follow-up plan after the surgery. The three modes of voice restoration are discussed at this point.

When the patient is ready to start voice rehabilitation, the speech therapist explores with the patient the three modes of voice restoration and the mode most suited to the patient. Regular sessions are needed and the speech therapist also works closely with the patient to improve other aspects of communication, for example, articulation and rhythm of speech.

Post-laryngectomy patients may often find communication frustrating at the beginning. However, with proper guidance and support from the medical team (consisting of doctors, nurses and speech therapists), communication becomes natural again.

SPEECH AND SWALLOWING DIFFICULTIES AND MANAGEMENT INPATIENTS WITH NPC POST-RADIATION

Treatment of cancer in the head and neck region usually involves radiation therapy, either administered alone or in combination with surgery and/or chemotherapy. Nasopharyngeal cancer (NPC) is a disease known to respond well to chemotherapy and radiotherapy, especially in the early stages.

Effects of radiation on speech and swallowing function may vary; patients will be affected to some degree with varied presentations over time. Usually these problems are not picked up until several months or years after its onset.

During this period of time the patient is at risk of developing nasal regurgitation, coughing during meals and episodes of aspiration pneumonia, symptoms of which suggest worsening of their swallowing function.

Common complaints by patients with NPC after radiation suggesting presence of speech and swallowing dysfunction include:

- Dry mouth (xerostomia)
- Altered taste sensation
- Voice change (i.e. hypernasality, hoarseness).
- Poor speech intelligibility

- Bad breath (halitosis)
- Restricted mouth opening (trismus)
- Tongue tremors (fasciculation)
- Food or liquid coming out from nose
- Food sticking in throat
- Requiring drinks to wash food down
- Coughing and choking while eating/drinking.
- Taking longer time to finish a meal
- Avoiding certain foods

Patients with the above complaints should then be referred to a speech therapist who would then assess and manage the speech and swallowing difficulties accordingly. Ideally, the speech therapist should evaluate all patients before, during, and after radiation to determine any changes in the patient's swallowing status and to start appropriate exercises as well as evidence-based swallowing strategies as needed.

There are two main objective assessment tools used by speech therapists to ascertain a patient's swallowing status and function. Videofluoroscopy for swallowing (VFS) is recognized as the gold-standard evaluation because it captures the entire oropharnygeal swallow. This allows for identification of specific characteristics of the swallowing disorder, which is necessary to determine appropriate interventions to be used and their effectiveness subsequently verified.

The fibreoptic endoscopic evaluation of swallowing (FEES)is a video-endoscopic tool that is sensitive to detect residues, laryngeal penetration, and aspiration, and avoids radiation exposure. Unlike VFS, it does not show the oral phase.

Common findings of VFS/FEES inpatients with NPC post-radiation:

- Decreased base of tongue movement to posterior pharyngeal wall resulting in reduced bolus propulsion into pharynx.
- Reduced laryngeal elevation and laryngeal vestibule closure resulting in high incidence of laryngeal penetration during swallow.
- Reduced epiglottic retroflexion resulting in reduced laryngeal vestibule closure.
- Reduced pharyngeal contraction resulting in residue along pharyngeal wall post swallow.
- Upper esophageal sphincter dysfunction
- High incidence that penetration and aspiration is silent.

Information gathered from VFS and/or FEES will allow the speech therapist to tailor effective speech and swallow rehabilitation exercises specific to the patient. Therapeutic interventions may include:

- Dietary modifications (e.g. fluids to help flush solids, or need for thickened fluids, blended diet) *vs.* need for alternative feeding via nasogastric tube or PEG.

- Postural strategies (e.g. head positioning).
- Swallowing maneuvers that are evidence based such as super-supraglottic swallow and the Mendelssohn Maneuver.
- Therapeutic exercises that target strength and range of movement for jaw, lips, tongue, larynx, and neck.
- Speech tasks working on improving intelligibility.
- Referral to ENT for vocal cord medialization, botox, and/or UES dilatation and hearing aids for hearing loss.
- Referral to prosthodontist for prosthetics to improve speech intelligibility and facilitate swallowing function (e.g. palatal lifts to manage velopharyngeal incompetence or palatal lowering device).
- Referral to dietician for nutritional advice.

It is therefore important to understand the need to diagnose and manage swallowing difficulties, since unrecognized dysphagia may lead to multiple health problems such as repeated admissions for aspiration pneumonia and poor nutritional and hydrational status. Coughing and choking during meals, prolonged eating time, and the limited range of foods that can be swallowed can also lead to social isolation thus affecting the patient's quality of life. As such, the speech therapist together with the patient's primary physician and other medical professionals play a significant role in maximizing optimum management inpatients with NPC post radiation.

References

1. Heiko Schoder *et al.*, *J Nucl Med* 2006; 47: 755-762.
2. Goerres, G.W. PET and PET/CT of head and neck tumours. In Clinical molecular Anatomic Imaging. (ed) G.K. van Schulthess.
3. Schneider, H.J., *et al.*, Hypopituitarism. *Lancet*, 2007, 369 (9571): pp. 1461-70.
4. Toogood, A.A., Endocrine consequences of brain irradiation. *Growth Horm IFG Res.*, 2004. 14 Suppl. A: pp. 5118-24.
5. Darzy, K.H. and S.M. Shaler, Hypopituitarism as a consequence of rain tumours and radiotherapy. *Pituitary*, 2005. 8(3-4): pp. 203-11.
6. Littley, M.D., *et al.*, Hypopituitarism following external radiotherapy for pituitary tumours in adults. *Q J Med*, 1989. 70 (262): pp. 145-160.
7. Lam, K.S., *et al.*, Effects of cranial irradiation on hypothalamic-pituitary function-a-5-year longitudinal study inpatients with nasopharyngeal carcinoma. *Q J Med.*, 1991, 78(286): pp. 165-76.
8. Van Aken, M.O. and S.W. Lamberts, Diagnosis and treatment of hypopituitarism: an update. *Pituitary*, 2005, 8(3-4): p. 183-91.
9. First year after Head and Neck Cancer: Quality of Life. Ellen R Gritz *et al. Journal of Oncology*. Vol. 17(1): 1999: 352-360.
10. Voice rehabilitation after total laryngectomy and ostoperative radiation therapy. William M. Mendenhall, *et al. Journal of Clinical Oncology*, Vol 20, (10), 2002: pp. 2500-05.

11. Aspiration rate following chemoradiation for head and neck cancer: and underreported occurrence. Nguyen N.P. *et al. Radiother Oncol* 2006 Sep; 80(3): 302-6.

12. Impact of dysphagia on quality of life after treatment of head and neck cancer. Nguyen NP *et al. Int J Radiat Oncol. Biol Phys.* 2005 Mar 1; 61(3): 772-8.

13. Impact of swallowin therapy on aspiration rate following treatment for locally advanced head and neck cancer. Nguyen, N.P. *et al. Oral Oncol* 2007 Apr; 43(4): 352-7.

14. Patient-controlled methylphenidate for the management of fatigue inpatients with advanced cancer: a preliminary report. Eduardo Bruera *et al. Journal of Clinical Oncology* 2003; 21(23): 4439-43.

B. SINGAPORE NATIONAL HEART CENTRE

The National Heart Centre (NHC) Singapore is a regional referral centre for cardiovascular disease, which provides one-stop comprehensive services for patients with heart, lung and chest problems. The centre has the largest number of internationally qualified cardiovascular doctors in Singapore.

Besides expertise in the treatment of highly complex cases with high success rate, NHC is also a training and education centre for cardiac specialists and health care professionals as well as an active research and development centre for cardiovascular diseases.

NHC is the first heart hospital in Asia to receive the prestigious Joint Commission International (lCl) accreditation, a testament to the high quality care and excellent outcomes, which we offer to our patients at competitive rates.

Heart disease is a major killer in Singapore and in many countries. Many suffer from heart disease without knowing and seek medical attention too late. At NHC, we are dedicated to providing excellence in health care as the national and regional referral centre for cardiovascular disease through cost-effective and best care possible at the best value. This will be achieved through our clinical services, teaching, research and training.

MAJOR HEART DISEASES

Coronary Artery Disease

Plaque that accumulates in your coronary arteries causing chest pain, heart attack and stroke.

The coronary arteries are narrowed from atherosclerosis (gradual buildup of fatty deposits) which block the flow of blood to the heart.

Arrhythmia

Abnormal heart rhythm.

Hypertension

A condition in which the blood pressure is raised, also known as high blood pressure.

Hyperlipidemia

High cholesterol level.

COMMON PROCEDURES

Coronary Angioplasty (Balloon Angioplasty and Stenting)

This treatment for severe blockages of the coronary arteries reopens narrowed coronary arteries using special devices such as catheters and stents. Often stents are placed into the area where the blockage occurs to keep the artery from narrowing again.

NHC performs a high volume of complex multi-vessel angioplasty procedures using the full range of special devices such as intravascular ultrasound (IVUS) techniques, drug eluting stents and distal embolic protection devices to deliver good outcomes for its patients.

Pacemaker or Automated Implantable Cardiovascular Defibrillator (AICD) Implantation

Patients with abnormal heart rhythms, which cause significant symptoms or those who are at risk of a more serious arrhythmia or arrhythmia complications may need to undergo a pacemaker or AICD implantation to help to restore their heart rhythm.

Coronary Artery Bypass Graft Surgery (CABG)

CABG is carried out to restore the flow of blood to areas of the heart where the coronary arteries have become blocked. This is done by using healthy blood vessels from another part of the body such as the arm, leg or chest wall. They are then surgically re-attached to bypass the diseased artery such that the blood can flow beyond the blocked artery. The procedure can be performed conventionally or, in selected cases, using minimally invasive techniques.

Valve Repair and Replacement Surgery

A valve that is not functioning correctly can be repaired or replaced. During the surgical repair of valve defects, the valve leaflets are reconstructed so that they can close properly. For badly damaged valves, the valve leaflets are replaced with an artificial valve. The depth and breadth of the experience of NHC surgeons with a broad variety of cases allows them to handle these more complex operations with success rates comparable to top international standards.

Thoracic Surgery

General thoracic surgery, including state-of-the-art, minimally invasive surgery, is done at NHC. Surgical procedures encompass all aspects of the disease spectrum in the chest cavity. NHC is also the first centre in Singapore to offer such comprehensive care in surgery, radiotherapy and chemotherapy in conjunction with the NCCS. In addition, NHC also provides emergency trauma care to patients with chest injuries.

SERVICES AT A GLANCE

Investigative Procedures	*Medical Therapeutic Procedures*	*Surgical Procedures*
• Ambulatory Blood Pressure Monitoring • Ambulatory Electrocardiogram (Holter monitoring) • Cardiovascular Magnetic Resonance Imaging (CVMRI) • Chest X-Ray • Duplex Ultrasound (Vascular Investigation) • Echocardiography (Stress Transoesophageal Echo) • Electrocardiogram (ECG) • Exercise Stress Treadmill Test • Multi-Slice Computed Tomography (MSCT) • Myocardial Biopsies • Nuclear Stress/Rest Perfusion Scans • Rest-redistribution Thallium Imaging • Rest Gated Blood Pool Scans • Signal-averaged ECG (SA-ECG) • Transtelephonic ECG • Upright Tilt Test	• Coronary Angiography/ Cardiac Catheterization • Electrophysiological Study • Intraaortic Balloon Counterpulsation • Intravascular Ultrasound Imaging • Pacemaker/Lead Extraction • Percutaneous Balloon Valvuloplasty of Mitral, Aortic and Pulmonary Valves • Percutaneous Cardiopulmonary Bypass • Percutaneous Coronary Intervention (PCI)—Angioplasty, Stent Implantation and Rotablator Treatment • Percutaneous Device Closure of Atrial Septal Defect (ASD) and Patent Foramen Ovale (PFO) • Permanent Pacemaker, Biventricular Pacing and Implantable Cardioverter-Defibrillators (ICD) Implantations • Pressure Wire Measurement • Radiofrequency Ablation of Atrial Fibrillation and Other Arrhythmias Rotational Coronary Atherectomy	• Abdominal Aortic Aneurysm Surgery • Binventricular Assist Device (BIVAD) • Complete Muscle Sparing Thoracotomy • Congenital Heart Disease Surgery • Drainage of Empyema • Endoscopic Vein Harvest • Endovascular Stent Graft Surgery for Aortic Aneurysms • Extra-Corporeal Membrane Oxygenation (ECMO) for acute cardio r espiratory failure • Heart Transplantation • Left Ventricular Assist Device (LVAD) • Left Ventricular Reconstructive Surgery (Dor or Saver Surgery) • Lung Cancer Multi-Modality Therapy (Complete workup and full consultation with oncology and pulmonology consultants, prior to surgical treatment) • Lung Reaction for Cancer of the Lung • Lung Transplantation for Advanced Lung Disease • Lung Volume Reduction Surgery (LVRS) for Chronic Obstructive Pulmonary Disease (COPD) • Maze Surgery for Atrial Fibrillation

- Mediastinoscopy for Staging of Lung Cancer
- Minimally Invasive (Endoscopic) Thoracic Sympathectomy
- Off-pump-Beating Heart Surgery
- Peripheral Vascular Arterial Surgery
- Repair of Pectus Excavatum
- Resection and Reconstruction of Chest Wall Tumour including Locally Advanced Breast Cancer
- Resection of Mediastinal Tumours
- Robotic-Assisted Surgery
- Surgery for Acute and Chronic Arterial Disorders
- Thoracic and Thoraco Abdominal Aorta Surgery
- Total Oesophagectomy for Cancer of Oesophagus/Other Disorders
- Trachea-resection and Reconstruction
- Valvular Heart Surgery including Valve Repair and Replacement Surgery
- VATS Pleurodesis for Spontaneous Pneumothorax
- VATS Thymectomy for Myasthenia Gravis
- Video-Assisted Thoracoscopic Surgery (VATS)

CARDIAC INVESTIGATIVE PROCEDURES

There is a wide range of investigations available to determine if there is heart disease, the type of disease if present, severity of the disease and the most appropriate treatment.

Investigative Procedures

- Ambulatory Blood Pressure Monitoring
- Ambulatory Electrocardiogram (Holter monitoring)
- Cardiovascular Magnetic Resonance Imaging (CVMRI)
- Chest X-ray
- Duplex Ultrasound (Vascular Investigation)
- Echocardiography (Stress, Transoesophageal Echo)
- Electrocardiogram (ECG)
- Exercise Stress Treadmill Test
- Multi-Slice Computed Tomography (MSCT)
- Myocardial Biopsies
- Nuclear Stress/Rest Perfusion Scans
- Rest and Exercise Gated Blood Pool Scans
- Rest-redistribution Thallium Imaging
- Signal-averaged ECG (SA-ECG)
- Transtelephonic ECG
- Upright Tilt Test

CARDIAC INTERVENTIONAL AND SURGICAL PROCEDURES

Coronary heart disease, heart failure and arrhythmias (abnormal heart rhythms) can be managed. They range from medical therapy, interventional procedures to open-heart surgeries.

Interventional Procedures

- Coronary Angiography/Cardiac Catheterisation
- Percutaneous Coronary Intervention (PCI)—Angioplasty, Stent Implantation and Rotablator Treatment
- Percutaneous Device Closure of Atrial Septal Defect (ASD) and Patent Foramen Ovale (PFO)
- Percutaneous Balloon Valvuloplasty of Mitral, Aortic and Pulmonary Valves
- Intraaortic Balloon Counterpulsation
- Intravascular Ultrasound Imaging
- Pressure Wife Measurement
- Percutaneous Cardiopulmonary Bypass
- Rotational Coronary Atherectomy

Electrophysiology and Pacing Procedures

- Electrophysiological Study
- Pacemaker/Lead Extraction
- Permanent Pacemaker, Biventricular Pacing and Implantable Cardioverter-Defibrillators (ICD) Implantations
- Radiofrequency Ablation of Atrial Fibrillation and Other Arrhythmias

Cardiac Surgery

- Conventional Coronary Artery Bypass Graft Surgery
- Off-pump/Beating Heart Surgery
- Congenital Heart Disease Surgery
- Maze Surgery for Atrial Fibrillation
- Left Ventricular Reconstructive Surgery (Dor or Saver Surgery)
- Heart Transplantation
- Valvular Heart Surgery including Valve Repair and Replacement Surgery
- Robotic-Assisted Surgery
- Endoscopic Vein Harvest

Thoracic Surgery

- Complete Muscle Sparing Thoracotomy
- Video-Assisted Thoracoscopic Surgery (VATS)
- Drainage of Empyema
- Lung Resection for Cancer of the Lung
- Lung Transplantation for Advanced Lung Disease
- Lung Volume Reduction Surgery (LVRS)for Chronic
- Obstructive Pulmonary Disease (COPD)
- Mediastinoscopy for Staging of Lung Cancer
- Minimally Invasive (Endoscopic) Thoracic Sympathectomy
- VATS Pleurodesis for Spontaneous Pneumothorax
- Resection and Reconstruction of Chest Wall Tumour including Locally Advanced Breast Cancer
- Resection of Mediastinal Tumours
- Total Oesophagectomy for Cancer of Oesophagus/Other Disorders
- VATS Thymectomy for Myasthenia Gravis
- Trachea-resection and Reconstruction
- Repair of Pectus Excavatum

Aortic and Peripheral Vascular Surgery

- Abdominal Aortic Aneurysm Surgery

- Peripheral Vascular Arterial Surgery
- Thoracic and Thoraco Abdominal Aorta Surgery
- Surgery for Acute and Chronic Arterial Disorders
- Endovascular Stent Graft Surgery for Aortic Aneurysms

Mechanical Heart Assist Device

- Left Ventricular Assist Device (LVAD)
- Biventricular Assist Device (BIVAD)
- Extra-Corporeal Membrane Oxygenation (ECMO) for Acute Cardio Respiratory Failure

Lung Cancer Multi-Modality Therapy

- Complete workup and full consultation with oncology and pulmonology consultants, prior to surgical treatment.

Many investigative tests are available today to diagnose heart or vascular disease. NHC has the latest equipment and experienced doctors to make reliable diagnoses and recommend the most appropriate treatment for the patients.

Multi-Slice Coronary Tomography Angiogram (MSCT)

This is a non-invasive 3D heart imaging test that helps determine whether either fatty or calcium deposits have built up in the coronary arteries, which supply blood to the heart muscle. This test has been found to be particularly useful in asymptomatic patients with higher risk for coronary disease, patients with atypical symptoms but at lower risks of coronary disease, or patients with unclear stress-test results.

Electrophysiological Study (EPS) and Catheter Ablation

EPS is a specialised technique where electrical catheters are introduced percutaneously to the heart to study irregular heartbeats called arrhythmias. This will determine the exact cause of the arrhythmia and help decide on the best treatment option. In suitable cases, catheter ablation can be performed. This uses the catheter to locate the abnormal focus or circuits and these can then be destroyed by radiofrequency energy, curing the patient of his arrhythmia permanently.

Cardiac Catheterisationl Coronary Angiography

Cardiac catheterisation is a procedure where a catheter is introduced into the heart via peripheral arteries or veins. The catheter is passed into the chambers of the heart to get detailed information about the heart and coronary arteries.

Coronary angiography is a procedure that uses a special dye (contrast medium) and x-rays to see how blood flows through the heart. It is usually done in conjunction with cardiac catheterisation.

NHC sees patients with heart problems ranging from narrowed coronary arteries, congenital heart disease, angina, abnormal heart rhythm, valvular heart disease and heart failure. The doctor will prescribe the most appropriate treatment strategy. This could range from medical therapy to interventional or surgical procedures to treat their underlying heart disease.

Percutaneous Coronary Intervention—Coronary Angioplasty and Stenting

This treatment for severe blockages of the coronary arteries reopens narrowed coronary arteries using special devices such as balloon catheters and stents. Often stents are placed into area where the blockage occurs to keep the artery from narrowing again.

NHC performs a high volume of complex multi-vessel angioplasty procedures using special devices such as intravascular ultrasound (IVUS) techniques, drug eluting stents and distal embolic protection devices to deliver good outcomes for its patients.

Pacemaker Implantation

Patients with abnormally slow heart rhythm can result in recurrent giddiness or fainting. Such patients require a permanent pacemaker which will then prevent the heart from stopping.

Implantable Cardioverter Defibrillator (ICD) Implantation

Patients with abnormal heart rhythms can cause significant symptoms or sudden death. The ICD is able to detect this and treat the patient immediately thus preventing the patient from dying suddenly from an arrhythmia.

Coronary Artery Bypass Graft Surgery (CABG)

CABG is carried out to restore the flow of blood to areas of the heart where the coronary arteries have become blocked. This is done by using healthy blood vessels from another part of the body such as the arm, leg or chest wall. They are then surgically re-attached to bypass the diseased artery such that the blood can flow beyond the blocked artery. The procedure can be performed conventionally or, in selected cases, using minimally invasive techniques.

Valve Repair and Replacement Surgery

A valve that is not functioning correctly can be repaired or replaced. During the surgical repair of valve defects, the valve leaflets are reconstructed so that they can close properly. For valves which are badly damaged, the valve leaflets are replaced with an artificial valve.

The depth and breadth of the experience of NHC surgeons with a broad variety of cases allows them to handle these more complex operations with success rates comparable to top international standards.

REMOTE ACCESS TO CARDIAC TOMOGRAPHY (CT) REPORTS

NHC has launched the 64-slice Toshiba Aquilion Multidetector Computed Tomography (CD, which features ViTAL Connect, a first in Southeast Asia outside Japan, at its facility.

ViTALConnect is a web-based diagnostic tool that allows access and analysis of clinical images at multiple locations. This means that the clinicians can access not only CT reports but manipulate real time CT data from a remote location with just a standard laptop computer and a secured internet connection. This greatly improves our workflow efficiency as it cuts down the need for doctors to travel between hospitals and departments.

Dr. Terrance Chua, Deputy Director and Head of Department of Cardiology at NHC comments, ViTALConnect gives us the capability to confer with the entire medical team at the same time. I can be at home or even in the US, and still be able to access patients' CT information by simply logging onto a Web address.

The 64-slice Toshiba Aquilion Multidetector CT is also the first 64-slice CT system with 350ms rotation in South East Asia, providing better temporal resolution (12.5% faster than other sites).

The other advantages of the Toshiba Aquilion54 includes:

- Quantam detector design delivers 54 simultaneous acquired 0.5 mm thin slices. This translates to improved clarity and resolution of scanned images.
- 64-slice data acquisition in cardiac scans; this implies that the entire heart can be covered in a few heartbeats.
- 3D-CTA of the arterial vascular system without venous contamination is assured.
- Provides up to 40 msec temporal resolution. This translates into faster scan speed, clearer and more accurate images.
- The 1.8 m scannable range accommodates scanning of trauma patients without the need to reposition.
- The sure Technologies are specifically designed to provide the best image quality at the lowest possible x-ray dose.

Dr. Cheah Foong Koon, Acting Head for Cardiac Radiology at NHC says, "Cardiac CT is an advanced imaging service that requires the hybrid specialized knowledge of imaging techniques and cardiovascular anatomy and physiology. In this particular collaboration, we are glad to be able to combine the expertise of these two disciplines—cardiology and radiology—for the benefit of patients, in terms of more accurate diagnosis leading to better treatment and management plans."

Accurate Cardiac Imaging at the NHC

The Nuclear Cardiology Laboratory of the National Heart Centre recently acquired a new gamma camera capable of reducing scanning time without loss of image quality. The CardioMD (Philips Corporation) is a cardiac-specific gamma camera with a small footprint that saves space, causes less claustrophobia and is more patient friendly.

Recent developments in the nuclear imaging community have improved the image quality of nuclear scans as well as reduced the time taken to acquire these images. The development of this Wide Beam Reconstruction (WBR) has opened doorway to improved resolution and cutting the acquisition time by up to half.

Proprietary software development by Alilips Medical Systems (Astonish) has been shown to improve image quality and reduce scanning time by reducing the total counts required, because of reduced signal-to-noise ratios.

Astonish uses an iterative 3D Ordered Subset Expectation Maximum (3D-OSEM) algorithm which has built-in correction for resolution recovery, scatter and attenuation correction. This has been shown in both phantom and clinical studies to improve resolution without compromise to quality. Future directions for this new equipment would be to perform fusion cardiology, whereby functional imaging will be incorporated into anatomical imaging by coronary CT Angiography.

Our initial experience with the new equipment and software is encouraging. We have performed standard imaging, and both half-time and half-frame imaging utilizing the Astonish software in over 50 patients. The results have been good, giving the interpreter more confidence in reporting the images. It is envisaged that this new equipment will result in improved through-put time, patient compliance and comfort and improved accuracy in data interpretation.

THE SURGICAL TREATMENTS FOR ISCHEMIC HEART (STICH) TRIAL

The STICH trial is a multi-centre international randomized trial sponsored by NIH (National Institutes of Health), USA.

The aim of the trial is to determine the optimal treatment of patients with coronary artery disease and poor heart function (LVEF <35%). It is especially pertinent in this day and age as it has been more than 20 years since the last randomized trial of surgical treatment for heart failure [the landmark Coronary Artery Surgery Study (CASS)]. Since then, there has been a lot of advances in the medical treatment of heart failure (e.g. aspirin, statin therapy, ACE inhibitors, new generation beta blockers, etc.).

There is some observational data from the CASS registry that inpatients with poor heart function and predominantly heart failure symptoms, the long-term survival in the medically treated and surgically treated patients may not be different. However, there other studies that suggested otherwise (e.g. Duke University database).

The current literature on the optimal treatment for patients with coronary artery disease and poor heart function with heart failure is mostly retrospective, single-centre based or underpowered with too few patients. With the number of heart failure patients reaching epidemic proportions, it is apparent that some modern evidence-based guidelines be developed for the treatment of this group of patients and hence a large multi-centre randomized trial like STICH is extremely important.

There are two hypotheses that the trial aims to examine.

Hypothesis 1—the coronary revascularization hypothesis—postulates that coronary revascularization and intensive medical therapy improves the long-term survival versus intensive medical therapy alone. The surgical ventricular reconstruction hypothesis—Hypothesis 2—is that inpatients with anterior akinesia, left ventricular shape and size optimization by surgical ventricular restoration plus coronary artery bypass grafting plus intensive medical therapy improves long-term survival. This *versus* coronary artery bypass grafting and intensive medical therapy without surgical ventricular reconstruction.

The patients recruited were divided into three strata; stratum A—patients eligible for medical treatment and ineligible for surgical ventricular restoration, stratum B—patients eligible for medical treatment and surgical ventricular restoration, and stratum C—patients who were ineligible for medical treatment and eligible for surgical ventricular reconstruction (see attached table). The other secondary endpoints examined in the study include cardiac morbidity, resource utilization, quality of life and exercise capacity.

There are also secondary hypothesis on whether cardiac imaging to assess the amount of ischaemic myocardium would identify patients who would benefit from myocardial revascularization. The trial design was such that 2800 patients were to be recruited from 90 centres in 15 countries over a 3-year period, and each patient was to be followed up for 4 years.

STICH trial enrollment was completed on 4 May 2007. 2,136 patients were recruited from 127 centres in 26 countries over 1,584 days. NHC was ranked 29 out of the 127 participating centres in terms of number of patients recruited.

In fact, NHC recruited the 781st patient in the CABG arm of the trial on 1 June 2006 which meant that STICH trial became the largest surgically treated heart failure trial in history, exceeding the number of patients recruited in the landmark CASS trial.

NHC was awarded a bronze award for patient recruitment in the STICH trial and was the country that recruited the most patients in South East Asia.

Dr. Chua Yeow Leng, Dr. Lim Chong Hee, Dr. Tan Teing Ee and Dr. Tan Ru San were appointed to the Hypothesis 1 working group of the STICH trial. We look forward to the conclusion of the trial in 4 to 5 years' time when the follow-up period would have been completed and the evidence provided would be substantial to guide treatment selection to this group of patients.

It will have a significant impact for us as it has been estimated 60,000 Singaporeans suffer from heart failure (with the commonest cause being coronary artery disease) and it has a prevalence of 6-8% of patients above the age of 65.

PERCUTANEOUS AORTIC VALVE IMPLANTATION

What is Aortic Valve Stenosis?

The aortic valve controls the direction of blood flow from the left ventricle to the aorta. When in good working order, the aortic valve does not impede the flow of blood between these two spaces. Under some circumstances, the aortic valve becomes narrower than normal, impeding the blood flow. This is known as aortic valve stenosis, or aortic stenosis.

Causes

The common causes of aortic stenosis include degeneration (aging process) and bicuspid aortic valve. As individuals age, calcification of the aortic valve may occur and result in stenosis. This is especially likely to occur in people with a bicuspid aortic valve, and even in those with perfectly normal valves, due to age-induced 'wear and tear'. Typically, aortic stenosis due to calcification of a bicuspid valve occurs in people in their 40s-50s, whereas that due to calcification of a normal valve tends to occur later—in people of age 70s-80s.

Aortic stenosis is a common problem. Approximately 2% of people over the age of 65, 3% of people over age 75, and 4% percent of people over age 85 have the disorder.

Symptoms and Treatment

Patients with mild or moderate degrees of aortic stenosis are often asymptomatic. When the disease progresses to the point when the patient starts to have symptoms such as angina, syncope or heart failure, the prognosis of the patient with medical therapy alone is poor. For such patients, surgical aortic valve replacement (AVR) provides dramatic improvements in symptoms and life expectancy.

Unfortunately, many patients with severe aortic stenosis do not undergo surgery, despite proven benefits of this therapy. Such patients frequently have multiple medical problems, such as advanced age, renal failure and calcified aorta, which increase the morbidity and mortality associated with surgery. Balloon aortic valvuloplasty (ballooning of the aortic valve) was developed in the 1980sas an alternative treatment. Although this technique provided relief of symptoms, the results were not durable, and its current role is mainly for palliation or as a bridge to definitive surgery.

A percutaneous (without open heart surgery) alternative to surgical valve replacement was first explored in an animal model by Andersen *et al.* It was not until 10 years later in 2002 that the feasibility of percutaneous AVR was demonstrated in humans by Cribier *et al.* using a transvenous transseptal approach.

Currently, there are two devices in the market for use in humans: The Edwards Lifesciences Edwards-Sapien Transcatheter Heart Valve (Fig. 1), a stainless steel balloon-expandable device which can be deployed from the transapical and transfemoral (transarterial, retrograde) approaches. The other device is the CoreValve (Fig. 2) which is a nitinol self-expandable device, currently deployed via the transfemoral approach, and very recently the transapical approach.

Successful percutaneous aortic valve implantation was associated with a significant improvement in the left ventricular function, and functional class (symptom status). Improvements were sustained at mid-term follow up (2-3 years) Importantly, the lack of late valve failure during clinical and serial echocardiographic follow suggests durability sufficient to offer significant benefit.

Conventional open heart surgery remains the first-line therapy for symptomatic aortic stenosis. However, percutaneous valve replacement is a viable alternative to conventional open heart surgery in selected high-risk patients with severe symptomatic aortic stenosis, We hope to make this technology available in the near future to Singaporeans.

PERIPHERAL ARTERIAL DISEASE

Peripheral arterial disease (PAD) is a major cause of limb loss in Singapore. However it does not receive as much attention as diseases involving the other vascular beds: namely, coronary artery disease and cerebrovascular disease. Yet it is a good predictor of heart attack and stroke risk.

How does PAD develop?

PAD develops when arteries in the legs become clogged with plaque—such as fatty deposits and cholesterol—that limits or completely blocks blood flow in the legs. This causes muscle pain in the calves, thighs, and buttocks.

Like atherosclerosis, PAD is caused by the buildup of fatty deposits—called plaque—in the arteries. Having blocked arteries can keep oxygen-rich blood from reaching the muscles when they need it most. This lack of oxygen causes the pain. PAD can increase your risk of heart attack and stroke. But the good news is that PAD can be easy to diagnose and is treatable.

With pain limiting their movements, the patients move gradually from an active lifestyle to a sedentary one. This results in immobility and a shorter life expectancy due to the increased risk of high blood pressure, heart attack, and stroke.

The risk factors for PAD include hypertension, high cholesterol, and diabetes—all of which are common illnesses in our population. One-third of diabetics over the age of 50 develop the disease.

Another high-risk activity, such as smoking, brings on the disease much sooner. So PAD patients, who otherwise would be in their late 70s or 80s, could start to feel symptoms as early as their 50s or 60s.

Symptoms and Treatment

The symptom involves intermittent claudication, or momentary limping because of pain. For example, when a patient with a blockage in his leg walks 100 metres, he starts developing pain in the calf muscle of the affected leg. He stops and rests for a few minutes; the pain goes away and he can go another 100 metres before it comes on again.

In the most extreme cases, if left unchecked, it can cause ulcers, gangrene, and amputation.

One way to prevent that is by checking their ankle and arm pressures during routine clinic consultations, which should be the same. The ankle-brachial index (ABI) is calculated by dividing ankle pressures by arm pressures. A value of 0.9 to 1 is normal. If it comes back as 0.5, that implies that the patient has significant disease.

Specific management of PAD involves:

1. *Lifestyle changes*: These include quit smoking; eating a balanced diet that is high in fibre and low in cholesterol, fat and sodium; and exercise.
2. Management of other related health problems, such as high blood pressure, diabetes or high cholesterol.
3. Practice good foot and skin care to prevent infection and reduce the risk of complications.
4. *Medications*: Medications may be recommended to treat conditions such as high blood pressure (anti-hypertensive medications) or high cholesterol (statin medications). An antiplatelet medication such as aspirin or clopidogrel (Plavix) may be prescribed to reduce the risk of heart attack and stroke.
5. *Intervention*: More advanced PAD can be treated with interventional procedures such as angioplasty (to widen or clear the blocked vessel), angioplasty with stent placement (to support the cleared vessel and keep it open), or atherectomy (to remove the blockage). In some cases, surgical procedures such as peripheral artery bypass surgery may be performed to re-route blood flow around the blood vessel blockage.

Despite the availability of health care in Singapore, PAD is still "under-diagnosed" for several reasons. One being that checking the arm and ankle pressures is not as routine as it should be.

In the US, the determination to increase awareness has recently led to Increased training for vascular medicine specialists for routine ankle-brachial check-ups and early detection for treatment.

The goal of therapy is to improve blood supply to their leg muscles so that patients maintain their functional level of activity. Once patients become couch potatoes, it's hard to get them off the couch. They need to be kept active to maintain their health.

Services at NHC Vascular Lab

NHC Vascular Laboratory is equipped with two state-of-the-art duplex ultrasound machines to provide diagnostic services for patients from the wards and outpatient clinics. Apart from the peripheral vascular system (veins and arteries) of the limbs, examination of the carotid arteries, renal arteries, and abdominal aorta can also be carried out. The laboratory also conducts graft surveillance of venous fistulae and peripheral reconstructive surgery.

AUTOMATIC IMPLANTABLE CARDIOVERTER DEFIBRILLATOR

The Past

The concept for an Automatic Implantable Cardioverter Defibrillator (AICD) was first conceived by Dr. M. Mirowski in 1966 in Israel, when his friend and colleague, Professor Harry Heller who was diagnosed with recurrent ventricular tachycardia, died from sudden cardiac death two weeks after diagnosis. It was not until 4 February 1980 that the first AICD was implanted in a human being at the Johns Hopkins Hospital. The first patient was a 57-year old woman with documented coronary artery disease. She had a history of acute myocardial infarction and recurrent syncope with documented ventricular fibrillation and had failed multiple drug testings. The procedure was performed under general anaesthesia, required a thoracotomy and performed by the surgeon, Dr. LeviWatkins. The original defibrillation leads were epicardial patches that were sutured to the outer surface of the heart with the pulse generator implanted in the abdomen. The device was successfully implanted without complications. Eventually, in 1985, the Food and Drug Administration (FDA) approved the AICD for commercial sale in the United States.

The Present

The invention of the transvenous defibrillation lead along with the downsizing of the pulse generator allow for AICD implants to be performed less invasively, thereby enhancing patient safety and reducing the convalescent time. Currently, AICD is performed by cardiologists and no longer requires a thoracotomy. The procedure is performed under sedation with the pulse generator implanted prepectorally in the left infraclavicular region and the defibrillator lead implanted transvenously and anchored in the right ventricular apex. Defibrillation threshold testing may be performed prior to wound closure. The total procedure time ranges from 1-2 hours and the patient is discharged the following day.

Indications for AICD have also evolved radically from its initial implantation inpatients with resuscitated cardiac arrest and expanded to implantation in individuals who are at risk for developing sudden cardiac arrest but have not yet had ventricular tachycardia, ventricular fibrillation or resuscitated cardiac arrest. Data for the use of AICD as a primary prevention therapy in multiple patient populations is robust. The landmark

MADIT II trial in 2002 demonstrated a relative risk reduction of 31% in all cause mortality inpatients with chronic ischaemic heart disease and used only ejection fraction (of less than 30%) as the main determinant of risk of sudden cardiac death. The SCD-HeFTtrial also similarly demonstrated a mortality benefit inpatients who are on optimal medical therapy with mild to moderate heart failure. It showed a 23% reduction in all cause mortality in the cohort of patients with AICD implanted when compared to the cohort without AICD implanted.

At the National Heart Centre Singapore, there has been more than 320 AICD implanted since 1999. In the last five years, there has been a consistent 10 per cent increase in the number of implants performed year on year. In addition to the conventional indications for AICD implant, we also offer AICD implant as an electronic bridge to heart transplant inpatients who are already on the waiting list so as to better their chances of acquiring a heart. Other more unconventional sites of AICD lead insertion such as placement of the AICD lead via a transilliac approach may be offered to patients with a combination of vascular access problem, and in those where an epicardial lead is not a viable option.

The Future

Many exciting developments are occurring in the field of AICD development. In particular, the two eagerly anticipated forefronts are that of remote monitoring and leadless AICD. The remote monitoring system allows for unidirectional communication between the device and the clinician so that details such as battery status and recent therapy deliveries can be sent to the clinician via the use of home-based transmitters or phone lines. Patients thus no longer need to make frequent trips to the clinician's office. In a leadless ICD system, there would no longer be transvenous insertion of the defibrillating lead. Instead the defibrillating lead is introduced subcutaneously. This reduces complications that arise as a result of the transvenous lead such as lead fracture and subclavian vein thrombosis. Anticipated advancements in the electronic components, memory storage abilities and capacitor technology also would create smaller devices that are more automatic with more storage data yet longer lasting.

References

Chiam PT, Ruiz CE. Percutaneous Transcatheter Aortic Valve Implantation—Assessing Results, Judging Outcomes and Planning Trials: The Interventionalist Perspective. *J Am Coll Cardiol Interv* 2008 Aug (in press).

Cribier A, Eltchaninoff H, Bash A, *et al.* Percutaneous transcatheter implantation of an aortic valve prosthesis for calcific aortic stenosis: first human case description. *Circulation* 2002; 106: 3006-8.

Eltchaninoff H, Tron C, Bauer F, *et al.* [Aortic bioprosthesis implanted percutaneously: three year follow up]. *Arch Mal Coeur Vaiss* 2007; 100: 901, 904-8.

Ruiz CE, Laborde JC, Condado JF, Chiam PT, Condado JA. First Percutaneous Transcatheter Aortic Valve-in-Valve Implant with Three Year Follow Up. Catheter Cardiovasc Interv 2008 Aug 1; 72(2): 143-8.

APPENDIX 2 *(Contd.)*

C. SINGAPORE NATIONAL EYE CENTRE

INTRODUCTION

The Singapore National Eye Centre (SNEC) is becoming a referral centre for cornea transplants, especially difficult ones.

Last mouth, a Canadian boy who had lost one eye to a rare disorder of the body's mucous membranes, called Stevens-Johnson syndrome, and who was close to losing the other one, came here and had a successful transplant.

A man from Thailand, who was unable to get rid of an eye infection which had baffled doctors there and in the United States, also turned to Singapore.

One reason for their seeking treatment here: the SNEC is one of a handful of places in the world that is focusing on a new kind of cornea transplant, whereby only part of the cornea is replaced.

Professor Donald Tan, its deputy director and director of the Singapore Eye Research Institute, says the new lamellar transplant gives better vision with lower risk of rejection.

There are two types of lamellar transplants—one changes only the top and the other the bottom layer of the cornea. If only the top layer *is* changed, there is almost zero risk of rejection, said Prof. Tan.

There is a 10 to 40 per cent risk of rejection in a normal cornea transplant. When only the bottom layer is changed, the top is kept intact and no stitching is needed to keep the transplant in place. This allows for faster recovery and lower rates of astigmatism, or blurriness.

Lamellar transplants are more challenging and take twice as long to do, said Prof. Tan, but the results justify the extra work.

More than 200 cornea transplants are carried out in Singapore in a year. About two-thirds of the donated corneas come from overseas.

Most of the operations are carried out at the SNEC. Last year, it did 194 transplants, up from 168 in 2005. A third of the patients were foreign. Lamellar transplants accounted for 26 per cent of its transplants u/l 2005, but Increased to 42 per cent last year.

For the past three years, Prof. Tan has been running courses on such transplants in the United States, and will do another one this year. Eye specialists from around the work I are also corning to Singapore to learn this and other techniques.

Dr. Jerry Tan, an eye specialist in private practice who carried out eight cornea transplants last year, described lamellar as still very new with no long-term outcomes.

But someone has to blaze the trail and "people like Donald are needed to do these very brave heroic procedures," he said.

There are very few doctors in the world who call do it well, Dr. Tan said adding that it was not something for which the private sector was geared up.

Such "experimental" techniques are best done in an institutional setting which are better at dealing with complications should they arise.

Another "experimental" technique which Prof. Tan pioneered here is to insert part of a blind patient's tooth into his eye to give him some vision. Since the first case involving a Thai youth in 2004, 19 patients two Singaporeans and 17 foreigners—have successfully regained their sight this way, with two more on the waiting list.

Prof. Tan has been asked by other eye specialists to form an Asian Corneal Society to be based in Singapore, to promote clinical standards, research and education in cornea transplants and eye-banking. Ophthalmologists from India, China, Japan, Taiwan, Korea, Thailand, the Philippines and Australia will gather here early this year for its inaugural meeting.

PRESBYOPIA TREATED

Those with presbyopia might now find a new and permanent solution to their condition—if they want to participate in a global clinical trial that is being conducted in Singapore.

Presbyopia usually affects those 40 years old and above and is commonly referred to in Mandarin as "lau hua yan" as the eye loses the ability to focus on near objects with age. The crystalline lens in the eye loses elasticity over time making focusing difficult.

The Singapore National Eye Centre (SNEC) now offers what appears to be the only effective treatment so far for the condition—the AcuFocus Corneal Inlay (ACI). Results so far have shown it to be effective with high patient satisfaction, says Chan Wing Kwong, senior consultant and head of Refractive Surgery at SNEC.

The current solution is Lasik, which does not provide satisfactory results and frequently causes distortions in vision.

Dr. Chan describes ACI as "revolutionary and ground-breaking."

The technique uses a simple optical phenomenon—the "pin-hole effect." A doughnut-shaped disc is implanted under the cornea of the eye to create a smaller aperture for light to enter the eye, thereby increasing the depth of field of vision.

The procedure does not involve tissue removal and takes a total of five minutes. Improvement in vision is immediate.

In fact, Dr. Chan notes that visual quality continues improving over time as the patient adjusts to the implant. Also, it need only be done in the dominant eye as the other one will adapt.

Twenty-four patients who have had the implant for three months already can now read words 1 mm high, better than what they saw with reading glasses.

Some side-effects include dimmer vision and slightly narrower visual field. Slight deterioration of far vision also occurs. But it is difficult for the patient to observe these changes, Dr. Chan said.

The treatment is expected to be commercially available in Singapore by 2009. It is estimated to cost between S$1,300 and S$1,900 per eye, comparable to the cost of Lasik, although patients can't use Medisave to pay for it as yet.

SNEC is the only trial centre for the ACI in Asia. It has 35 patients so far and is looking to enrol more.

CYTOMEGALOVIRUS IRITIS

You may suffer from inflamed, irritated eyes and be prescribed eye drops to sooth your woes. Such a condition used to be diagnosed as Iritis. And while some are acute, erupting suddenly, many patients would have chronic inflammation of the eye for years.

A Singapore National Eye Centre (SNEC) study has discovered that a common virus may be causing the condition.

The centre's head of Ocular Inflammation and Immunology Service, Associate Professor Chee Soon Phaik, found that 41.7 per cent of patients who suffer from iritis are infected with the cytomegalovirus, which—up till recently—had been associated with HIV-patients who are prone to retinal infections.

"We used to just see infections in the retina until we saw a chronic infection in the cornea," said Assoc Prof. Chee.

Many such patients also have iritis. But it was only in 2003 when the first iritis patient tested positive for cytomegalovirus that a worrying trend started to emerge.

Since then, Assoc Prof. Chee has seen 70 cases of iritis patients testing positive for cytomegalovirus. Of these, 40 per cent—who are usually in their 20s and 30s—have acute iritis, which may develop into glaucoma. The rest—typically males over 57 years old—have chronic iritis.

While not debilitating, patients with the infection are normally prescribed steroid eye drops, which have been found to aggravate the situation, requiring a transplant later.

Treatment for cytomegalovirus is expensive, with non-subsidized antiviral drugs costing some $200 per tablet. In three months, a patient can spend as much as $11,000.

Still, the rate of relapse is 75 per cent.

SNEC's 70 patients are still undergoing treatment, and the centre is pioneering research on such infections and its treatment.

Currently, there have been a few case studies of cytomegalovirus of the eye worldwide and data suggests that Asians are more prone it.

SURGERY TELECAST

Singapore took another step to becoming one of Asia's top eye centres yesterday, with a live telecast of eye surgery to doctors at Aravind Eyecare System, India's largest eyecare provider.

Also sitting in on the two-hour transmission were more than 40 eye doctors from Shanghai, who are on a study programme at the Singapore National Eye Centre (SNEC).

Associate Professor Donald Tan, director of the Singapore Eye-Research Institute and deputy director of the SNEC, did a corneal transplant with a new $500,000 state-of-the-art laser.

Prof. Tan said the laser cuts the cornea cleanly and this can make a significant difference in eyesight quality for the recipient. Hand-cut corneas tend to have slightly jagged edges.

Singapore does about 200 cornea transplants a year. The next tele-surgical conference, scheduled for next year, will show eye doctors here what the Indian eye centre is capable of.

Aravind, based in Tamil Nadu state, does 220,000 major eye operations a year, making it the biggest eyecare provider in India, and possibly the world, said SNBC director Ang Chong Lye.

The SNEC signed a memorandum of agreement with Aravind, that includes working together on research projects and treatment of glaucoma.

The SNEC is also working with German laser company 20/10 Perfect Vision to improve its laser equipment, Prof. Tan has asked for a laser machine that will enable surgeons to slice a 0.5 mm-thick cornea in half, so only the top or bottom half can be used. In 30 per cent of transplants, only the top layer of a cornea is needed. If a laser does a neat cornea slice, this 30 per cent can use just the top half and avoid rejection.

In the case of those who need just the bottom half, it can be slipped, under the existing top and avoid the need for stitches, which can distort the cornea. Replacing only the bottom layer also preserves nerves, ensuring continued sensation rather than eye numbness.

LARGE MOLE IN THE EYE OPERATED

- A young girl who once had a black mole covering almost the entire white of her left eye now looks just fine.
- Doctors took stem cells from 10-year-old Mercy Mohen's own eye, grew them in the laboratory and created a patch to repair her damaged conjunctiva, the thin surface layer of the eye.
- The Singapore doctors are the first in the world to harvest the stem cells—master cells that can replicate them.
- They have filed a patient for their pioneering effort, which they had used to help Mercy, who was born with the mole.
- She could see, but doctors were worried because the mole was growing into the cornea, the transparent part of the eye in front of the eyeball.
- Until recently, she could not have had her mole removed as it wuld have left too much of her eye raw and exposed.
- After the operation last year, Mercy kept looking at herself in the mirror, admiring her eye which now looks normal, said her father, Mr. Mohen Ambrose.

- The doctors who worked this miracle on her are from the Singapore Eye Research Institute (Seri).
- The method sounds deceptively simple. Doctors took a tiny amount of stem cells from the conjunctiva high up under Mercy's eyelid.
- In the laboratory, they grew these cells into a sheet over 100 times the size of the original bit of cells measuring about 2 sq. mm.
- After they removed the mole, they stitched this sheet over the exposed areas in the white of her eye.
- Head of the ophthalmology department at the National university of Singapore, said the conjunctiva stem cell technique has been used on 24 patients here in the past two years.
- But the technique is still on clinical trials and is not yet available to everyone.
- Most of the patients had fleshy growths covering their corneas, a common eye problem called pterygium.
- The third most common eye problem treated here, it affects on ein 10 people over the age of 40, though not all need surgery.
- If the growth covers a large part of the iris, or if it is fast growing, doctors would cut-off the growth and patch it up with conjunctiva from another part of the eye.
- Associate Professor Tan, said the results are optimistic, though the fleshy part regrows in about a third of the patients on the stem cell treatment.
- It recurs in 5 to 35 per cent of patients who are not on the stem-cell treatment.
- Nevertheless, this is a significant advance in the treatment of eye disease.
- The team hopes to have better outcomes in the future.
- They also hope to start work on growing retina from stem cells as well as bio-engineering various layers of the cornea for transplant.
- The retina lies at the back of the eye and translates what the eye sees to the brain.
- If they succeed, it could damaged corneas.
- The team, which hopes to publish its work in medical journals soon, will present their findings to about 600 eye specialists from 37 countries who will gather here next month for a four-day eye research meeting.
- Seri and the Association for Research in Vision and Opthalmology (Arvo) are organizing the Meeting on Research in Vision and Opthalmology jointly.
- Arvo meetings are considered the foremost eye research gatherings in the world, say eye doctors, and had never been held outside the United States before.

HIGHLIGHTS

SNEC HONOURED WITH THE PRESTIGIOUS MINISTER FOR HEALTH AWARD

- For drawing a link between fusarium keartitis (a rare fungal corenal infection) and the Bausch and Lomb Renu Moistureloc contact lens solution, a team of ophthalmologists and other health care professionals led by Prof. Donald Tan, Deputy Director, Singapore National Eye Centre (SNEC), were bestowed the first Minister for Health Award in July 2006.
- Comprising 16 experts from Singapore Eye Research Institute (SERI), Singapore General Hospital, the Ministry of Health, the Health Sciences Authority, Tan Tock Seng Hospital and National University Hospital, the team was the first in the world to point out the connection between the infection and the contact lens solution, braving controversy. This averted an epidemic of potentially blinding infections. Bausch and Lomb eventually recalled the product globally in May 2006.
- The clinicians received praise from the Minister for Health, Mr. Khaw Boon Wan, for their courage in taking the lead to sound the alert worldwide. Director of Medical Services, Ministry of Health, Prof. K Satkunanantham, also commended the clinicians for their alertness in identifying changes in the pattern of diseases.
- In the June 2006 issue of the Journal of the American Medical Association (JAMA), the teams' findings were published in an article: "An Outbreak for Fusarium Keratitis Associated with Contact Lens Wear in Singapore."

CELEBRATING A DECADE OF OUTSTANDING RESEARCH

- 2007 marked the 10th anniversary of SERI. Under the visionary guidance of the institute's founding director, the late A/Prof. Chew Sek Jin, and his successor, Prof. Donald Tan, SERI has grown from strength to strength and established a reputation of being the leading eye research centre in the region.
- The two directors had worked ceaselessly to secure grants and develop sophisticated laboratories and a research clinic, which now occupy two levels in the SNEC building. Today, SERI has some 30 laboratory based research staff and 39 researchers engaged in clinical research projects. It has also established a comprehensive network of clinician-researchers in affiliated institutions and hospitals in Singapore.
- Ongoing research alliances that SERI has forged with renowned international institutions include Johns Hopkins University in the US, Moorfields Eye Hospital in UK, Lions Eye Institute in Australia, and other collaborating centres in Asia.

- Going one step further to synergise international expertise on vision science research, SERI hosted the inaugural Asia-Association for Research in Vision and Ophthalmology (ARVO) meeting in 2007—a biennial meeting aimed at highlighting major basic science, clinical and translational aspects of vision and ophthalmic research. Previously held in Singapore in 2003 and 2005 under the banner of SERI-ARVO, the meeting has been renamed Asia-ARVO to reflect ARVO's commitment to partnering SERI and countries in Asia to raise awareness of vision and ophthalmic research.

ADVANCING INTER-COMMUNITY MEDICAL EFFORTS

In March 2007, Singapore National Eye Centre embarked on a landmark 3-Dimension High-Definition (3D-HD) telemedicine experimentation together with Asahikawa Medical College (AMC) of Hokkaido, and Chulalongkorn University Hospital in Bangkok. The experimentation featured the transmission of live ophthalmic surgery using transforming 3D-HD technology across three countries.

Earlier in June 2006, an international faculty led by Clinical A/Prof. Ong Sze Guan of SNEC and Prof. Akitoshi Yoshida of AMC performed complex surgery at the SNEC operating theatres which was transmitted live in 3D-HD to a record 1,500 ophthalmologists from nearly 50 countries attending the Asia-Pacific Academy of Ophthalmology congress at Suntec International Convention and Exhibition Centre, Singapore.

As one of the two principal investigators for this new technology experimentation, SNEC has contributed to Singapore's status as a international hub for ophthalmology.

In April 2006, SNEC launched its first publication entitled "Clinical Ophthalmology—An Asian Perspective." Co-authored by 69 SNEC faculty and collaborators from Harvard Medical School and the University of British Columbia, the book showcases SNEC's track record of clinical excellence and focuses on the diagnosis and treatment of major eye diseases in Asia. It contains gems from the cumulative experience of its ophthalmologists, clinician-scientists and researchers.

Award	Recipient(s)
Inaugural Minister for Health Award	SNEC, jointly with experts from six other health institutes
Work-Life Excellence Award 2006	SNEC
American Academy of Ophthalmology (Special Recognition Award)	Prof. Arthur Lim, Founding Medical Director and Emeritus Senior Consultant, SNEC
American Academy of Ophthalmology (Achievement Award)	Prof. Donald Tan
American Academy of Ophthalmology —Ophthalmic Photographers' Society Awards	SNEC Ophthalmic Photographers
GCEO Excellence Awards 2007	A/Prof. Wong Tien Yin, SNEC

THROUGH THE EYES OF LOVE

SNEC regularly initiates and participates in community projects as part of good corporate citizenry. SNEC became the first corporate charity of the Care Corner Family Service Centre (Queenstown) with the launch of the "Through the Eyes of Love" project. The Centre is combined to building resilience in families and individuals in times of crisis and difficulties and expanding their resources and coping abilities.

In December 2006, SNEC organized the 7th National Eye Care Day in conjunction with the eye departments of Changi General Hospital, Tan Tock Seng Hospital, National University Hospital and Jurong Medical Centre. More than 3,300 members of the public aged 45 years and above received free eye screening during the one-day event. The event continued to be a major educational initiative aimed to promote public awareness of common blinding conditions and the importance of preventive eye care.

SNEC also participated in the President's Challenge Health Relay 185. Our staff joined over 1,200 participants from other health care institutions to complete a 24-hour 185 km run to raise funds for the needy.

EDUCATION

Towards Better Eye Care

August 2006 saw the uniting of ophthalmology communities in ASEAN and Europe towards the advancement of ophthalmology, vision sciences, eye care and the management of eye hospitals and centres. This was brought about by a noteworthy Memorandum of Understanding signed between the ASEAN Association of Eye Hospitals (AAEH), of which SNEC is a founding member, and the European Association of Eye Hospitals (EAEH), to collaborate in benchmarking of best practices, quality improvement initiatives, ophthalmic centre administration, education and research.

The pioneer intake of the Advanced Diploma in Optometry offered by Singapore Polytechnic in conjunction with SNEC graduated in July 2006. First launched in 2004, the part-time course was specially designed to meet the need to upgrade the technical skills and knowledge of qualified optometrists in line with new challenges in the optical industry.

RESEARCH

Moving Ahead in Ophthalmic Research

Scientists from SERI led by A/Prof. Aung Tin and geneticist Dr. Eranga Vithana discovered a new eye disease gene, SLC4A11, that causes blindness in children. Mutations in the identified gene cause congenital hereditary endothelial dystrophy (CHED). The discovery of the gene significantly impacts on identification and treatment of CHED, and could facilitate gene replacement therapy in the most accessible part of the eye.

The findings were published in the prestigious Nature Genetics, ranked first of 120 journals in genetics.

SERI organised the 11th International Myopia Conference where eminent ophthalmologists, research scientists and optometrists presented and discussed the latest findings in myopia research. Over the next three years, SERI, together with the National University of Singapore, will embark on a new study involving 3,000 children aged six months to six years to examine the issues of myopia. This is the second study undertaken jointly by the two institutions.

WORKLAND PER ANNUM

Day Surgeries	28,137	26,815
Specialist Outpatient Clinic Attendances	253,972	246,811

STAFFING (AS AT END MARCH)

Total	465	442
Doctors	82	72
Nurses	133	131
Health Sciences Professionals	61	54
Others	189	186

COMMON EYE AILMENTS IN ASIA

PRESBYOPIA

Commonly called 'old age vision', this occurs when the lens (focusing mechanism of the eye) loses its elasticity. It affects most people after 40, and results in blurred images for near work like reading this booklet, despite the eye's efforts to focus.

To counter the problem, the lens needs to be altered or assisted. The choice of correction depends on lifestyle and occupational factors. The cheapest, safest and easiest option is spectacles. Refractive surgery is also popular but has been proven ineffective as a long-term solution.

One innovation comes from the University of Arizona which is developing 'switchable bifocals', glasses that allow users to switch from near-to far-sighted vision with the press of a button. These are meant to replace todays 'split bifocals', which require looking down to read and up for distance.

Researchers hope to also replace the switching button with an infrared sensor that detects distance and automatically adjusts the focals.

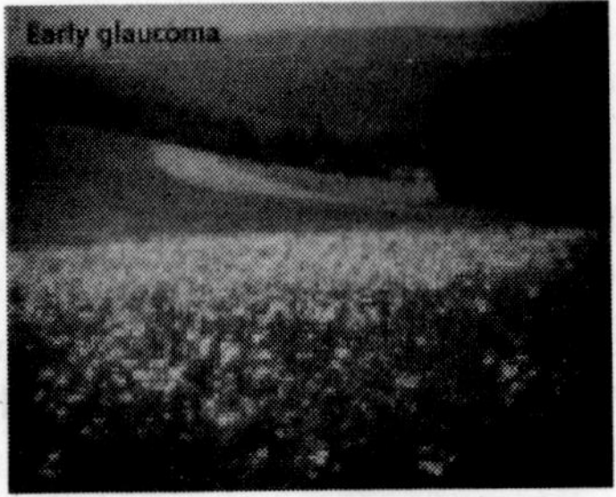

GLAUCOMA

Glaucoma is the leading cause of blindness in Hong Kong and a close second to cataracts in the Philippines. It happens when excess fluid and pressure inside the eyeball damages the optic nerves, and can lead to blindness if left unchecked.

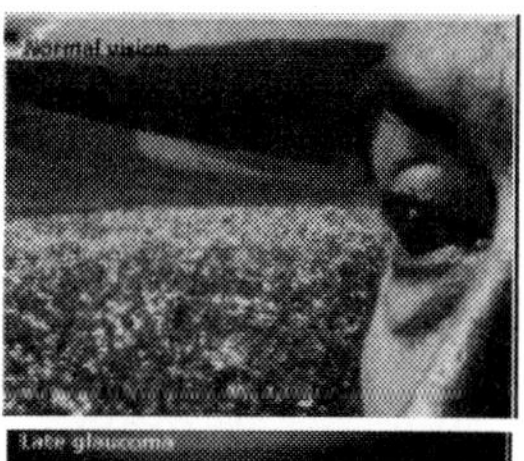

This degenerative eye disease affects the middle-aged or older, and comes in two forms. The first form is painless, revealed only by a slowly narrowing field of vision. Victims are often unaware of their gradual loss of Sight until it is too late. The onset of the other version is accompanied by acute pain.

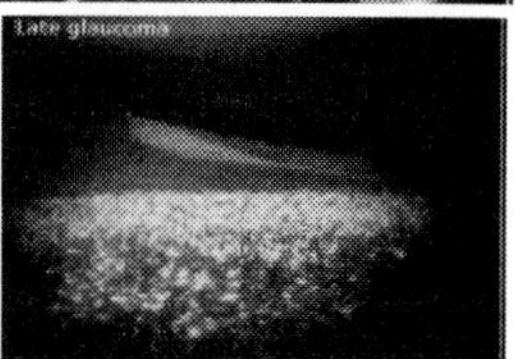

There is no cure for glaucoma, but early diagnosis can halt its progress. Depending on the type of glaucoma, treatment can take the form of either medications, laser therapy or surgery.

RETINAL DETACHMENT

The retina transforms light entering our eyes into information for our brain, but it can become separated from its rightful position. Detachment can lead to loss of sight if not treated promptly.

Detachments arise from a tear in the retina, enabling fluid from the vitreous to enter the space under the retina. It may be caused by short-sightedness, previous eye surgeries or injuries. A previous detachment in the other eye or a family history of detachment also increases the risk.

This condition is diagnosed from sudden onsets of numerous floaters and flashes, and partial blurring of vision. The good news is, over 90 per cent of detachments can be reattached.

"If a tear is found before the retina detaches, laser photocoagulation is applied around the tear to seal its edges and prevent fluid from seeping under the retina," says Dr. Doric Wong, head and senior consultant of vitreo-retinal services.

CATARACTS

The eye's transparent lens clouds up as people age. A clouded lens is called a cataract, which prevents enough light from entering the eye and blurs our vision. Cataracts are the leading cause of reversible blindness in the world, with over 20 million victims.

Although cataract is usually age-related, it can be caused by other factors like long-term intake of steroids, illnesses like diabetes, or injury. If it interferes with daily life, surgery is the answer. An operation involves making a small cut on the eye, removing the cloudy lens, and then replacing it with an artificial lens that will last a lifetime.

Cataract surgery has become faster, more efficient and safer with the latest technology, according to Dr. Zainah Alsagoff, deputy head and consultant of the cataract and comprehensive ophthalmology service at the SNEC. Latest advancements include smaller incisions, ultrasound instruments in place of manual ones, and procedures that do not need stitches.

Intraocular lenses (IOLs) replace the defective natural lens after surgery. The most widely used is monofocal IOLs, which only provide good distance vision. Multifocal IOLs that enable both near and far sight have been developed, but not everyone is suited for their implantation.

CORNEA BLINDNESS

An estimated 45 million people worldwide are blind and 135 million are visually impaired. Blindness in Asia is traditionally triggered by corneal afflictions, trauma, leprosy, and nutritional deficiencies in children.

Although improvements in health standards and sanitation are decreasing its prevalence, doctors are seeing more cases attributed to age, accidents, previous surgeries, and contact lens-related corneal diseases.

A widespread cause of corneal scarring is infection caused by trauma or improper use of contact lenses. Intensive antibiotics can treat the infections from contact lenses. In most cases, scars will surface and permanently hamper vision, broaching the need for a corneal transplant.

Normal corneal transplants, or Penetrating Keratoplasties (PK), replace the entire central cornea. A less invasive method is Lamellar Keratoplasty (LK), a partial corneal transplant that only removes the infected parts of the cornea. The surgeon does not penetrate the eye, thereby reducing surgical complications and reducing the risk of rejection after an LK to virtually nothing.

DIABETIC EYE DISEASE

Diabetic Eye Disease is the result of high blood sugar levels and damages the small blood vessels in the retina. Bleeds and leaks ensue, leading to damaged eyesight.

A gradual and painless blurring of vision marks the onset of this condition, and its risk increases with the duration of diabetes. About 60 per cent of diabetics carrying the condition for 15 years or more face the prospect of complete blindness. Successful treatment of Diabetic Eye Disease hinges on early detection and remedy. Diabetics should adhere to a good diet, medication and annual eye checks.

Laser photocoagulation can be used in the condition's early stage to seal leaking blood vessels and discourage the growth of new ones. In its later stages, more complex surgery is needed.

AGE-RELATED MACULAR DEGENERATION

The macula is that tiny spot on the retina responsible for small details and colour. Macular degeneration causes the loss of this central vision. The condition is linked to ageing—hence the name Age-related Macular Degeneration (AMD).

There are two types of AMD. The more common Dry AMD occurs when central vision slowly declines due to the loss of retinal cells. Wet AMD is caused by abnormal blood vessel growth that can cause bleeding or fluid leaks beneath the retina. This leads to distorted vision and eventually vision loss.

Although its cause is still unknown, AMD has been linked to high blood pressure, overexposure to ultraviolet rays, and possibly a diet low in antioxidants, vitamins and minerals. Early detection is crucial because lost vision cannot be regained.

A few options are available for Wet AMD

Laser photocoagulation—the abnormal blood vessels are destroyed with heat, but tills also damages normal retinal cells and affects vision.

Photodynamic therapy—a light-sensitizing drug is used to close off the abnormal blood vessels.

Anti-angiogenesis therapy—the eye's vitreous cavity is directly injected with drugs like Macugen, Lucentis or Avastin to destroy abnormal vessel growth 'Bionic eyes' may be common in three to five years. These retinal prostheses will fit into the eye to stimulate the retina and restore sight. This breakthrough is currently being researched for blindness due to age-related macular degeneration or retinitis pigmentosa.

WAYS TO KEEP EYES HEALTHY

REST OFTEN

Take regular breaks (every 40 minutes) from focused work like long hours in front of the computer. Walk around and look at far-off objects for a change. You can also lubricate your eyes with artificial tears to help them feel more comfortable.

LISTEN TO THEM

When your eyes are weary or itchy, they're telling you they need a break.

PROTECTION NEEDED

Sunglasses protect the retina from harmful ultraviolet rays. Blue wavelengths are the culprits, and the best filters are glasses in the amber, orange, or brown shades. (Ask for 100 per cent UV protection) They should be worn whenever it is sunny, especially in high glare areas like near water or snow: A wide-brimmed hat is also effective for blocking glare. Some form of eye protection is also vital in jobs involving machinery and flying particles.

QUIT SMOKING

Along with other harms, smoking increases the risk of macular degeneration and optic nerve damage.

TALK TO YOUR FAMILY

Sometimes eye problems are inherited. If you are diagnosed with a condition, share that information with your family and get their eyes examined. Early diagnosis and treatment of all eye conditions can minimize sight loss.

REGULAR CHECKUPS

Everyone should have an eye exam before the age of five to check for child-related eye problems. Many problems can be treated if detected early. One compulsory exam in the 20s and two in the 30s is ideal. After 40, check your eyes every two to four years; and after 65, one to two years. Persons with a family history of eye conditions or diabetes should have more frequent exams.

DIET RIGHT

At least 12 glasses of water daily prevents puffiness in the eyes. Research has identified the following nutrients as essential to healthy eyes.

INSIGHTFUL NUTRITION

Nutrient	*Benefits*	*Sources*
Vitamin E	Its antioxidant properties help protect the eyes against the development and progression of cataracts.	Whole grains, nuts and legumes; polyunsaturated oils (vegetable oils); monounsaturated oils (olive oils)
Vitamin C	As above	Fruits and vegetables (Especially citrus fruits, melons and broccoli)
Zinc	The US National Eye Institute has found that zinc slows AMD progression	Meat, poultry, fish, and dairy products
Carotenoids (Lutein and Zeaxanthin)	Latest trials suggest they protect against cataracts and AMD	Fruits and vegetables (particularly dark leafy greens and those that are yellow or green).

APPENDIX 3

NARAYANA HRUDAYALAYA HEALTH CITY, BANGALORE

Bangalore—the Silicon Valley and business-processing outfit of the east is rapidly becoming the health care destination of the world. Besides the excellent weather around the year, and the cosmopolitan environment, Bangalore is fast evolving into the intellectual capital of the world. The city was recently chosen by GE as the research center of the future with the creation of the Jack Welch Research Center—a dream destination for every Indian super-specialist from the West to settle down in. With the Indian Space Research Organization, based in Bangalore, planning a health satellite, Bangalore will become the world's back-office for high-tech health care delivery. With the backing of biotechnology and pharmaceutical giants like Boon and IT giants like Infosys and Wipro, Bangalore is all set to redefine health care

The Beginning

Asia Heart Foundation (AHF), a non-profit, charitable organization was founded by a group of heart specialists to establish high-tech hospitals in developing nations. Apart from assisting in commissioning the B.M. Birla heart Research Institute, Kolkata in 1989 and the Manipal Heart Foundation, Bangalore in 1997, the AHF decided to promote its won hospital in Kolkata, a 150-bed heart hospital, Rabindranath Tagore International Institute of Cardiac Sciences (RTIICS) in the year 2000. The AHF went one step further in realizing the potential of Bangalore being the health care destination of Asia by creating Narayana Hrudayalaya, a first-of-its-kind cardiac care hospital. Shankaranarayana Constructions (SNC), synonymous with its construction expertise in dams, roads, highways and power projects in India, made this dream a reality.

The Story behind it All

Celebrating its 50th Anniversary, SNC requested the AHF to setup a heart hospital. A hospital that would be the largest in the world, state-of-the-art in every aspect and capable of handling every surgical procedure of the heart. To make this feat achievable no constraints were set in terms of size, equipment or finance. The best in every field were employed with the aim of providing quality patient care.

Located in Bangalore's Bammasandra Industrial Area on Hosur Road (NH-7), Phase-I of the hospital is spread over 25 acres with a built-up area of over 2.5 lakh sq. ft. Presently, it has 500 beds with 10 operating rooms with the capacity to perform up to 25 heart surgeries in a single day. With the onset of Phase-II, Narayana Hrudayalaya will sprawl over an impressive 100 acres. The structure will accommodate 780 beds, 30 operating rooms to perform 75 heart surgeries a day. Besides the hospital, it will also accommodate a teaching institute cardiologists, cardiac surgeons, cardiac anaesthetists, nurses, health technicians and health care specialists. The entire project will have 5000 beds called the "Health City" with Speciality hospitals for every disease.

Coronary Artery Bypass Grafting (CABG) and Redo Coronary Artery Bypass Grafting

Indians are genetically three times more susceptible than Europeans to have a heart attack. In India, the bread winner of the family most often is the victim of an attack.

At Narayana Hrudayalaya 60% of the surgeries carried out are Coronary Artery Bypass Grafting (CABG) and Redo Coronary Artery Bypass Grafting.

Having carried out over thousands of Coronary Artery Bypass Grafting and Redo Coronary Artery Bypass Grafting operations, the team of experts at Narayana Hrudayalaya are amongst the most experienced in the world when it comes to performing CABG, Redo CABG and specifically Coronary Artery Bypass Grafting without using a heart-lung machine. Complete arterial graft using internal mammary artery and radial arteries too form one of our core competencies.

Dr. Praveen Kumar is one of the world's most experienced doctors in performing CABG's and Redo CABG's.

DOR's Procedure

Left Venticular Volume Reduction Operation and Carotid Endarterectomy

Dr. P.V. Rao, Chief of the Heart and Lung Transplantation Programme in Narayana Hrudayalaya strongly believes that terminal heart failure, mainly due to ischaemic cardiomyopathy and left ventricular aneurysms can be corrected by his favorite technique called DOR's Procedure along with Coronary Artery Bypass Grafting operation. With over 200 left ventricular volume reduction surgeries to his name, he is one of the most experienced in the world in this procedure. He has also conducted a large series of carotid endarterectomies to improve blood supply to the brain, along with bypass grafting operations.

Blue Babies

Heart Operations on Children with Heart Diseases

India is home to the largest number of children in the world, and the largest number of children with heart diseases in the world as well. Approximately 3 lakh children every year are affected by heart diseases in India. Dr. Colin John, head of the pediatric and adult surgical programmes is one of the most experienced cardiac surgeons in the world specializing in operating on children, especially those suffering from complex heart problems such as Tetralogy of Fallot (TOF) or in simple terms 'Blue Babies'.

Heart Surgeries on Newborn Babies

Narayan Hrudayalya gets referrals from over 13 countries for surgeries in complex heart diseases. Especially in newborn babies, barely a few hours old. Dr. Rajesh Sharma is one of the most experienced surgeons in the world, in arterial switch operations performed for the Transposition of the Great Arteries. He also specializes in Double Switch operations for congenitally corrected transpositions, performed at very few centres in the world.

Ross's Procedure and Aortic Aneurysm Surgey

An ideal valve to replace a human value is another human valve, 30 years ago. Dr. Ronald Ross at Guy's Hospital, London, demonstrated on operation, which was subsequently called Ross's Procedure. This procedure ultimately became the ideal operation for patients with an Aortic Valve Disease. Dr. Devi Shetty who was trained in cardiac surgery at Guy's Hospital, London, has had the best results in this complex heart operation, performing over 100 procedures with a 100% success rate. He also is one of the most experienced doctors in the world in performing operations like Bental Procedure for Aortic Root Aneurysm and Aortic Arch Replacement surgery for Dissecting Aneurysm of Aorta, Pulmonary Endarterectomy for Chronic Pulmonary Embolism and Coronary Artery Bypass .Grafting on beating hearts.

Cardiac Surgeons

Dr. Shekahar Rao, MS; MCH, DNB. A Consultant Cardiac Surgeon, had his education at leading medical institutions in India viz. St. John's Medical College, Bangalore, Post Graduate Institute for Medical Education and Research, Chandigarh and Sri Chitra Lirunal Institute of Medical Sciences and Technology, Trivandrum. He subsequently did his advanced fellowship training in cardiovascular surgery at the Mayo Clinic, USA. Prior to joining Narayana Hrudayalaya, he was the Senior Consultant and Head of the Department of Cardiothoracic and Vascular Surgery at the Sri Sathya Sai Institute of Higher Medical Sciences, Puttaparthi and Bangalore. He brings with him a background of expertise and experience in both congenital and acquired cardiac surgery and currently focuses on pediatric and adult congenital heart diseases.

Dr. Sanjay B. Dhaded, MS; MCH, FIACS, FICC. A Consultant Cardiac Surgeon with Narayana Hrudayalaya, Dr. .Sanjaya did his specialization at Seth G.S. Medical College and King Edward Memorial Hospital, Mumbai. He brings with him the experience of being a lecturer with the Department of CVTS, KEM Hospital, Mumbai. He has had specialized training in beating heart coronary surgery at centers in Italy and Germany and has a keen interest in minimal access surgery. He was a consultant Cardiac Surgeon with the Manipal Heart Foundation before joining Narayana Hrudayalaya.

Dr. Avery Mathew, MS; MCH. A Consultant Cardiac Surgeon with Narayana Hrudayalaya, Dr. Mathew trained at Kasturba Medical College. He spent 5 years with Apollo Hospital in Chennai before moving to St. Vincenfs Hospital, Sydney to work with adult cardiac surgery and cardio-pulmonary transplants. His fortelies in Aortic Aneurysms besides Coronary Artery and valve Surgery. He was a Consultant Cardiac Surgeon with the Manipal Heart Foundation before joining Narayana Hrudayalaya.

Dr. Julius Punnen, MS; MCH. An alumnus of Kasturba Medical College, Manipal, Dr. Punnen joined Dr. Devi Sheely's team in 1997 at The Manipal Heart Foundation, Bangalo moved to Narayana Hrudayalaya as a consultant cardiac surgeon. Having trained at prestigious hospitals like the Children's Hospital, Westmedal and St. Vincent's Hospital, Sydney, he brings with him the experience of having worked with both children and adults with cardiac complications as well as Cardia-Pulmonary transplantations. He has set-up the Homograft Heart Valve Bank in Narayana Hrudayalaya.

Dr. Kuldeep Kumar, MS; MCH. A trained Cardio Thoracic surgeon from The Medical College, Calicut, Dr. Kuldeep has worked extensively with the Madras Medical Mission and the Leeds General Infirmary in England. He has also worked at the Zhikder Medical College, Dhaka and the Manipal Heart Foundation before joining Narayana Hrudayalaya as a Consultant Cardiac Surgeon. His core interests lie in Coronary Bypass Surgery, LV Aneurysms Surgery and Aortic Aneurysm surgery.

Dr. B.R. Ravindra Setty, MS; MCH. (CVTS). An alumnus of the Mumbai University, Dr. Setty was trained at Austin and Repatriation Medical Center, Melbourne and Alfred Hospital, Melbourne in complex Arterial Coronary Artery Bypass Grafting and artificial hearts, ventricular assist devices and heart and lung transplants. He worked at the Manipal Heart Foundation before joining Narayana Hrudayalaya as a Consultant Cardiac Surgeon.

Interventional Cardiology

Dr. Pradeep Sheety strongly believes in primary interventions on an acute heart attack. He is in charge of the postgraduate training programme for cardiologists in interventions on the heart and post graduation courses like DNB in Cardiology and Fellowship in Interventional Cardiology through the National Board of Examination, New Delhi and the Rajiv Gandhi University of Health Sciences, Karnataka.

Interventional Electrophysiology

Dr. Ravikoshore is one of the most experienced doctors in invasive Electrophysicology of the heart which treats rhythm disturbances of the heart, commonly termed 'palpitation'. His core competency lies in AICD implantation for serious rhythm disturbances of the heart and biventricular pacing for terminal heart failure. He also conducts training programmes for young cardiologists in the field of Electrophysiology.

Endovascular Interventions

More and more Aneurysms of the Aorta are becoming amendable by Endovascular Stent Graf insertions, entirely avoiding a major surgical procedure. Dr. Sanjay Mehrotra besides being very active in Coronary Interventions has a special interest in performing endovascular treatment of Aortic diseases. Narayana Hrudayalya is one of the largest centres in the world dealing with diseases of the aorta, surgically and with endovascular treatment.

Cardiology

Dr. P.V. Suresh, MD; DM. A consultant in cardiology, Dr. Suresh trained in cardiology at PGIMER, Chandigarh and was later associated with the Manipal Heart Foundation Besides being an Interventional cardiologist, he is also active in the field of Paediatric Interventions, Paediatric Echocardiography and Pacemaker Implantations.

Dr. B.K. Mahala, MD; DM. An alumnus of SCB Medical College, Cuttack, Dr. Mahala was a Consultant Cardiologist with the Manipal Heart Foundation before joining Narayana Hrudayalaya in 2001. He is currently a Consultant Cardiologist and the Director of the Echocardiography Programme at Narayana Hrudayalaya. In addition to Interventional Cardiology, his interests include teaching and complex Echocardiography.

Dr. Sunita Maheswari, ABP; ABPC, (USA) A Consultant Paediatric Cardiologist certified by the American Board of Paediatric Cardiologist, Dr. Maheswari is trained in trans catheter interventions in children with heart diseases, an area she works in at Narayana Hrudayalaya. An acclaimed author, she was honoured with the American Heart Association Young Clinician Award.

Dr. Bagirath Raghuraman, MD; DNB (Gen. Med); DM (Cardio). After completing his DM at Sri Jayadeva Institute of Cardiology, Bangalore, Dr. Bagirath trained in Advanced Management of Cardiac Failure and Cardiac Transplantation at Papworth Hospital, Papworth, Cambridge, United Kingdom. He set-up India's first ever Heart Failure Clinic for the management of heart failure inpatients at Narayana Hrudayalaya, where he works as a consultant Cardiologist.

Super Speciality Training Programme

Dr. K. Muralidhar, MD. An alumnus of PGIMER Chandigarh, Dr. Muralidhar had his training in Cardiac Anaesthesia at Sri Chitra Tirunal Institute, Trivandrum and Glenfield General Hospital, Leicester; UK. He joined Dr. Devi Shetty in 1989 at the B.M. Birla Heart Research Center; Kolkata and later at the Manipal Heart Foundation before joining Narayana Hrudayalaya, Bangalore. Besides being a Senior Consultant in Cardiac Anaesthesia and Chief of Anaesthesia services, he is also the Director for

Post-Doctoral courses. Credited to his name are innumerable research papers in his field. He is also a faculty member of the University of Minnesota and the Rajiv Gandhi University of Medical Sciences.

Dr. George Cherian, MD; DM; FACC; FAMS; FRCP; FAHA. A distinction holder from The Christian Medical College, Vellore, Dr. Cherian completed his training at Vellore and fellowship at the Massachusetts General Hospital, Harvard University, Hammersmith Hospital and the Royal Postgraduate Medical School, London. He was the past president of the Cardiology society of India and was a professor and head at Christian Medical College, Vellore, a visiting professor of UCLA, an advisor to the World Health Organization, the Armed Services of India and the author of over 200 journals and books. Dr. Cherian, a professor in Cardiology at Narayana Hrudayalaya, also trains young aspirants in cardiology.

Dr. P.S. Jairaj, MS (Gen. Surgery); FRACS. Dr. Jairaj began his career in Australia and became a professor of cardio thoracic surgery at the Christian Medical College Vellore in 1978. In 1990 he established the open heart surgery unit in the Sultanate of Oman at the Royal Hospital, Muscat He was a professor at St. John's Medical College, before joining Narayana Hrudayalaya as a professor to train young surgeons.

Dr. T.V. Chandrashekar, DA (Lond); FFARCSI. Prior to joining Narayana Hrudayalaya as a Consultant Cardiac Anaesthetist, Dr. Chandrashekar worked in the UK and Saudi Arabia as a consultant Anaesthetist. Today he is the co-ordinator for paramedical courses conducted at Narayana Hrudayalaya Institute of Medical Sciences. His interests lie in hypnosis, organizing haemodialysis and photography. Naryana Hrudayalaya conducts various super-speciality training programmes in heart-related procedures in affiliation with the National Board of Examinations, New Delhi, the Rajiv Gandhi University of Health Sciences, Karnataka, and the Paramedical Board, Karnataka.

Anaesthesiologists and Intensivists

Dr. Sanjay banakal, MD. A senior Consultant Anaesthesiologist with Narayana Hrudayalaya Dr. Sanjay completed his post-graduation at the Kasturba Medical College, Manipal. He underwent further training in anaesthesia in the United Kingdom and in cardiac anaesthesia at the B.M. Birla Heart Research Center, Kolkata. Before joining Narayana Hrudayalaya he was a lecturer in the Department of Anaesthsiology at Kasturba Medical College and St. John's Medical College, Bangalore.

Dr. Keshava Murthy, MD (Anaes); DA; DNB (Anaes). A Consultant Cardiac—Anaesthesiologist with experience spanning nearly decade, Dr. Murthy worked at the Tata Memorial Hospital Mumbai and as a Cardiac Anaesthesiologist at the Meenakshi Mission Hospital and Research Center, Tamil Nadu. His core competence at Narayana Hrudayalaya lies in paediatric Cardiac Anaesthesia.

Dr. Rajneesh Garg, MD. A Consultant Cardiac Anaesthesiologist with Narayana Hrudayalaya, Dr. Garg is an alumnus of the prestigious All

S. No.	Name of Course	Board/University	Duration of the course	Eligiblity
1	2	3	4	5
1.	DNB in Cardio Thoraic Surgey	National Board of Examination, New Delhi	3 years	Ms (Gen.Surg)*
2.	DNB in Cardiology	National Board of Examination, New Delhi	3 year	Ms (Gen.Surg.)*
3.	Fellowship in Cardiac Anaesthesia	National Board of Examination, New Delhi	2 years	MD (Ane.)*
4.	Fellow in Critical Care medicine	National Board of Examination, New Delhi	2 years	MD*
5.	Fellowship in Interventional Cardiology	National Board of Examination, New Delhi	2 years	DM (Card.)*
6.	Fellowship in Paediatric Cardiology	National Board of Examination, New Delhi	2 years	MD (Paed.)*
7.	Fellowship in Paediatric Cardiac Surgery	Rajiv Gandhi University of Health Sciences, Karanataka, Bangalore	1½ years	MCH (CT-Surgery)
8.	Fellowship in Cardiac Anaesthesia	Rajiv Gandhi University of Health Sciences, Karnataka, Bangalore	1 years	MD (Anae)*
9.	BSc. Perfusion Technology	Rajiv Gandhi University of Health Sciences, Karnataka, Bangalore	3 years	PUC (PCB)
10.	B.Sc. Nursing	Rajiv Gandhi University of Health Sciences, Karnataka, Bangalore	3 years	IPUC (PCB) 45%
11.	Diploma in General Nursing	The Indian Nursing of Council and Karnataka Nursing Council, Karnataka	3 years	II-PUC
12.	Post Basic Diploma in Cardio Thoracic and Vascular Nursing	Karnataka Nursing Council, Karnataka	1 years	GNM/B.Sc.
13.	Para Medical Courses Diploma in :		2 years	I-PUC
	Medical Laboratory Technolgoy		3 years	ISSLC

(Contd.)

(*Contd.*)

14. X-Ray Technology		2 years	II-PUC
		3 years	SSLC
15. Physiotherapy		3½ years	II-PUC
16. Operation Theatre Technolgoy		2 years	II-PUC
		3 years	SSLC
17. Medical Record Technology	Para Medical Board, Government of	2 years	II-PUC
	Karnataka, Bangalore	3 years	SSLC
18. Post-graduate Diploma in Hospital Mgt.	Narayana Hrudayalaya	2 years	Graduate
19. Certificate Course in CCSD Technology	Narayana Hrudayalya	1 years	II-PUC (PCB)
			SSLC

India Institute of Medical Sciences, New Delhi. With experience spanning nearly a decade, he holds special interest in the field of intra-operative trans-esophageal echocardigraphy.

Dr. Ratan Kumar T. Gupta, MD; DNB (Anaes). A trained Cardiac and Neuro Anaesthesiologist Dr. Gupta was in-charge of post-cardiac surgical intensive care at the Chitra Tirunal Institute for Medical Science and Technology in Trivandrum before moving to Bangalore. After a stint at the Manipal Heart Foundation in Bangalore, he moved to Narayana Hrudayala as a Consultant Intensivist. His area of focus is Fibreoptic Bronchoscopy and Echocardiography.

Dr. Cajetan Mario Francis Tellis, MD (Paediatrics). A post-graduate from St. John's Medical College, Bangalore, Dr. Tellis worked in Lucknow as a Registrar in General Paediatrics. He completed his fellowship in Paediatric Cardiac Critical Care at the Manipal Heart Foundation, Bangalore. He has been working with Narayana Hrudayalaya since its inception.

Telemedicine

One of the largest Telemedicine Networks in the world, sponsored by the Indian Space Research Organization (ISRO), the Narayana Hrudayala Telemedicine Network runs through 26 locations in an outside the country, offering video consultation round-the-clock, primarily for heart patients from remote areas. The network has been instrumental in treating over 12,000 patients in the last two years, entirely free of cost.

The ECG Network

Using ordinary telephone lines, a large number of Family Physician's clinics are networked with Narayana Hrudayalaya for early diagnosis of heart attacks.

Narayana Institute of Neurosciences

Dr. Thimappa Hegde, MBBS, MCH (Neura). The director of the Narayana Hrudayalaya Institute of Neurosciences is renowned for being a multifaceted personality with many accomplishments to his name. He acquired his training in Neurosurgery at the prestigious National Institute of Health and Neurosciences (NIMHANS), Bangalore. On completion of his training, he served on the faculty of NIMHANS and rose to the position of Additional Professor of Neurosurgery. He worked in NIMHANS for over 20 years and during his tenure he was instrumental in initiating stereotactic and functional neurosurgery. Dr. Hegde has performed several thousand neurosurgical procedures Dr. Hegde's interests include stereotactic and functional surgery, spinal surgery and fusions, trauma, neuro-endoscopy and neuro-oncology.

Narayana Institute of Neurosciences

Dr. Arvind Bhateja trained in General Surgery at the KEM Hospital,

Mumbai and then completed his training in Neurosurgery at NIMHANS. His areas of interest include spinal surgery, neuro-oncology, pediatric neurosurgery, neurotrauma, neutro-endoscopyand sterotactic and functional surgery.

Dr. H.V. Madhusudan. Completed his training in neurosurgery at NIMHANS in 200. He then worked as a consultant at the Sri Satya Sai institute of Higher Medical Sciences at Bangalore. He furthered his education in the US, where he completed fellowships in spine surgery in Arizonal and in Gamma Knife and Neuro-oncology at the renowned Roswell Park Caoncer Center in Buffalo, New York. His areas of interest include spinal surgery, stereotactic surgery, neuro-endoscopy, neuro-oncology and gamma knife surgery.

Dr. Rajesh K.N., MBBS, MD (Gen Medicine), DM (Neurology). Completed postgraduation in General Medicine from Bangalore Medical College. He underwent training in DM-Neurology at G.B. Plant Hospital, New Delhi. He has also worked as a Senior Resident in the Department of Neurology and Department of Neuro Rehabilitation at Nimhans. His areas of interest include Electrophysiology and Neuro Rehabilitation.

Lab, Blood Bank and Imaging Services

Dr. T.N. Raguunath. A consultant Biochemist current heading the department of Laboratory medicine at Narayana Hrudayalaya, completed his post-graduation from the University of Detroit Michigan, USA. Dr. Raghunath has had extensive laboratory experience both in the USA and India. He is responsible for the quality of Lab services of Narayana Hrudayalya.

Dr. N. Prem Anand Nagaraja. A consultant Microbiologist and the Chairman of the Hospital Infection Control Committee, completed his MD in Medical Microbiology from JIPMER, Pondicherry. He has over 14 years of experience in the fields of Clinical Microbiology and Infection Control both in India and abroad. He also heads the Homograft Laboratory, Central Sterile Supplies, Hospital Waste Management, Antibiotic Polices and Surveillance. The 3M Center for Excellence was started under his guidance and he has since then been involved in teaching practices in Hospital Infection Control for nurses, CSSD staff and hospital administrators. He is also the Principal, Narayana Hrudayataya Institute of Paramedical Science and the clonical co-ordinator for research projects.

Dr. T.S. Sreedhar Murthy MD (Pathology). A Consultant Pathologist and Blood Bank Officer at Narayana Hrudayalaya, completed his MD in pathology from the Bangalore Medical College and gained extensive experience in the field of transfusion medicine, tissue typing and cross matching from Rotary Blood Bank, Bangalore. He is currently the head of the regional blood bank center at Narayana Hrudayalaya.

Dr. Abhijit Bandyopadhyay, MBBS, DRM, DNB. A Consultant in Nuclear Medicine at Narayana Hrudayalaya, Dr. Abhijit completed his MBBS at the Calcutta National Medical College, DRM at Tata Memorial

Hospital, Mumbai and further completed his DNB in nuclear medicine at Jaslok Hospital, Mumbai. He worked at Hinduja, Mumbai and Bombay Hospital, Mumbai before joining Narayana Hrudayalaya.

Yeshasvini Micro Health Scheme (YMHS)

Narayana Hrudayalaya, in association with the Government of Karnataka, created the concept of a farmers' health scheme "Yeshasvini", which was subsequently launched by the State Co-operative Department. Yeshasvini offers all types of operations of the stomach, brain, gallbladder, spine, bones, kidneys and heart, entirely free of cost to 1.7 million farmer's families across the state of Karnataka for a monthly payment of just Rs. 5. In just one year, over 9,100 patients underwent various operations and over 36,000 people underwent free outpatient consultation in the 92 recognized hospitals across state of Karnataka under this scheme.

Today Yeshasvini is being launched by many state Governments of India under various names.

The Government of Karnataka is in the process of launching a micro health scheme for the teachers of Karnataka, in association with the Department of Education to cover 3.5 million people.

Rabindranath Tagore International Institute of Cardiac Sciences (RTIICS)

A 150-bed heart hospital spread over 6 acres of land on the eastern metropolitan bypass of Kolkata, the Rabindranath Tagore International Institute of Cardiac Sciences (RTIICS) was built under the banner of the Asia Heart Foundation, in association with the Government of West Bengal.

Today RTIICS is recognized as the largest heart hospital in Eastern India, with an average outpatient consultation of 300 patients a day. It also performs 30 cathlab procedures and 6 major heart surgeries, everyday.

Armenian Church Trauma Center

The Armenian Church Trauma Center, a 200-bed center, deals with Poly Trauma, Orthopaedic, Vascular and other trauma-related specialities with services in nephrology.

R.C. Agarwal Memorial Hospital, Tinsukia, Assam

Constructed to reach out to the underprivileged heart patients of Assam, the R.C. Agarwal Memorial Hospital is a 50-bed modern hospital set-up to treat virtually every type of cardiac emergency. The hospital is linked to Narayana Hrudayalaya, Bangalore and the Rabindranath Tagore International Institute of Cardiac Sciences, Kolkata.

Rotary Narayana Sankara Nethralaya, Kolkata

It is the dream of every citizen in Eastern India suffering from eye diseases to visit Sankara Nethralaya, Chennai (Madras). The Rotary Narayana Sankara Nethralaya in Kolkata was created in association with Sankara Nethralaya, Chennai (Madras) to serve the needs of these people.

Today, it is the most technology compliant eye hospital in Eastern India. This state-of-the-art eye hospital, spread over 3 acres of land, is situated in the heart of Salt Lake City, Kolkata.

Affiliate Hospitals CSI Hrudayalaya, Bangalore

Naryana Hrudayalya, in association with the Church of South India set-up a 12-bed Coronary Care Unit (CCU) called CSI Hrudayalaya. At the CSI Hospital in Bangalore Contonment, the unit is managed and run by cardiologist at Narayana Hrudayalalya, round the clock, with OPD and diagnostic facilities.

CSI Hrudayalaya, Bangalore

CMH Hrudayalaya was set-up in association with the Chinmaya Mission of Bangalore Chinmaya Mission Hospital, Indiranagar, Bangalore. A 14-bed Coronary Care Unit with OPD and diagnostic facilities, it is managed and run by the Senior Consultants of Narayana Hrudayalaya predominantly to treat heart attacks.

Sahakarna Hrudayalay, Kannur, Kerala

Sahakarna Hrudayalay, Kannur, Kerala is promoted by the Kerala State Co-operative hospital complex, under the Chairmanship of the Honourable Minister for Co-operation, Government of Kerala. This is 150-bed super speciality heart hospital with 4 operating rooms and 2 cardiac cathlabs, one of Kerala's largest heart hospitals created for the common man.

Narayana Hrudayalaya Outreach Programme

Narayana Hrudayalaya condusts heart camps in rural areas, Screening hundreds of heart patients with a mobile diagnostic lab donated by the Ashraya Hastha Trust, Bangalore. Every camp draws 200 to 600 heart patients. Those who suffer from major cardiac problems undergo treatment at Narayana Hrudayalaya, free of cost or at subsidized rates.

Patients in these camps undergo virtually every type of non-invasive investigation like ECG, Echodoppler, Treadmill with the help of the mobile cardiac diagnostic lab.

Over 500 such camps were conducted by the Asia Heart Foundation and Narayana Hrudayalaya in remote parts of India, Bangladesh, Sri Lanka and Nepal in the last 14 years.

Thrombosis Research Institute (TRI)

Prof. Dr. Vijay V. Kakkar, a pioneer in thrombosis research from England set-up the Thrombosis Research Institute as a part of the Thrombosis Research Institute of London, to conduct various research activities about the pre-disposition of Indians on early coronary artery disease. The Institute is on a mission to produce a vaccine that will prevent premature atherosclerosis, a contributing factor for heart attacks among young adults.

Narayana Hrudayalaya Charitable Wing

The Narayana Hrudayalaya Charitable Wing raises finance for heart operations of the underprivileged from various individuals and philanthropists. To date the wing has helped save thousands of lives. For details contact lakshmi Mani, Manager, Charitable Wing.

Hospital Management System

Narayana Hrudayalaya has collaborated with SN Informatics, a Bangalore-based IT solutions company focused on providing total solutions in health care. After 2 years of interactive exercises, the hospital today uses an integrated hospital management system developed by SN Informatics. The solutions are designed to cover all areas of activities, from patient management and laboratory management to material management and telemedicine. The solutions have enabled Narayana Hrudayalaya to offer quality, cost-effective medical care. The Hospital Management System today stands certified by Microsoft.

SN Informatics offers software for hospital management and telemedicine to charitable organizations free of cost as a mission to bring health care to the masses.

Our partners in the International Outreach Programme

Children's Heart Link, USA. This a Minnesota-based charitable organization which has helped Naryana Hrudayalaya organize free heart valves and medical disposables. It also arranges training programmes of the hospital's specialists in the US and their medical visiting faculty to Narayana Hrudayalaya.

GOPIO, Malaysia. The Global Organization of People of Indian Origin is a partner of Narayana Hrudayalaya's efforts to reach out to the under privileged heart patients of Malaysia. In association with GOPIO, the hospital is in the process of setting up a modern charitable cardiac diagnostic lab at Pearl Court Kuala Lumpur, linked with the Telemedicine Network at Narayana Hrudayalaya.

SACIM, Mauritius. The Society of Aid to Children Inoperable in Mauritius (SACIM) has organized heart operations on nearly 100 children in association with Narayana Hrudayalaya. The hospitals association with the SACIM spans over a decade.

Ganashastha, Dhaka. Ganashanstha is one of the largest health care NGOs in Bangladesh. Narayana Hrudayalaya offers training programmes to cardiology students of Ganashastha University, Dhaka, Bangladesh.

Indo-Tranzanian Friendship Hospital, Tanzania. Narayana Hrudayalaya is in the process of setting up the world's first telemedicine medical hospital at Arusha, Tanzania through satellite connectivity, aimed at offering cardiac care to the underprivileged heart patients of Africa.

Interhealth Technologies, Benmore, South Africa. This South African organization, under the directorship of Kevin Thomas, arranges for heart patients of African countries to be treated at Narayana Hrudayalaya.

Narayana Hrudayalaya (NH), means God's Compassionate Home, in Sanskrit. Situated in the South Indian city of Bangalore, best known as India's Silicon Valley, almost everything about this heart hospital was unique, from its buildings and equipment to the doctors, nurses, and their treatment and care of patients. At the entrance to the main foyer of the hospital was a circular Chapel, equally divided into four independent quadrants, each a place of prayer and meditation for the four main religious faiths of its patient population—Hindus, Muslims, Christians, and Sikhs. Depicting the unity of human faith, the four streams naturally converged at the center of the chapel. (Tarun Khanna, V. Kasturi Rangan, Merlina Manocaran, 2005).

Founded in 2001 by Dr. Devi Prasad Shetty, NH had grown rapidly in four years to house 500 beds, 10 fully commissioned operating theatres (OTs), two cardiac catheterization laboratories and its own blood and valve banks. The pediatric intensive therapy unit which consisted of 50 beds, was one of the largest in the world with 40% of all procedures performed at NH being pediatric treatments. Since its opening, the hospital had completed over 11,228 open-heart surgeries (OHS), half of which were pediatric. In 2004 alone, it performed 4276 surgeries, of which 1,467 were on children. To complement the surgeries, NH also performed 5,430 catheterization procedures that year.

To provide affordable cardiac care to the masses, NH followed a hybrid strategy of attracting paying patients by virtue of its reputation for high quality, but combined this appeal with a relentless focus on lowering its costs of operation wherever possible, so that a larger number of people could afford to seek treatment. The surplus gained from paying patients was used to subsidize procedures that were performed at, or below, cost for patients who, could not afford the full fee. In 2004, the proportion of patients who paid NH's full price to those that could not afford to pay, was about 60:40.

The break-even price for a typical OHS at NH was approximately Rs. 90,000 (US$2,000) for adults and Rs. 130,000 (US$2,800) for children. At a price of Rs. 110,000 (US$2,400) for a regular package involving OHS (inclusive of surgery and hospitalization charges), NH's charges were the lowest in the country where the average cost of OHS in a private hospital was Rs. 250,000 (US$5,500). At the upper end, patients who opted for executive wards paid Rs. 140,000 to 195,000 (US$3,100-$4,300); this package provided private rooms instead of general wards, although treatment and care across all packages was identical. The prices of various procedures at NH and comparative prices at other Indian hospitals.

In addition, the hospital offered a scheme called Karuna Hrudaya, which allowed financially constrained patients to pay Rs. 65,000 (US$1,400) per OHS, with NH absorbing the remaining costs. For patients who could not afford this package, the Narayana Hrudayalaya Trust, a charitable organization with offices within the hospital, helped to arrange funds from a general corpus or by specifically seeking donations from a list of individuals and organizations.

Dr. Devi Shetty, looking a full to years younger than his 50 years, proceeded to layout his vision for the future of the hospital:

"We have only completed Phase I. In Phase II, we will have over 100 acres of facilities. We are planning on 800 beds, 30 operating rooms, and 20,000 surgeries a year. Besides the hospital, we will build a teaching institute for cardiologists, cardiac surgeons and other health care specialists," he said.

The Indian Health Landscape

With an estimated population of 1.08 billion in 2003 (of which approximately 400 million were under 18), India was the world's second-most populous country after China. Its reported per capita income in 2003 was US$600 (US$2,900 per capita income on a PPP basis). While economic growth was impressive since the late 1990s (India registered an average 6% GDP growth between 1999 and 2003), the distribution of income remained highly skewed. More than 250 million people lived below the poverty line and the richest 20% was estimated to hold close to 50% of household income.

In 2003, the Indian government spent approximately 1% of its GDP on public health care (the equivalent of US$4 per person a year), which placed it at one of the lowest public health care spending in the world (see Exhibit 7 for comparative health statistics). Private spending was several times higher and the overall expenditure on health was estimated to be 5% of the GDP, compared to the Asian average of 6.3%. While there had been improvements in life expectancy (from around 40 years at the time of independence (in 1947) to 64 years in 2003), general indicators of health and nutrition remained poor. The National Nutrition Monitoring Bureau estimated that 85% of the Indian population and 47% of children under three years of age did not receive enough nourishment.

With over 15,000 hospitals (the second highest number in the world) and nearly 600,000 physicians (the fourth highest number in the world), it appeared that India's health care system was well equipped. However, the actual number of physicians per 1,000 population was only 0.5 (comparable to 2.7 in the USA) and since approximately 70% of doctors were located in urban areas while the same proportion of the population still lived in the rural areas, actual access to health care was limited by inconvenient and expensive travel.

While public health care was mostly free, the high incidence of corruption at government hospitals (stories were told of having to bribe the security guards at hospitals even to visit a patient) lowered the cost differential between public and private health care. In addition, public hospitals and clinics were notoriously understaffed and under-equipped. In an article on the public health system in India, Dr. Atul Gawande, a surgeon at Boston's Brigham and Women's hospital, described a hospital in Nanded (about 400 miles of Mumbai) that had just 500 beds and nine general surgeons to service a population of 2.3 million people: " . . . the

TABLE I

Comparative Health and Health Care Stataistics

	India	*Karnataka*	*U.S.*	*China*
Population (million)	1,027	53	288.4	1,276
Life expectancy (years), 2002	64	64	77	71
Intant Mortality Rate (deaths per 1,000 births), 2002	67	55	77	71
Public Health expenditure (% of GDP), 2001	0.9	0.7	6.2	2.0
Private Health expenditure (% of GDP), 2001	4.2		7.7	3.4
Per capita health expenditure (PPP USD), 2001	80		4,887	224
Overall spending on health care as % of GDP, 2003	6.0		14.1	5.0
No of physcians per 1,000 Population	0.5	0.4	2.7	1.6
No. of hospital beds per 1,000 population	0.9	0.3	3.4	2.3
Population without access to improved water source (%), 2000	16			25
Children under weight for age (% under 5) 1995-2002	47			11

Source: Medical Markets Fact Book, 2004, Human Development Report, 2004, "Health Care in Karnataka," Hinduonnet.com.

TABLE 2

Volume of Procedures at NH

	Inpatients	*Outpatients*	*Catherization Lab Procedures*	*Surgeries*
Apr. 2001—March 2002	4,242	9,875	2,116	1,842
Apr. 2002—March 2003	7,226	10,863	3,367	2,742
Apr. 2003—March 2004	10,262	15,382	4,777	3,570
Apr. 2004—May 2004	2,029	3,466	821	714

Source: Narayana Hrudayalaya.

faucets don't work . . . examinations take place behind a thin rag curtain with gaping holes in it," he wrote. Everyone he asked said they would borrow money or sell their possessions to access private health care and according to Dr. Gawande, "even the Prime Minister does not go to his government's hospitals."

TABLE 3

Comparative CABG Volumes

	Cleveland Clinic (Ohio)	Mayo Clinic (Minnea-polis)	Mass General Hospital (Boston)	NH
No. of GASO surgeries a year	1,151	2,500a	1,000	3,570
Average surgeries a day	3	7	3	10
Number of cardiac surgeons	11	9	9	18
Average surgeries per surgeon	105	278	111	198
Rank by U.S. News and World Report (2004)b	1	2	5	—

Source: Hospital web sites, *U.S. News and World Report, 2004.*
a Overestimated—Web sites gives figures for all cardiac surgeries.
b Ranking for "Heart and Heart Surgery."

Given that less than 14% of the population was supported by health insurance, treatment was an option only for the rich or those able to borrow to pay the bill. A report by McKinsey and Co. estimated that the richest 7% in the country accounted for 30% of spending in private health care and over 40% of inpatient spending, reflecting the skewed access to private health care.

Ironically, India's private health care industry, while closed off to the country's majority, was gaining popularity among foreigners. With improving quality and technology at Indian private hospitals, the concept of medical tourism was spreading with an estimated 150,000 foreign patients receiving treatment at Indian hospitals in 2003. The low cost of treatment at Indian private hospitals (relative to developed countries) was an attraction—for instance, OHS could cost up to US$70,000 in the United Kingdom and US$150,000 in the USA, but was just US$3,000-$10,000 at the best Indian hospitals. Dr. Shetty related the story of a friend who operated on a British patient in India: "He [the patient] said there's every chance an Indian would operate on him in the United Kingdom, so why not get operated by an Indian in India?"

The Demand for Cardiac Care in India

Heart disease was one of the most common illnesses in India—approximately 2.4 million people needed heart surgery every year, although due to lack of affordable treatment, only 60,000 surgeries were performed. The prevalence of the disease had significant implications on its workforce—it was estimated that 28% of the 5 million Indians who died of cardiovascular disease every year were under 65 years and almost 25% of heart attacks occurred among the under-40 population. Congenital heart disease was a particular concern-around 224,000 newborns in India was affected by heart disease every year and the rural population was particularly susceptible due to poverty and unhygienic conditions that worsened the condition.

Research showed that Indians were particularly at risk of heart disease, with the Indian subcontinent contributing 45% of the global burden of coronary artery disease. Dr. Shetty said:

"Indian genes are three times more vulnerable to heart disease. The average age for heart attacks in the West, for instance, is 65 years, whereas in India, it is 45. When I was a student in London, it was normally a young son who brought his elderly father in for bypass surgery. In my practice in India it is more often the elderly father who brings his son in."

Operations Strategy at NH

The operations strategy at NH followed the dual principle of highest quality at the lowest cost consistent with that quality. There were absolutely no compromises when it came to the quality of the hospital's facilities, equipment, and support services. The 500-bed hospital was housed in a modern setting with spacious areas for all amenities, beginning with the check-in counter, to surgical and treatment wards. Equipment costing Rs. 35 crores (US$7.8 million) was imported and all supplies were obtained from vendors who provided the highest quality. Simultaneously, since Dr. Shetty's vision was to provide health care at an affordable price to the masses, the operations attempted to drive unit costs lower through a high level of capacity utilization and productivity.

Calling his strategy "the Wal-martization of health care," Dr. Shetty and his team-leveraged their strong reputation in cardiac care to perform a high number of procedures. NH performed approximately 19 OHS and 25 catheterization procedures a day, almost eight times the average at other Indian hospitals. The volume of procedures completed allowed the unit cost of surgery to be significantly decreased. Dr. Shetty explained: "While other hospitals may run two blood tests on a machine each day, we run 500 tests a day—so our unit cost for each test is lower. And this works with all our processes. Also, because of our volumes, we are able to negotiate better deals with our suppliers. Instead of buying expensive machines (like other hospitals), we pay the supplier a monthly rent for parking their machines here-and then we pay them for reagents that we buy to run the machines—and they are willing to do this because our demand for the reagents is high enough to make up the profits for them."

Careful dealing with suppliers also helped maintain low costs: "We don't sign long-term contracts," explained Dr. Nitish Shetty, the medical superintendent who headed the hospital's administrative affairs. "We negotiate every purchase because prices in India are very flexible and we don't want to be locked-in to use a supplier who suddenly becomes expensive." By keeping the administrative team lean, NH also avoided the usual problem of corruption that plagued other corporate hospitals where suppliers had to bribe administrative staff to reach the purchasing manager, thus pushing prices higher.

While the Calcutta hospital and NH had separate purchasing departments (the two hospitals were owned by different entities), there was enough communication between the two departments to increase their bargaining power. The hospitals enjoyed 30%-35% discounts on medical supplies, the largest cost component, since they (together with two smaller units also owned under the banner of AHF) made up approximately 10% of the cardiac care market in India.

In addition, NH embraced new technology as another way to reduce costs. Instead of performing chest X-rays with film that cost Rs. 50 and required processing, the hospital used digital X-rays that did not incur recurrent costs. The hospital had also implemented comprehensive hospital management software for its operations, which helped maintain minimum inventory and allowed quicker processing of tests—such advances were said to have increased the hospital's efficiency which in turn drove overall costs lower.

"The irony of health care in India is that while this country boasts world-class pharmaceutical companies that manufacture drugs for the developed world (e.g. Ranbaxy Laboratories Ltd; Dr. Reddys Lab Ltd [the latter is listed on the NYSE] and CIPLA7), the access of the Indian population to medicine is severely limited by high prices," lamented Dr. Shetty. Approximately 10% of health care costs in India was attributed to prescription drugs, compared with 11% in the USA. "An Indian over the age of 60 (the retirement age in the country) could spend Rs. 2,000-3,000 a month on medicines alone, and this is a large sum for most," added Dr. Shetty. At NH, the prescription drugs made up approximately 8%-10% of the cost of cardiac surgery.

In 2004, Biocon Ltd, an Indian company that developed biopharmaceuticals for sale in developed countries, introduced cardio-diabetes products as part of its first line of generic drugs. NH started using the drugs, which were estimated to be up to 80% cheaper than the market rate for similar medication. "We are a cartel," claimed Dr. Shetty, "our connections to other heart hospitals means at our suggestion, they too will start to use these products." Again, this reflected a relentless emphasis on costs at NH.

The core cost-savings, as explained by Dr. Shetty, was the staff salaries: "Compared to hospitals in the West which spend up to 60% of their revenues on staff salaries (including surgeons' fees), the comparable percentage for salaries at NH is only 22%. This does not mean our doctors are poorly paid-rather, they work much longer hours (doctors at NH work an average of 12-16 hours a day) and perform more procedures." Also, unlike other Indian hospitals, NH's doctors received fixed salaries and not a percentage of the revenues they generated.

From its first day of operation, NH had a sufficient mix of paying and nonpaying patients to sustain its charitable mission. "We have never had to turn away a patient for lack of funds," stated Sreenath, a chartered accountant by profession, who had been with NH since it opened. The mission of providing below-cost care (where necessary) required careful planning and internal financial controls and to this end, the finance department employed a unique daily accounting system where all revenue and costs for the day (including prorated salaries, cost of medical supplies, etc.) were accounted for.

Telemedicine

A major component of Dr. Shetty's ambition to provide cardiac care to the rural poor was the use of telemedicine. Since cardiac specialists were rare in remote areas, heart attack victims usually turned to general practitioners (GPs) who sometimes prescribed incorrect treatment due to lack of knowledge and/or facilities to correctly diagnose the problem. Dr. Shetty explained: "If a patient with chest pains walks in to see a GP, the doctor usually thinks it is indigestion so he'll be given an antacid and sent home . . . 24 hours later, the heart fails and it may be too late."

Sensing the need for immediate treatment and care in rural areas, Dr. Shetty set-up nine coronary care units (CCUs) across India, linked to NH or RTI (depending on proximity). Each CCU was equipped with beds, medication, computers, electrocardiogram (ECG) machines, video-conferencing devices and technical staff who were trained to operate the equipment. In addition, NH trained the GPs at the CCUs to perform checks on patients and administer treatment. With help from S.N. Informatics, a software development company located in Bangalore, NH also created a software program that allowed ECG images to be scanned and transmitted via a web connection.

When a patient visited a CCU, the GP on duty first took an ECG which was transmitted to a specialist at NH or RTI. With the patient and the GP on the screen, the specialist then diagnosed the condition and advised the GP on the appropriate treatment. Patients who needed to be kept under observation stayed overnight at the CCUs and specialists at NH and RTI conducted daily virtual checks on their condition. In serious cases, the patient, once stabilized, was transferred to NH or RTI for surgery. In very remote areas where video conferencing facilities could not be set-up, a network of around 100 family physicians were still able to use the software to transmit ECG images for diagnosis at NH.

Although telemedicine was not a new concept in India in 2001 (the Apollo Group of hospitals started using telemedicine earlier), NH and RTI made up the country's largest network and were the only hospitals in India that provided the service free. The cost of setting-up of the CCUs was funded by AHF, as were the staff salaries and operation costs. Almost from the beginning, the project was supported by the Indian Space Research Organization (ISRO), a government agency which adopted telemedicine as a community project and provided connectivity for the CCUs free of charge.

ISRO's technology allowed telemedicine to operate by satellite connection thus providing clearer images than the more expensive (and less reliable) phone lines—"the patient must see the compassion on the doctor's face," said Dr. Shetty.

In addition, the government of the state of Kamataka (in which Bangalore is the capital city) was so enthusiastic about NH's work that the state planned to sponsor a further 29 CCUs. NH continued to monitor all CCUs closely—for instance, when they discovered that a CCU did not keep stock of streptokinase (an injection that had to be administered within six hours of a heart attack), the hospital set a policy of daily "virtual" rounds of CCUs to ensure all systems were working and ready.

"Telemedicine gives ordinary doctors the opportunity to accomplish extraordinary things," Dr. Shetty said. Between 2001 and July 2004, the NH facility performed 9,591 tele-consultations and the CCUs had 4,077 in-patients, many of whom would not have received treatment otherwise. The telemedicine units were also linked to a clinic in Malaysia, a children's cardiac facility in Mauritius and a medical school in Hanover, Germany, with plans for new connections with Bangladesh, Tanzania and Pakistan. And Dr. Shetty believed the concept could be extended across other medical areas. "If the patient does not require surgery, then the doctors may not need to touch him—once thousand of CCUs are networked, telemedicine can be self-sustaining for a few rupees per patient."

While the telemedicine project utilized government infrastructure (i.e., the support by ISRO and the state government), the initial concept originated and was implemented via efforts at NH. To Dr. Shetty, this reflected the need for individuals and the private sector to take the initiative in areas where the government was typically held responsible. Dr. B.C. Bommaiah, a cardiologist at the hospital agreed, although he added the need for the right attitude on the part of doctors to implement such initiatives. "Not all doctors will agree to take responsibility for patients that they do not meet in person," he said. "But our doctors will care for someone they see on the screen."

Mobile Cardiac Diagnostic Lab

Both NH and RTI also organized outreach camps for cardiac diagnosis and care. Each weekend, two buses were sent out to rural areas, up to 800 km away from the hospitals in Bangalore and Calcutta. Each bus was staffed with at least three doctors, including an experienced cardiologist and two technicians trained to perform echo cardiograms. In order to ensure that the best possible diagnosis could be made onsite, the buses were outfitted with echocardiography equipment, a treadmill, a defibrillator, ECG machines, equipment needed for resuscitation in emergencies, and a generator to ensure the machines could be used in rural areas with irregular power supply. The first two mobile diagnostic labs were donated by the family of Mr. K. Dinesh, one of the founders of Infosys Ltd.

The outreach camps were organized by local associations (e.g., the Lions Club or Rotary Club) who advertised the day-long event in advance and arranged for patients to attend. On average, each camp screened 400 people a day, none of whom were required to pay either the hospital or the organizers. When a diagnosis indicated that the patient required medical intervention, he was advised to visit NH or RTI, where the procedure was performed at or below cost price with help from the NH charitable trust.

Training the Next Generation

In addition to their clinical work, the doctors at NH were also actively involved in training the next generation of specialists. NH ran 19 post-graduate programs for doctors and other medical staff, including diplomas in Cardiac Thoracic Surgery, Cardiology and. Medical Laboratory Technology. The hospital also offered the country's only formal training program for pediatric cardiac surgery, reflecting the rich expertise of NH's doctors in pediatric care.

In 2005, NH was scheduled to offer India's first Diploma in Cardiology, in collaboration with the Indira Gandhi National Open University (IGNOU). This program was Dr. Shetty's solution to bridging the gap between the 18,000 doctors graduating from India's medical schools each year and the 180 newly trained cardiologists and cardiac surgeons each year. Aimed at producing intermediate-level specialists, the program would require MBBS-qualified doctors (the Indian equivalent to an M.D.) to spend two years training at NH or at 50 other recognized heart hospitals in India.

A higher supply of cardiologists was expected to drive the costs of care lower, a concept which Dr. Shetty believed was extendable to other areas of health care. In nephrology, for instance, the requirement for trained nephrologists to operate dialysis machines was part of the reason that treatment was expensive. If India were to allow trained technicians to operate the machines (as is the case in the USA), or (as Dr. Shetty envisioned) offer a Diploma in Nephrology that would provide intermediate training, more doctors would be able to offer treatment to patients, thus lowering the cost of access to treatment.

Beyond training doctors, a separate department at the hospital coordinated the training of nurses. The 700 nurses at NH were required to complete a year of training which included a minimum six-month period in a critical care unit. As a result of intensive instruction, NH nurses were known across the state for their abilities and dedication; a writer to a Bangalore newspaper once likened each of them to Florence Nightingale. The downside to the excellent training, though, was the high turnover as skilled nurses sought better opportunities overseas. Ms Rohini Paul, the director of Nursing said, "Although we pay the highest salaries (in Bangalore), we lose many of our nurses because the skills they learn here will earn them better pay abroad; but this does not worry us, since there are so many more nurses waiting to join."

In addition to training nurses to be specialized in cardiac care, the college of nursing which was housed within NH offered degree and diploma courses for trainee nurses. To encourage students from poor remote areas who would benefit most from these educational opportunities, NH arranged to guarantee bank loans taken by the students to cover fees and living expenses. In return, the trainee nurses worked at the hospital during their course and for up to two years afterwards, thus supplying much-needed manpower.

The Insurance Scheme—Yeshasvini

The passion to serve the masses also drove Dr. Shetty to develop an insurance program called Yeshasvini. With an established name in Karnataka for his work in cardiac care, Dr. Shetty was approached by a milk cooperative for an endorsement of its product. As he learnt about the membership of the cooperative and their demographic profile, however, it occurred to Dr. Shetty that this could be the opportunity he had been seeking to access a clustered and organized group of middle to low income people, with poor access to health care.

Armed with this vision, the team at NH set-up a health insurance scheme for 1.7 million farmers and their families in Karnataka. Yeshasvini was launched in 2002 for farmers belonging to various state cooperatives-all farmers who had been members of a cooperative for at least a year were eligible to participate, regardless of their medical histories. For Rs. 5 (US$0.11) a month, cardholders had access to free treatment at 150 hospitals in 29 districts of the state for any medical procedure costing up to Rs. 100,000. See Exhibit 15 for a breakdown of procedures performed at NH alone under this scheme.

Prior to the scheme, it was estimated that the average occupancy of hospitals in Karnataka was only 35% although the state boasted 30 private medical colleges, each with over 500 beds, actual occupancy was low reflecting the lack of afford ability rather than a lack infrastructure. While micro-insurance schemes had existed in various forms in developing countries, the efforts were often unsystematic, resulting in little success. Recognizing this, Dr. Shetty chose to utilize the existing government infrastructure, in the form of state-controlled cooperative societies of Karnataka. In particular, the Principal Secretary of the Cooperative Department, Government of Karnataka, Mr. A. Ramaswamy, lent his support to the project and arranged for the involvement of then-Chief Minister, Mr. S.M. Krishna. Yeshasvini was launched as a state program, with the government contributing Rs. 2.5 for every Rs. 5 paid by the farmers.

By collecting the insurance fees up front for a year, the Yeshasvini Trust (which was created to own the scheme) was able to minimize initial need for funds. Research by the NH team estimated that only 8% of the policyholders would require medical procedures, thus the total funds collected was expected cover the cost of treatment for those in need. In order to keep the upfront collection costs to a minimum, the State government made available the infrastructure of its post offices (operated by the government) to collect the Rs. 5 premium, track monthly payments, and issue a "Yeshasvini member card." The initial task of getting the hospitals to participate and selling the idea to cooperatives was conducted by the Trust, but the daily operations were later handled by a third-party administrator, which also coordinated payment to hospitals.

The first year records of the scheme indicated that the majority of claims administered were for noncardiac treatment (the most common use of the scheme was for gynecological problems). Hanuman Prasad, who worked with the insurance team at NH, pointed out Yeshasvini was mostly used for low-cost treatments (approximately Rs. 2,000) which people would otherwise have forsaken since there was little money to spare to treat nonlife threatening conditions (see Exhibit 16 for the types of procedures performed under this scheme). In its first year, nearly 9,000 people underwent various operations and a further 35,000 received outpatient treatment across the state. By early 2005, the scheme included a quarter of the cooperatives 10 million members.

As in telemedicine, the insurance scheme relied on using government infrastructure but most of the planning and implementation was contributed by the NH team. "People are more willing to trust government agencies," explained Hanuman Prasad. "If we had started this as a private organization, there may have been less interest." Still, Dr. Shetty's and NH's reputation in the state helped gamer support for the program, both among the farmers and the hospitals. In particular, the hospitals which already had low utilization, could see the benefits of participating in a trustworthy scheme that would increase their patient flow without additional costs.

The success of Yeshasvini subsequently prompted Dr. Shetty and his team to consider new avenues for similar programs-for instance, plans were underway to administer an insurance scheme for teachers in Kamataka. Dr. Asha Naik, who was on the initial team for Yeshasvini, felt that the learning and publicity from Yeshasvini would make the second scheme easier to launch: "Since people have heard of Yeshasvini, there is greater awareness of the importance of health—of course, there are some things that we will do differently now. We need to use smart, digitalized cards to prevent fraud in using the scheme."

Spurred by this success, Dr. Shetty aspired to build on the insurance program to organize self-help groups in the state. One possibility was to have communities of 200 families living in a common area to band together to increase their purchasing power. "We are using health care as the carrot," said Dr. Shetty. "We want to encourage them to come together to purchase medicine but they should see that this is the same concept for other items. If 200 families want to buy television sets, they will have a higher bargaining power than each family buying it individually."

While Yeshasvini, the telemedicine program and other outreach schemes (including the mobile cardiac unit) were funded by AHF, a nonprofit organization, Dr. Asha Naik pointed out that the distinction between these programs and Narayana Hrudayalaya Pte Ltd (the private company that ran the hospital) were mere technicalities. "We have different legal vehicles for the work we do but everything is linked to Dr. Shetty and it's all his ideas that we are implementing," she said. Certainly these programs, while appearing distinct, were all part of Dr. Shetty's dream to "cure the world's poor for less than a dollar a day," starting with the Indian state of Karnataka.

The Plan for Health City

Having built NH into a reputable and profitable hospital, Dr. Shetty was keen to extend the concept of affordable health care to other specialties with NH serving as the "backbone" hospital. Dr. Shetty offered this rationale: "We have reached a plateau in cost-reduction by increasing our volume of surgeries—the yearly increase in procedures is now small but our resources are still underutilized—our machines, sterilization department, blood bank, etc. can be used by other hospitals within Health City and this will drive unit costs even lower."

To this end, NH started non-cardiac units, with the plan to house each specialty in new buildings that were being constructed in the 35 acres around the hospital. The neurosurgery unit was started in May 2004 with three surgeons and within 10 months, had completed 320 operations. A 500-bed orthopedic and trauma hospital was expected to be ready by end 2005, while another building was being constructed to house the existing neurosurgery unit and a planned pediatric unit.

In addition, the Emami National Institute for Bone Marrow Transplant (named after the Emami Group of Companies of Calcutta who fully funded the equipment) was started in 2004 as the state's largest bone marrow transplant unit. The unit was headed by Dr. Sharat Damodar, a hematologist trained in bone marrow transplant and who was already working with the cardiac team at NH. Once again, Dr. Shetty managed to reduce the cost of bone marrow transplant from the national average of Rs. 1.2 million (US$27,000) to Rs. 400,000 (US$8,900), this time by leveraging the hospital's existing infrastructure. The blood bank, for instance, had previously discarded unused blood after 10 days (as it was unsuitable for cardiac surgery) but could now utilize blood for up to 26 days after collection, in transplant procedures. In addition, the investigations performed for the bone marrow transplant utilized the existing equipment at NH, thus adding little fixed costs.

The plan, according to Dr. Shetty, was to build a total of 10 hospitals in a common area, with each hospital housing one or two specialties. The hospitals would be self-sufficient within each specialty (thus each building would have its own OTs, intensive care units, etc.) but would draw on common facilities such as blood banks and laboratories that were already established at NH. By employing specialists in each field who would be able to perform high volumes of surgeries and by leveraging the under-utilized common facilities, Dr. Shetty expected to offer tertiary health care at below-average costs. For instance, the cost of brain surgery at NH was expected to be Rs. 45,000 (US$1,000) while major spine surgery would cost Rs. 25,000 (US$550) at NH, approximately half the cost at other Indian hospitals. .

FREQUENTLY ASKED QUESTIONS

Q. You claim that India will be the largest provider of cardiac care in the world by 2006. Are you mad?

Not at all. India is already the largest producer of doctors, nurses—and heart patients—in the world. With economic liberalisation, the world is increasingly becoming boundaryless. Very soon economic realities will prevail. With painfully long waiting lists and high costs of surgery, the days are not far away when poor patients from all over will come here for heart surgery. One of my friends had an emergency case with a British tourist in Goa. After performing an angiogram, the patient was told he needed surgery which he could get done here or in the UK. He preferred to undergo the surgery here. "There's every possibility that an Indian would operate on me there", he said. "So why not get operated by an Indian in India?" We'll hear more such cases.

Q. Given the waiting lists in Britain, would you consider taking people from there?

Certainly. It will be inevitable in a few years. Some insurance company will com forward to provide the connecting link. After all, it's a matter of life—and that at the fraction of the cost in developed nations.

Q. Since coming back from Guy's, you've helped thousands of poor patients get state-of-the-art cardiac care. What motivated you to take on such a massive task?

I came back home to Kolkata (Calcutta), which is essentially a microcosm of India, a magnified village with well-equipped hospitals but extremely poor people unable to afford modern health care. This stopped me from getting cast in a typical doctor's mould. I was lucky enough to become Mother Teresa's personal cardiac surgeon, and five years of close association with her and her work changed my life. If I hadn't returned to Kolkata and not seen so much misery, maybe I wouldn't have taken up the cudgels this way.

Q. Why is heart care so important in India that it needs special projects and extra cash?

Indians are genetically prone to heart disease: they are three times more vulnerable than Americans or Europeans. In England, the average age of my patients was 65 years. Here it is 45.

Q. How easy it is to get those funds?

Believe it or not, it's not difficult to arrange for funds when your cause is noble. When I look back just three years ago on how funds came in for the Rabindranath Tagore International Institute of Cardiac Sciences in Kolkata, my resolve to spread the charitable health care approach gets stronger. After initial help from a construction businessman (whose father I had operated on) to build a cardiac diagnostic laboratory, there were grants from the corporate sector and soft loans for equipment from Tata Finance. One of my patients, a stockbroker, donated £72,000 as working capital. These helped get the building finished and start the hospital, by which time the Armenian Church came forward with an amazing £500,000. After inspecting us, they were so impressed they increased the amount to £ 1 million for a neurosurgical, renal and vascular trauma centre. Within six months we will have the largest trauma centre in eastern India. My plans have never suffered for lack of funds.

The medical fraternity has accused you of stealing the media limelight as the only Good Samaritan in town. Does that offend you?

I don't expect every one to be supportive of my activities. I am continually inspired by Albert Schweitzer's words that when you are working for man, don't expect him to remove stones from your path, expect him to put more there. I am one of the few privileged people in the world who at the early ago of 47 has everything a man can ask for. I don't want anything more in life for my personal gratification. Yes, health care is full of politics, but fortunately I've never been a victim as I never practised medicine for my personal gain. I began as a social worker and am continuing that way.

Q. Why isn't this cash coming from international bodies? Shouldn't they be promoting free or subsidised health care generally?

If there is one organisation that can be squarely blamed it is the WHO. Headquartered in Geneva, separated from reality, it runs its global activities with help from government representatives who are mostly bureaucrats. In the countries I travel to, bureaucrats are a class of people who are experts in nothing but authorities on everything. They are not best-suited to guide planning at the WHO. One of the WHO declarations was "Health for all by 2000." How can a global body make that kind of statement when a country like Zambia does not have an echo-Doppler, without which you cannot detect any heart problem, or when one cannot find a single functioning ECG machine in many African countries?

Q. That doesn't sound too good . . .

It gets worse. The WHO has saddled most governments with grants and soft loans, not donations. Millions of pounds are given which are ill-spent either on buying expensive equipment which tends to be left unused or on expanding the physical infrastructure. I have met people from the government who say they don't know how to spend the money. Then comes the repayment, when the axe falls on the taxpayers.

Q. So what should happen?

Shift the WHO headquarters from Geneva to any Third World country where it would be able to assess the problems without any filters. Subsidised health care should be extended to all possible areas.

Q. So have you given up on politicians?

Apart from the WHO, I have stopped blaming the politicians and bureaucrats. We are better placed to bring about changes by being outsiders, not by being a part of the system. All that the government can do is to stop being an obstacle. If it decides to be a bystander, things will fall in place. My belief is that within ten years, the government health care systems in all Third World countries will fold up. The government will not be able to pay even salaries, never mind offering health care. In that situation, organisations like ours should come forward to take over and manage it in a professional manner.

Q. For the past six months you've been running telecardiology units at your Bangalore and Kolkata hospitals which link to coronary care units (CCUs) in remote parts of eastern India. How's it going?

The first eight hours after a heart attack is the golden period for treatment and few district hospitals have the expertise and the equipment to manage cardiac emergencies. So we set-up CCUs in remote areas of northeastern parts of India which are the most backward. These units have been linked to my two specialised hospitals in Kolkata and Bangalore through ISDN lines. We have trained doctors from district hospitals in critical care management and echocardiology. Patients who didn't have access to cardiac care can now go to their nearest CCU, where doctors, with guidance from specialists at these two base stations, will provide treatment. We can also make final interpretations of ECG, echocardiograph and other reports through telecardiology. We saw 600 patients in the first seven weeks.

Q. Are there any areas of cardiac care which are specially well suited to this treatment-from-a-distance?

All kinds of diagnoses can be made through telecardiology. One the initial reports are analysed and if the patient requires just medication, not surgery, it will be provided by our experts from here. If the patient needs surgery, he will have to undergo that in his home country or he is welcome to come to us. As the telecardiology network expands and matures, we'll train doctors to provide advanced services in the local CCUs. Paedifatric heart care is another area of concern because 1 in 140 children born anywhere in the world requires heartcare.

Q. You're extending telecardiology to Mauritius, Bangladesh and Malaysia, Why?

In these countries, either affordable cardiac care is not available for the underprivileged, or cardiac care itself is a scarce service. I regularly get patients from these countries, and many times we feel that the patient need not have travelled all that way. Sometimes newborn babies or toddlers are brought to us only to find that either they do not require an operation or they can wait for a few years. Similarly, a patient whose coronary arteries are found to be blocked after investigation through a link-up facility can be advised on the future course of action. If they want to avoid surgery in their home country because that country is just too poor, they can be called to Bangalore and operated on at a third of the cost. The NGOs we're working with might even arrange for some funding.

Q. This must all get very expensive. After all, the hospital at Bangalore will equip CCUs with instruments and train personnel while the NGOs will only bear local administration expenses

In my 12 years of running the hospital in India I've seen that people are increasingly becoming more giving. The opening up of the global economy has created at lot of wealth among middle-class people. It used to be that wealth was accumulated over long periods, often by not-so-legitimate means. But now the people who have become rich do not have to read newspaper to understand poverty. And when good people become wealthy, money gets spent on better causes.

Q. But I've heard there's a difference in the economics of running your hospital.

Yes, it's very different. In Western hospitals, about 60 percent of the revenue is spent on salaries, while in government hospital in India, 90 percent goes on salaries. By contrast, in our hospital only 12 to 13 percent is spent on salaries. That doesn't mean our doctors are being exploited. Since their output is ten times more, unit operating costs are very low. To earn a given salary in another hospital, a doctor would have to perform one operation a day. With us he might have to operate on five patients. We also work with zero inventory, so the burden lies with the supplier. And since we are the largest consumers of medical disposables, we procure them at a discount of 30 to 35 percent.

Q. You've moved incredibly fast in 12 years, two big heart hospitals and research centres, one heart foundation, 9000 operations—4000 of which were on children—plans for mobile ECGs to every GP in Karnataka. . . What's next?

There's so much to be done. I dream of having a CCU in every government—run district hadequarter hospital and linking them to the Bangalore and Kolkata hospitals. Starting from a small village near Bangalore, I want to show the world that some kind of health insurance is possible for the poor who cannot currently dream of heart care.

Q. How would that work?

The idea is to make these poor people believe that just as they spend money on rice, milk and kerosene, they will have to spend a minimal amount, say 10 to 15p a month, even when they are well, towards health insurance. While the rich have private health insurance, the poor need organised health care. Today, no health service in government hospitals in India is free, least of all cardiac care. It is subsidised for the poorest of the poor but the quality of service offered is deplorable. We are discussing health insurance with some insurance companies.

Q. Besides cardiac care, what fascinates you?

Nothing. I dream, breath and live health-care. And I am fortunate to have found a team that shares my dream.

An electronic between specialists at city hospital and coronary care units (CCUs) in rural communities. The telemedicine programme, called the Integrated Telecordiology and Telehealth Project (ITTP), is the largest of its kind in India—and a model for Asia.

In India, there's barely on qualified doctor per 2000 rural dwellers. Before the first telemedicine CCUs began operating in June 2001, 50 per cent of patients seeking help at district hospital died without specialist advice. That's beginning to change dramatically.

"We have treated over 11,000 patients and the death rate has dropped to less than five per cent," says Dr. Alok Roy, Shetty's long-time partner and Vice-president of the ITTP. Shetty alone has consulted on more than 8500 telemedicine cases.

"Dr. Shetty is a visionary," says K. (Dinesh, co-founder of INFOSYS, one of India's largest software companies. Australian cardiac surgeon Colin John agrees. "Dr. Shetty and his telemedicine team have given specialists the tools to reach out to underprivileged people around the world."

Devi Shetty is an astorishingly busy man, performing two to three open-heart surgeries in 14-hour days, six days a week. During his 16-year career, he and his team of surgeons have performed 17,000 life-saving operations.

A week later, the system faced its greatest test. An unconscious 60-year old man was carried into the unit with plummeting blood pressure and a rapid pulse. His ECG showed ventricular tachycardia, which can swiftly lead to cardiac arrest and death.

The medical officer had seen such patients before, but with no way to treat them, they had all died. Now the on duty cardiologist in Calcutta ordered him to apply electric-shock paddles to the heart.

The patient didn't respond. "Increase the power," ordered the cardiologist, watching his vital signs by video. This time, the man's heart was jolted into normal rhythm.

That evening there was rejoicing in the Telemedicine Centre. "We need no other proof," a jubilant Roy told Shetty. Then the pair sat down to figure out the next step.

The stumbling block was India's unreliable and expensive phone lines, which could disconnect at a critical moment. Only satellite communication, run by the Indian Space Research Organisation (ISRO), would be up to the task. "Why don't we talk to them?" Shetty asked.

He made his pitch to the then ISRO Chairman K. Kasturirangan, explaining that the connection had to be good enough for high-quality images. "The patient must see the compassion on the doctor's face." "It is going to revolutionise health-care delivery to poor areas around the world."

Kasturirangan was excited: The ISRO had carried out a few telemedicine experiments, but nothing on this scale, or with the potential to help so many. "I will give you any connectivity you want," he said.

The ISRO installed the main dish outside Dr. Roy's office window and similar dishes at the telemedicine CCUs. Now the doctors would have a crystal-clear picture and no bill.

As world about the telemedicine Project spread, other states wanted in, offering to pay for equipment, manpower and running costs. Shetty and Roy agreed. Bring high technology to rural India had its own problems. Power fluctuations fried circuit boards in teleconferencing equipment; uninterrupted power supply with back-up batteries was installed to protect the units.

"We had to train the technicians at each station in basic repair and carry spares for the most common breakdowns," says Dr. N.K. Singh, director of the telemedicine programme. When angiograms took up to 90 minutes to transmit, an Indian company, Televital designed compression software to cut the time to five minutes. The entire system would operate 24 hours a day. Shetty insited that incoming ECGs be read within five minutes of arrival.

In July 2001, the second telemedicine CCU, at Bankura Sammilani Medical College Hospital in West Bengal, was inaugurated, and a third in August at the Tripura Sundari District Hospital.

Today 19 CCUs operate across India, and 27 more are being deployed across Karnataka State.

"Once thousands of CCUs are networked, telemedicine can be self-sustaining for a few rupees per patient," says Shetty. That's only the beginning. The telemedicine centre at Narayana Hrudayalaya has links to a clinic in Kuala Lumpur, a children's cardiac facility in Mauritius and a medical school in Hanover, Germany. Shetty is also planning centres in Bangladesh, Tanzania, Yemen, Pakistan and Zambia. Meanwhile, Shetty and his team rolled out Heart Care on Wheels, a bus with state-of-the echocardiography, colour doppler, a computerized treadmill and laptop computers. The diagnostic lab roams all over Karnataka, treating up to 500 patients a day and performing 150 ECG's. Onboard specialists communicate with Bangalore via satellite.

Last March Devi Shetty successfully performed open-heart surgery on four-year-old Pulak Nasar. After the operation, the parents sat with their son in the paediatric intensive care unit. "He's going to be fine," Shetty assured them. He has since heard Pulak is fishing and running around as any healthy boy should.

"Telemedicine lets ordinary doctors do extraordinary things," Shetty says, "It is going to revolutionise health care delivery to poor areas around the world."

(Hutchison, *Reader's Digest*, Feb. 2004).

Chain of Centres

Chain of telecardiology centres and heart clinics, now health Insurance for the poor. In the long entrance hall of Narayana Hrudayalaya are waiting hundreds of patients for help. For most of them it's like a gift to be treated in this hospital, that is one of the biggest in the world. Every two of three beds are reserved for the needy. Through a spacious prayer hall with a carved statue of God Vishnu, the Creator leads the way to the office of Dr. Shetty.

This director is at work, holding in his hands ECG of a man, sent to him on computer from Calcutta. Using a microphone and a web-camera he is now discussing the strategy for treatment with the patient. The patient, who couldn't have afforded to pay for a crucial Bypass operation in a usual hospital, now lies in one cardiological treatment center in Calcutta. This center thanks to an aid from Dr. Shetty is connected to the clinic in Bangalore via ISDN. "God bless the doctor," says the patient and his tears can be seen over the screen.

Heart surgeon Devi Prasad Shetty is famous all over India not only for these telecardiology treatments but also for building up a chain of heart clinics with heart foundation and trauma centers. In association with Asia Heart Foundation, Indian Space Research Organization and local organizations Dr. Shetty wants to export the idea of network of consultation centers to Bangladesh, Malaysia and Mauritius. He says, "the heart operations there are not affordable by the poor. I often get patients from these countries who either are unable to travel or don't really need an operation. Both the types can be helped through telemedicine."

International body like World Health Organization (WHO) should be more accessible for medical help to the needy countries. One of the WHO's declarations "Health for everyone by 2000" is away from reality, maintains Dr. Shetty, "when some of the African countries do not even a single working Echo-Doppler." He advises, WHO headquarters should be moved from Geneva to any Third World country where it can access the problems without filters.

Even if you take a quick look at Narayana Hrudayalaya hospital, you will notice the classrooms, where new colleagues are familiarized with hospital's philosophy. Dr. Shetty says, "Such a huge venture is impossible unless everyone sets in unconditionally."

It's 10:30 in the morning, the surgeon has already performed 2 operations and is preparing for another one: a usual routine for someone who has performed around 13,500 heart operations in 17 years of his career, of which 5000 were performed in babies.

On the way to OPD Dr. Shetty says, "What you have seen here in Bangalore is nothing compared to our assignments in recent future." According to him, the Public Health not only in India but also in many developing countries is on verge of collapse. The governments soon won't be able to pay up for the personnel. "Organizations like ours then have to bridge this gap, so that at least the basic medical facilities remain maintained."

As a religious man he believes "God doesn't confront us with problems without creating solutions for them. But while looking for these solutions one must not think only about oneself."

Nothing stops him from working his seemingly impossible project. He himself wants to facilitate health insurance for the poor, who can't afford private insurance. He states, these people save only a small sum every month and for insurance they would have to make an upfront payment. Hence they would never have a chance to get into a government hospital. He plans to finance his own scheme with the help of foreign patients. Within few years India would be an important provider of facilities for heart surgery, as it is the largest instructor of doctors and nurses. Dr. Shetty maintains, due to long waiting lists for heart operations and huge treatment costs in many western countries, many foreigners will have themselves treated on in India.

NH in Global Health

Globalization can help rein in America's soaring health-care costs. That's one reason he is studying Indian hospitals such as Narayana Hrudayalaya, founded by cardiac surgeon Dr. Devi Shetty. Some reasons for its low costs can't be easily replicated elsewhere. The land was owened by Shetty's family. The hospital's 25 foreign trained surgeons earn half what they could in the US. Outsize malpractice awards are rare in India, so insurance costs are low. But the hospital also operates for fee or anyone who cannot pay and on any infant younger than one month. For the rural poor, it runs 39 remote clinics and mobile-testing labs with satellite links that so far treated 17,000 patients.

Some the of the biggest savings come from its business model. In the U.S., the chief surgeon manages the entire patient process, from testing and diagnosis to supervising the operating room, recuperation, and billing. Narayana works more like an assembly line: The surgeons perform only surgery.

That may seem like a recipe for shoddy care. But Shetty asserts it actually translates into fewer mistakes because specialist focus on what they do best. The 1.35% mortality rate for coronary bypasses and 2.7% rate for aortic valve replacements reported by Narayana are roughly half the average of U.S. hospitals, according to federal statistics, though those aren't the only measures of quality care. "The importance of volume is not well understood in our industry." Shetty says. "A surgeon doing three or four operations a day does much better work than one doing three or four in a week." The factory approach also leads to economies of scale. The hospital uses all of its expensive CAT scanners and X-ray and magnetic-resonance machines to the max. "In the U.S., a lot of this infrastructure is used five days a week," says Shetty. "We use ours 14 hours a day, 7 days a week.

This raises intriguing questions. If Indian doctors can effectively diagnose and treat heart conditions in farmers in distant villages, why can't American consumers use videoconferencing to consult offshore specialists 24/7? Why can't an enterprising hospital chain bring Narayana's model to the US. Or at least set-up hospitals in Mexico or the Caribbean charging a fraction of US prices?

Health without Wealth

An ambitious cooperative health care scheme for the poor launched by the Karnataka Government allows its members to avail of major medical treatment free of cost at 83 hospitals in the state. Made Gowda, 53, a farmer from Mandya district near Bangalore, recently underwent a heart operation In Narayana Hrudayalaya, the city's largest heart hospital. Nothing unusual about the whole thing except for the fact that he paid virtually nothing for the surgery that normally costs between Rs. 1.2 lakh and Rs. 1.4 lakh. For the cost of a coffee in an upscale coffee bar, farmers and their families undergo different types of operations, including those of the stomach, gall bladder, uterus, eyes, heart and brain, free of cost.

Gowda is one of 17lakh farmers who paid just Rs. 5 every month under a cooperative sector scheme that allows them to have similar operations. His was one of the 6,000 surgeries carried out at the 780-bed Narayana Hrudayalaya under the Yeshasvini health scheme launched in the cooperative sector by the Government in June last year, basing it on an idea thought of by Narayana Hrudayalaya's founder and heart surgeon Devi Shetty. The members of the cooperatives involved in this scheme, mainly poor farmers, pay just Rs. 60 per annum. In return, they can avail of the best health care in the state. Says Shetty: "We cannot become a developed nation unless health care is made available to all strata in society. He adds, "We found the problem was not the infrastructure but the inability to pay for health care which was the real malaise."

And that was how he struck upon the Yeshasvini scheme that would, in the first phase, make modern health care available for free to 17 lakh farmers and their family. The scheme works because studies have shown that on average only 0.08 per cent of the people covered would require operations. This means the cost of their treatment is borne through the contribution of the others who do not need medical help. It is this concept that came to the rescue of farmers like Gowda and Jayamma for Anekal village in Bangalore who underwent hysterectomy—removal of the diseased uterus-for free. They could never have otherwise afforded the normal costs of the operations that are usually in the range of Rs. 15,000-20,000.

It all began when the Karnataka Milk Federation (KMF), a cooperative with more than two million members in Bangalore, invited Shetty. He had been asked to endorse a milk product but he took the opportunity to convince the KMF managing director to extend health benefits to all its members by paying a nominal Rs. 5 a month. It was at the same function that the surgeon got the opportunity to suggest this revolutionary health plan to Chief Minister S.M. Krishna. Krishna, in turn, introduced Shetty, to A. Ramaswamy, principal secretary in the department of cooperatives. So was born the Yeshasvini scheme with KMF members as its first beneficiaries.

Ramaswamy, who named the scheme Yeshasvini (victor, in Sanskrit), says that in the scheme a major chunk of the budget allocated for health care in a family goes to the earning male member, followed by children and women. The scheme, however, does not cover a married member's parents. It is now extended to most cooperative units in the state. And, it is supported by 83 hospitals across Karnataka which are paid by the scheme trust for the members' treatment. Maharashtra and Tamil Nadu Governments are in dialogue with the trust to include cooperatives in their states in this ambitious scheme. Shetty dreams of expanding Yeshasvini throughout the country.

Enthused by the initial success of the Yeshasvini health programme for farmers, the state Government decided to create a corpus of Rs. 100 crore in January this year with contributions from its coffers, profitable cooperative institutions, MNCs and other donors. State Cooperatives Minister H. Vishwanath ways that his target is to cover five million people. "Smart cards are being issued to those covered under this health plan. Farmers and farm workers can avail of medical benefits in the areas of cardiology, urology, gynaecology, orthopaedics, hernia and other general procedures," he adds.

Prema, a farm worker from Mandya, who was treated for a broken leg, says, "The treatment came at the right time for absolutely no cost at all." Chikkayya, a farmer who underwent a surgery for a debilitating backbone disorder, says, "The money I paid every month was half the price of a bidi packet. Now not only have I stopped smoking bidis, I am happy too."

For those like Prasanna, 21, from Tumkur district who had an open-heart surgery and valve replacement, the scheme is good news with a touch of sadness. "My father would have been living today if this scheme had been in effect, say, three years ago," he says.

The Yeshasvini scheme has attracted global attention with two major US bodies, Harvard and the Rockefeller Foundation, planning to study it closely and replicate it elsewhere, especially in African countries. The World Bank too has shown interest in the functioning of this health programme with the intention of finding more pragmatic solutions to low-cost, high-quality health care in the developing world.

It is good health care at affordable prices that matters most to Shetty. He dreamt big, but the rewards too have been promising.

Forbes Asia says

Yeshasvivi's contribution to India, and to the world, "is providing proof of the concept that at 5 rupees a month it is possible to provide health care to the poor," he says in his soft, plumy voice. A strong believer in the "Wal-Martization of Health Care", he has always relied on the "law of large numbers", be it reducing costs at his hospitals or initiating Yeshasvini.

Statistically, in a random population in India less than 1% require surgery. So the first milestone was enrolling very large numbers of people. Yeshasvini, run by a nonprofit trust, approached the local bureaucracy in Karnataka, which has 30,000 cooperatives in its system. These often pay premiums up front and settle with members later. The state government provided a fixed annual subsidy of 75 cents per person in the first year. (The payments have risen slightly or are computed differently as costs have escalated—Yeshasvini has an "adverse selection" of illness-prone members even with the large numbers cushion—but the price tag remains at less than $3 a year per patient.)

"Initially, working with 80 hospitals we proved that it's a viable business. Then we convinced other hospitals in the state, which have large unutilized capacities, that they could choose to do fewer surgeries at a higher cost or more surgeries at a lower cost, but with assured payment; says Dr. Shetty. Now the hospitals, he smilingly adds, cannot survive if they don't recognize Yeshasvini cardholders.

A country that produces the fourth highest number of physicians (600,000) in the world and has the second-largest number of hospitals (15,000) still fares rather bleakly on the health care front. Less than 2% of the population has private health insurance; government programs cover another 12%.

"Health insurance has rarely met with success in India," says David M. Dror, a professor who specializes in this field at Erasmus University in Rotterdam, the Netherlands. Dror has studied some of the 25 micro health insurance programs operating in India, which he says have had more success than commercial policy issuers.

"Yeshasvini is interesting to people because it covers 160 procedures and the network of hospitals includes the best available where they are located. People, even poor people, prioritize choice and quality health care," he argues. In July Dror launched a first-of-its kind micro-insurance academy in New Delhi.

Microinsurance itself can be commercialized. Most insurance majors like Zurich Financial Services, American International Group and Allianz are actively pursuing the strategy in emerging markets, including India, where they typically partner with domestic entities. Basically, micro marketing means linking to mass organizations or localities rather than peddling higher-premium products through agents to individuals.

Overall, the insurance market is booming in India, growing 28% in 2005-06. The health portfolio is the fastest-growing sector in non-life insurance, according to the Insurance Regulatory Development Authority in Hyderabad. In 2006-07 health premiums grew 42% to $740 million; it was a measly $115 million in 2001 when insurance-sector reforms began.

But, says Authority Chairman C.S. Rao, unavailability of credible actuarial data, which crimps product innovation, and high transaction costs for the insurers are inhibiting a mass market.

Dr. Shetty believes mass organizations have to playa larger role for the commercial sector to find this market viable. In a pilot program begun in 2005, he has teamed private insurer ICICI Lombard with the Biocon Foundation, a charity of wealthy entrepreneur Kiran Mazumdar-Shaw, to form Arogya Raksha Yojana, a program aimed at children and others in Karnataka who wouldn't be reached by Yeshasvini, as well as the slums of Kolkata. (In Karnataka it also covers two Tibetan settlements with help from Hollywood star Richard Gere's foundation, Healing the Divide.)

"We realized that retailing of micro health insurance was not easy," says Rani Desai, head of Biocon Foundation. While ICICI made a profit even in the first year, the program is now turning to self-help groups among the poor to build volume.

Yeshasvini has piggybacked on Dr. Shetty's charisma and NH's reputation. Will its early success therefore be transferable to similar endeavors? He thinks it will need to as governments in India realize the futility of shoring up health care infrastructure and turn to helping provide health insurance instead of health care itself to those in decrepit surroundings.

Shetty has ensured that his own hospitals provide three rates—general, charitable and Yeshasvini—to keep treatment affordable. For him Yeshasvini is just the beginning. He is already in talks with the two largest government-managed entities—the State Bank of India and the Indian postal department, both with more than 100 million depositors—for a custom-built insurance program. In the eastern state of West Bengal he has helped formulate a new micro health insurance product for several thousand primary and secondary school teachers.

Public sector National Insurance has teamed with teacher associations to use the government's $2.50 monthly health care allowance for teachers to instead provide health insurance to a teacher's entire family. The product will launch before year-end.

Poor people are weak in isolation, but in groups they gain strength as consumers, says Dr. Shetty. One gets a sense of that force if you glance at the Yeshasvini counter at NH-six days a week hundreds of villagers, partly in a queue, partly in a crowd, clamor for consultations. A mass market is being born.

Asia Heart Foundation

Asia Heart Foundation is a charitable trust, working in the field of health care.

We at AHF feel that it is important to develop a cachet of qualified medical graduates for the future, which will help India administer its health care system more effectively for the common man.

We believe children from rural India have the fire and zeal required to become outstanding heart surgeons, neurosurgeons and other specialized medical professionals in fields that require more commitment and dedication. We also feel that these children can be motivated to use their training in improving health care systems in their villages and small towns.

Towards this endeavour, we want to initiate a scholarship program for school students in West Bengal, through which we will be able to encourage young meritorious school students from rural India to take up the medical profession.

Our Role in this project

For Asia Heart Foundation this project is close to our hearts, as we believe that this is not just a question of helping others but helping our future. We are privileged to have created some of the best heart hospitals of India and to have brought high technology heart surgery to the level of a common man.

We proved to the world that by paying just Rs. 5 a month you can run the world's largest micro health insurance program, we made telemedicine a reality in association with ISRO and we introduced new techniques of treating various heart diseases. The scholarship program will give us a platform to share their aspirations to become doctors and also create a bond with these children that will extend beyond the time that they spend in the program.

Keeping this in mind we have set the ball rolling by starting this scholarship program, which will launch 150 rural students of on a journey to become qualified doctors. These 150 students in West Bengal is a start but can only begin to address the situation. In the future we will extend this program to 2000 students annually, making it 2000 more doctors for India every year. To do this we need your help, support and generous contribution. We want this program be launched only in West Bengal since West Bengal is close to our heart. Under Rajiv Gandhi Aroyga Raksha Yojna, Asia Heart Foundation has initiated a project to revamp the health care facilities in the 16 blocks of Amethi. The project covers the basic health care needs of 2.4 million people living in a 3800 sq.km. area. We are setting up a chain of primary health care centres in all the blocks of Amethi offering out-patient services that include consultation, medicines and telemedicine facilities with specialty centres at Narayana Hrudayalaya, Bangalore and RTIICS, Kolkata.

Our Units

- Rabindranath Tagore International Institute of Cardiac Sciences (RTIICS), Kolkata.
- Armenian Church Trauma Center, Kolkata.

- Manjulaben Mehta Kidney Hospital, Kolkata.
- Rotary Narayana Sankara Nethralaya, Kolkata.
- R.C. Agarwal Memorial Hospital, Tinsukia, Assam.
- Narayana Hrudayalaya, Bangalore.
- Narayana Nethralaya, Bangalore.
  Sparsh Orthoepedics and Trauma Centre, Bangalore.
- Narayana Institute for Advanced Research (Cancer Hospital), Bangalore.

APPENDIX 4

NARAYANA NETHRALAYA HEALTH CITY, BANGALORE

Our Mission

They at Narayana Nethralaya are committed to provide the best services in eye care through continual improvement of processes and systems through involvement of people continual improvement of processes and systems through involvement of people and state of the art technology.

India is rapidly becoming a destination for international medical tourism due to high quality professional care executed at reasonable and affordable rates. We believe in high quality patient care. Currently, we have highly skilled professionals to take care of our large patient base. We take pride in letting you know that we match our growing volume of work with improving quality.

We are now ready to shift gears to venture into research, specifically clinical and applied. Currently our efforts are directed towards groundwork towards this goal. We believe that by collaborating nationally and internationally with institutions that have advanced basic research capabilities, we can avoid reinventing the wheel. Interdisciplinary approach is not only the fashion, but a necessity today. Our long-term vision is to be recognized as one amongst the best research and academic institutions in the world.

Channelizing the variegated talents of this team of incurable optimists and dedicated and skilled eye care professionals towards creating a world class service structure is a major challenge and a pleasure.

We are now increasingly focusing on community eye care services other than just cataract surgery, paediatric eye health, ocular infections, steam cell applications, ocular complications of HIV/AIDS and basic science research. Our emphasis on knowledge management by using electronic medical records which facilitates evidence based eye care has lead us to investing heavily on medical informatics.

A Centre of Excellence

Narayana Nethralaya is specialty eye hospital in Bangalore, having two large units, one located centrally at Rajajinagar, and the other at the Narayana Hrudayalaya—Health City campus on Hosur Road.

Narayana Nethralaya was started in the year 1982 as an eye clinic at Srirampuram, Bangalore by our Chairman.

Dr. K. Bhujang Shetty: Recognizing the need to provide comprehensive eye care to the ever-growing number of patients, while at the same time offering the best in ophthalmic subspeciality services, Dr. K. Bhujana Shetty established Narayana Nethralaya as it is today in 1993.

The new eye hospital at Narayana health city is spread over 120,000 sq. ft, and has separate wings for various specialities and departments, which are fully equipped with the state of art diagnostic and therapeutic tools. This hospital proudly lodges a dedicated area for community eye care which caters to the needs of the financially under-privileged. Paediatric eye health is one of our thrust areas. Research expansion is one of our current priorities and we have a dedicated wing to facilitate this endeavor. Our thrust into basic and applied research simultaneously with state of the art diagnostics and therapeutics, in conjunction with some of the best minds in the Narayana Health city promises to allow us to make path breaking changes in treatment paradigms in the years to come.

Of note, is the serious effort being directed to switch over to Electronic Medical Records in a phased manner. A new department of medical informatics has been set-up to exploit information technology to improve patient care and create knowledge from data.

The National Board of examinations, New Delhi has recognized the hospital for training of candidates for the DNB course (ophthalmology) with an intake of 6 candidates per year.

Their programme gives vast learning experience in terms of clinical, surgical and continuing medical education programmes. Our consultants are responsible as thesis guides for mentoring the research work.

Areas of Clinical Care and Research

- Cataract and Refractive Lens Surgery
- Cornea and Refractive Surgery
- Vitreoretinal surgery
- Uveitis and Ocular Immunology
- Pediatric Ophthalmology and Strabismology
- Glaucoma
- Ocular Oncology and Oculopasty surgery
- Ocular Trauma
- Community Eye Health
- Telemedicine
- Neuro-ophthalmology
- Ocular Electrophysiology
- Ocular Genetics
- Ocular Microbilogy and Molecular Diagnostics

The Services

Cornea, Refractive Surgery and Ocular Surface Service

Well trained corneal surgeons provide "cutting edge" treatment for most corneal disorders. Modern innovations in keratoplasty like DALK and DSAEK for corneal endothelial disorders, Intacs® and Corneal Collagen cross linking, are now utilized here to manage hitherto difficult disorders like Keratoconus, Pellucid Marginal degeneration, and post-LASIK ectasia. The "Dr. Rajkumar Eye Bank" Affiliated to the Eye Bank Association of India, has done commendable work in eye banking and eye donation awareness. The refractive surgery services (for eliminating the need for glasses) utilize a combination of incisional and top for the line LASIK machines liked to wave front and Pentacam analyzers to deliver optimal patient satisfaction. Advanced ocular surface disorders can now be treated with Amniotic Membrance and Stem Cell Transplantation, where our consultants have considerable expertise.

Contact Lens and Vision Rehabilitation Centre

Services of the contact lens clinic include fitting of contact lenses for refractive errors such as myopia (short sight) and hypermetropia (long sight), RGP lenses for Keratoconus, and cosmetic contact lenses. A special group of patients—those with severe low vision who cannot be cured with surgery of medication—find support, treatment and low vision aids in the Vision Rehabilitation Centre. Low vision aids (LVA) are special devices used to help the patient with poor vision to utilize the residual vision in a more effective way and in certain cases, improve the vision. Services of the low vision aids clinic help the patient to see the world better with whatever residual vision the patient has.

Cataract, IOL and Refractive Lens Surgery Service

Cataract surgery is the most commonly performed surgery by any eye doctor world wide. Narayana Nethralaya is fully equipped with the most modern technology for performing sutureless cataract microsurgery. Apart from the standard procedures such as Phacoemulsification with foldable intraocular lens implantation, and manual small incision cataract surgery, our surgeons can comfortably perform surgeries for complicated cataracts, congenital cataracts and cataracts resulting from other eye disorders. Newer, state of the art refractive lens procedures include phakic IOL procedures inpatients who are unsuitable for LASIK are being performed at our institute. We are currently involved in a clinical trial that will compare newer types of intraocular lenses.

Uvelitis and Ocular Immunology Service

The Uveitis and Ocular Immunology Service provides a multidisciplinary approach to the treatment of ocular inflammatory disease and other infectious disorders. Experts here deal with diagonosis and management of complex infectious and autoimmune diseases of the eye as well as eye diseases associates with various other systemic medical disorders. The diagnostics are backed by a well equipped laboratory, pathology and molecular diagnostic services, and the consultants are conversant with appropriate intervention techniques. In addition, we have the experience with the latest treatments including the use of immunosuppressive and immunomodulation for autoimmune eye diseases.

We co-ordinate with the other subspecialities of ophthalmology and internal medicine efficiently to get the optimal treatment outcomes for patients with complex Uveitic disorders. Another field of specialization is HIV/AIDS associated ocular infections wherein we have a combined experience of having seen over a few thousand HIV/AIDS cases with ocular complications. We were the first in the world to have reported the association of serious eye problems with Chikungunya fever.

Vitreoretina Service

The Vitreoretina service at Narayana Nethralaya is a major referral center which deals with management of diabetic retinopathy and diabetic eye diseases, retinal detachment, ARMD, infections, trauma and various other retinal disorders. the intelligent use of the complete spectrum of the latest diagnostic equipment (FFA, ICG, Ultrasound B Scan UBM, Optical Coherence Tomography, and Visual Electrophysiological Tests. Such as ERG, multifocal ERG, EOG and VEP are effectively used by a team of highly trained retinal surgeons combined with modern surgical unit, to get optimal visual results. Clinical trials are underway to evaluate newer drugs and treatment options.

Glaucoma Service

The center offers state of the art technology to diagnose, monitor and manage all kinds of glaucoma and related disorders. Modern diagnostic tools for early diagnosis of glaucoma like newer automated perimeters, GDx-analyzer, OCT and HRT machines for retinal nerve fiber layer analysis and optic nerve imaging are available are available for the experts to diagnose glaucoma at initial stage itself and prevent patients from going blind. In addition to providing routine glaucoma management latest treatment modalities like laser and implant are use to manage complicated glaucomas.

Optical Services

Optical Services offers a full range of comprehensive optical services from routine to highly specialized eyewear. We offer a full line of optical lenses from the most basic single vision to the most technologically advanced lenses. Our skilled opticians have extensive experience filling difficult and unusual prescriptions while working closely with doctors from many of our specialty ophthalmology services.

Neuro-Ophthalmology and Ocular Electrophysiology Service

We also have a specialized head ache clinic which caters to patients with chronic headache. Neurological diseases such as strokes, brain tumors, multiple sclerosis are associated with a variety of eye diseases. Neuro-ophthalmology services in consultation with neurologists specialize in dealing with eye disorders associated with neurological disorders. We work closely with the Narayana Institute of Neurological Sciences at health city and provide the necessary support in diagnosis and management of patients with neurologic problems. The Visual Electrophysiology lab, approved by the ISCEV is a valuable diagnostic adjunct to a wide variety of neuro-ophthalmic and hereditary and acquired retinal disorders. The spectrum of tests include VER, ERG (flash full field, Pattern and Multifocal) and EOG. In addition, it is valuable in our ongoing research.

Orbit, Oculoplasty and Ocular Oncology Services

This is a unique subspeciality, treating diseases involving not only the eye, but the surrounding lids, socket, and lacrimal system. In addition to providing standard treatment to common oculoplastic problems, we go a step further. Orbital tumors and fractures are routinely dealt with. Socket reconstruction and cosmetic rehabilitation is done at our customized ocular prosthesis clinic. Endoscopic LASER-DCR is routinely done in selected cases to achieve better cosmetic outcomes. A unique area of expertise includes the ocular oncology service which provides the latest international treatment algorithms, many times drawing international specialist co-operation to get best results. The Botox clinic deals effectively with troublesome disorders like hemifacial spasm and essential blepharospasm.

Pediatric Ophthalmology and Strabismology Services

This department has grown to be a major referral centre for pediatric eye disorders. Adult patients suffering from squint and double vision are also dealt with. The paediatric ophthalmology wing at the Narayana Nethralaya at health city provides a very child friendly ambience, modern vision screening systems for infants and children are in use. Consultants here deal with an entire gamut of paediatric eye diseases including strabismus, amblyopia, cataract, glaucoma and pediatric eye cancer. Of note is the genetics and metabolic laboratory backup which ensures excellent diagnostic and research potential. The department provides appropriate therapeutic intervention for all stages of retinopathy of prematurity, a blinding disease of the premature newborn. Using the expertise of excellent anesthesiologists at Narayana Hrudayalaya, we are equipped to perform ocular surgeries with ease in newborns especially those with cardiac disorders. We also have facilities to provide vision stimulation and rehabilitation for children with low vision. Through our highly dedicated and organized school screening programs we have been able to provide the high quality eye care to the under privileged children of our society.

Eye Banking and Cornea Transplant Services

Corneal disease is a major cause of blindness responsible for 7.1% of blindness in India. Recent data reported that only 10% of the required 400,000 corneas are being procured annually.

Dr. Rajkumar Eye bank was inaugurated by the charismatic matinee idol Dr. Rajkumar 1994. A touching testimonial to his commitment to lead by example lead by example is in the fact that he willed his eyes. He motivated a large number of people, and following his unfortunate demise in April 2006, his family continues their support. He will always remain with us in our hearts.

This Eye Bank was established with the purpose of disseminating the importance of eye donation and to facilitate the collection, processing and distribution of eyes to patients having corneal blindness. State of the art eye bank with international standard tissue banking facility allows us to utilize eyes collected from donors.

Caring for Community

School Screening Camps

Recognizing the fact that visual morbidity in the young children is largely preventable, an organized approach is being followed in schools in Bangalore and beyond to detect visual problems in children.

Cataract and Eye Health Camps

We are proud to be able to serve the community at their doorstep. Patients in these camps undergo comprehensive eye examination, undergo cost effective cataract surgery with intraocular implants. We undertake cataract screening and base hospital surgery approach in and around Bangalore. In addition customized spectacles are distributed for refractive errors detected during screening. More than 375 camps have been held so far and nearly about 40 free surgeries are done per week. We are gearing up to increase the number of surgeries as our country has a large cataract backlog.

Pavagada Paediatric Eye Health Project

Pavagada is a remote talunk in Tumkur district is underserved in terms of health, education it is one of the most socio-economically backward area. water scarcity and Fluorosis being rampant. At the behest of Swami Japananda, our team has now joined hands with the ophthalmologists at the Sharada Devi eye hospital there to extend tertiary level eye care. A special effort is being made by our paediatric ophthalmologists to address the rather high incidence of eye disease in children of this place along with epidemiologists and genetic backup. The specialized treatment is done free of cost.

Ocular Complications of HIV/AIDS

HIV/AIDS affects the eyes in 50-75% cases, this is the leading cause of suicidal deaths in young HIV patients that servely impacts livelihood of thie individual as well as the family. All patients with HIV AIDS who need eye screening for related eye complications are evaluated by our specialists. This service is provide free-of-cost.

We aim to do a statewide epidemiological study to monitor and initiate corrective measures to tackle and minimize avoidable blindness in

HIV/AIDS patients. WE are currently trying to find funding resources for providing further care for these patients including medications and or eye surgeries.

Research

Having established a large patient base and credibility over the last two decades, our aim is move to the next level to become one of the best eye institutes in the country and be recognized internationally in the fields of patients care, scientific research, education and community work said Dr. Khannan M. Narayana Director, Strategic Planning and Research.

Innovative Research Activities

- Clinical Trials
- Polymerase Chain Reaction Laboratory
- Stem cell laboratory
- Narayana Nethralaya Library and informatics centre
- Electronic Medical Records
- Teleophthalmology Services
- Image Processing Laboratory
- Publications

Publications

2006-2007

1. Pai SA, Rohit S, Vijayan PB, Venkatasubramaniam G, Yadav NK, Shetty BK, Babu RB, Narayana KM. Clinical, anatomic, and electrophysiologic evaluation following intravitreal bevacizumb for macular edema in retinal vein occlusion. *Am J Ophthalmol.* 2007 Apr.; 143(4):601-6.
2. Mahendradas P, Ranganna KS, Rohit.S, Balu R, Babu RB, Narayana KM, Shetty BK. Ocular Manifestations Associated with Chikungunya. *Ophthalmology* 2007. (In press)
3. Rohit S, Babu RB, Suresh M, Samprathi AB, Shetty BK. Neuro-ohthalmic disorders presenting as a diagnostic surprise during pre laser in situ keratomileusis (LASIK) evaluation. J Cataract *Refract Surg.* 2007. (In press)
4. Mahendradas P Kamath G, Mahalakshmi B Shetty BK. Serpigenous choroiditis like picture due to toxoplasmosis. *Ocular Immunology and Inflammation.* (In press)

Molecular Diagnostics

Polymerase Chain Reaction Laboratory

It is an advanced technique used to diagnose the presence of infectious agents in tiny quantities of ocular fluid and other parts of the body. This lab is primarily intended to aid in diagnosis of infections in the eye and other organs in the body. This will have a large positive impact in clinical care and research into infectious causes of eye and systemic diseases. It is equipped with the state of the art PCR machines and is of WHO-GMP standards.

Stem Cell Laboratory

The decade has been recent advances in the field of regenerative medicine and the stem cell research providing great hopes for many currently untreatable medical conditions. Stem cell destruction due to chemical, thermal injury, drug allergy or autoimmune diseases leads to the limbal stem cell deficiency, characterized by corneal opacities and blindness. The limbal stem cell followed by transplantation in the patients.

Dr. Himanshu P. Matalia heads the stem cell research group. This puts us in the elite club of handful of laboratories in the world that are doing such research and also applying into clinical practice.

Index